Harriman

Trails

A Guide and History

By William J. Myles

Second Edition 1999

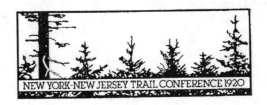

NEW YORK-NEW JERSEY TRAIL CONFERENCE 1920

Edited by: **Daniel D. Chazin**
Designed by: **Suzanne Antonelli**
Cover Design by: **Steve Butfilowski**
Cover Photograph: **Michael Warren**

View of Turkey Hill Lake from Long Mountain

Published by

The New York-New Jersey Trail Conference

G.P.O. Box 2250
New York, New York 10116

Library of Congress Cataloging-in-Publication Data

Myles, William J., 1913-
    Harriman trails: a guide and history / by William J. Myles. —
2nd ed.
       p.   cm.
    Includes index.
    ISBN 1-880775-18-2
    1. Hiking—New York (State)—Harriman State Park—Guide-
books. 2. Hiking—New York (State)—Bear Mountain State Park—
Guide-books. 3. Trails—New York (State)—Harriman State Park—
Guide-books. 4. Trails—New York (State)—Bear Mountain State
Park—Guide-books. 5. Harriman State Park (N.Y.)—Guide-books.
6. Bear Mountain State Park (N.Y.)—Guide-books.
I. New York-New Jersey Trail Conference. II. Title.

GV199.42.N652H375 1999
917.47'3—dc20   91-41530
                                              CIP

TABLE OF CONTENTS

INTRODUCTION

Writing this book has been a labor of love. It was inspired by reading the first (1923) edition of the *New York Walk Book*, written by Raymond Torrey and Frank Place. They combined a great enthusiasm for trails in the New York metropolitan area with an impressive ability to describe what they saw. Another, lesser, inspiration was Bill Hoeferlin's *Harriman Park Trail Guide* (1944). This handy little booklet gave trail distances and a list of scenic attractions, from Agony Grind to Witness Oak.

Through the years, as I hiked in Harriman Park, I became interested in stories about the trails, and of places I saw along the way. At last, I gave in to my friends' suggestions and decided to write a book. This, now, is the result: a detailed description of 225 miles of 43 marked trails, as well as 103 miles of 56 unmarked trails. Wherever possible, I have related the history of the trail — who made it, and how it changed through the years.

The trail descriptions are not intended to make it unnecessary to use a map and compass. Anyone hiking the trails in Harriman Park — especially the unmarked trails — should take along a compass and a map of the Park, and know how to use them. Throughout the book, references are made to Maps #3 and #4 of the New York-New Jersey Trail Conference, which cover the Harriman-Bear Mountain Trails.

In the course of writing this book, the author has had the help of many people. It was always a pleasant experience to become acquainted with these people, who willingly shared their knowledge. Most helpful was Jack Focht, Director of the Trailside Museum. Week after week, Jack carried down from the Park headquarters attic the correspondence files of Major Welch from 1912 to 1939. Thanks are also due to former PIPC Executive Director Nash Castro, who helped in many ways and made available the minutes of Commission meetings from 1909 to 1990, and to Bob Binnewies, the present Executive Director. Tim Sullivan, Chief Ranger, shared his closet-full of maps, and answered numerous questions about Park history.

The story of Doodletown was reconstructed with the help of Denzel Livingston and his wife Grace. Recently, Grace has been a part-time switchboard operator at Park headquarters. Also helpful was ex-Doodletown resident Elizabeth Stalter.

At the other end of the Park, in Sloatsburg, the author became acquainted with Marvel Becraft Babcook, Fred Waldron and Clarence Conklin. They all were interested, and willingly shared their memories. Meyer Kukle helped in many ways, especially with interviewing knowledgeable old-timers.

Mention must be made of the author's friends who helped to scout many faint trails that deserve to be remembered: Erwin Conrad, Jay Kadampanattu and David Sutter — all of the Union County Hiking Club. In addition, several friends — including George Neffinger, Frank Oliver, Tim Sullivan and James Ransom — took the time to review the manuscript and made many helpful suggestions.

Thanks are also due to the volunteers who typed the manuscript into the computer: Carole Coe, Mimi Davisson, Francine Foley, Michael Golub, Mark Gorbics, Patricia E. Guempel, Howard J. Dash, Kenneth King, Linda R. Kline, William G. Koellner, Donald J. Little, Bob Miller, Bill Pruehsner and Robert Spellman.

Finally, I want to thank our editor, Dan Chazin, for correcting many inconsistencies in my text and for providing precise measurements of the trails.

BILL MYLES

November 1991

PREFACE TO THE SECOND EDITION

Since the first edition of this book was published in 1992, a number of changes have taken place to the trails in Harriman/Bear Mountain Park. The Appalachian and Arden-Surebridge Trails near Island Pond have been rerouted, the White Bar Trail has been extended to the Johnsontown Road circle, the new Menomine Trail has been blazed to provide access for hikers from the Silvermine parking area, and the Diamond Mountain and Tower Trails have been combined into a single trail. All of these changes, and many others, have been incorporated into this second edition of my book. Additional historical information has also been added, and several mistakes have been corrected.

I would like to thank my editor, Dan Chazin, for his work in producing this second edition. Also, I want to thank Andy Smith, a ranger with the Park, for the information he provided regarding his family and the Pittsboro Trail, and Elizabeth "Perk" Stalter, author of a book on Doodletown, for much valuable information on the history of Doodletown. I am grateful to my friend Jay Winslow who produced, for this edition, beautiful black-and-white prints from original color slides. Finally, I want to thank Kay Bresee of the Appalachian Trail Conference who spent many hours making the necessary changes and corrections for this edition of the book.

BILL MYLES

July 1999

THE MARKED TRAILS

ANTHONY WAYNE TRAIL

Length: 2.8 miles
Blazes: white

Miles

0.0	Leave PG Trail at Turkey Hill Lake.
0.3	Cross Woodbury town line.
0.55	Old Route 6; go right.
0.6	Turn left off road.
0.7	Cross new Route 6.
1.05	Cross Seven Lakes Drive.
1.2	Cross 1779 Trail.
1.75	Cross Palisades Interstate Parkway.
1.9	Enter gate on left and go uphill on bike trail.
2.1	Go left on Beechy Bottom East Road.
2.45	Go left on older road.
2.5	Turn right, rejoining Beechy Bottom East Road.
2.55	Turn right, uphill.
2.8	End at Timp-Torne Trail.

The Anthony Wayne Trail (AW) starts on the Popolopen Gorge Trail (red dot on white) at the southwest end of Turkey Hill Lake. The lake — a reservoir which feeds Queensboro Lake — was built in 1933-34 by a unit of the Civilian Conservation Corps. The trail goes south through a valley, with Summer Hill on the left, toward Route 6 (Long Mountain Parkway). On the way, it crosses an old woods road (which was Long Mountain Road until 1919 and made into a fire trail in 1946), then turns right onto a once-paved road (Route 6 from 1919 to 1967; widened in 1936).

The path that the Anthony Wayne Trail has followed so far was once known as the Curtis Hollow Trail. That was before Turkey Hill Lake was made, when the trail went north through Curtis Hollow (now the lake) and across West Point land to the Forest of Dean Road. The old trail can still be seen, faintly, on the hillside at the northwest end of the lake.

On once-paved old Route 6, AW passes the remains of the picnic/car camping area that was built about 1920. The trail then leaves the old road and continues south, soon crossing present-day Route 6. On the far side and down the bank to the left it crosses a little stream and joins an old road (the 1946 fire trail). This is a region of wild grapes, wild roses and, unfortunately, piles of rubbish. The Anthony Wayne Trail then crosses Seven Lakes Drive at an abandoned comfort station. Behind the comfort station, a trail starts west to Cranberry Mine.

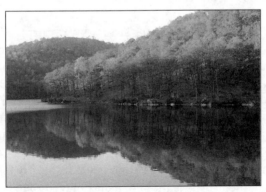

Turkey Hill Lake – Autumn reflection

In another 0.15 mile, AW crosses the route that General Anthony Wayne is thought to have taken in 1779 (now designated as the 1779 Trail). At 1.75 miles, it crosses the Palisades Interstate Parkway on an overpass and reaches the Anthony Wayne Recreation Area. This great playground, which gave its name to the trail, was first opened in June 1955. The trail was marked in 1960 by the Tramp and Trail Club.

AW now goes left through a gate and up toward West Mountain on a gravel road, blazed with blue-on-white plastic markers as a bike trail. It then turns left onto Beechy Bottom East Road, which it follows for 0.35 mile. The large water pipe along this trail comes from the water plant at Queensboro Dam. At 2.55 miles, AW turns right, uphill, and climbs the foot of West Mountain, to end at the Timp-Torne Trail (blue), 2.8 miles from the start.

Appalachian Trail

Length: 18.75 miles (Bear Mtn. Bridge to Route 17)
Blazes: white

Miles

0.0	Bear Mountain Bridge (toll booth at west end).
0.4	Tunnel under Route 9W.
0.75	Junction of paved paths behind Bear Mountain Inn.
1.25	S-BM Trail (yellow) leaves, left.
1.8	Turn right onto Scenic Drive.
2.6	Summit of Bear Mountain; Perkins Tower.
3.15	Turn left, down Perkins Drive.
3.65	Turn right, off Perkins Drive.
4.2	Cross Seven Lakes Drive.
4.45	Fawn Trail (red) begins, right.
4.65	Turn right, off bridle path.
4.9	West Mountain; view east.
5.0	Timp-Torne Trail (blue) joins.
5.1	View west.
5.65	View west.
5.8	T-T leaves, left.
6.35	Cross Beechy Bottom East Road.
6.55	Cross Anthony Wayne South Ski Trail.
6.65	Cross wooden bridge over Beechy Bottom Brook.
6.70	Turn sharp right; R-D Trail joins from left.
6.90	Cross Palisades Interstate Parkway.
7.05	Cross Owl Lake Road.
7.2	Cross 1779 Trail.
7.7	Black Mountain; views to south and east.
8.1	View of Silvermine Lake.
8.2	Cross fire road (ski trail).

9.1	William Brien Memorial Shelter; Menomine Trail begins, right.
9.9	R-D leaves, left.
11.1	Cross Seven Lakes Drive.
12.0	Stevens Mountain.
12.55	Cross old road.
13.25	Cross Arden Valley Road; R-D Trail joins.
13.75	Fireplace, right.
14.35	Hurst Trail (blue), left, to shelter.
14.45	R-D leaves, left.
14.95	Left on Surebridge Mine Road.
15.05	Leave road.
15.8	Long Path (turquoise) crosses.
16.2	Island Pond Mountain.
16.45	Lemon Squeezer.
16.55	A-SB joins briefly.
16.7	Briefly join "Crooked Road."
16.9	View of Island Pond to left.
17.0	Cross stone spillway.
17.1	Cross gravel road leading to Island Pond.
17.15	Turn left onto Island Pond Road.
17.25	Turn right, uphill.
17.65	Summit of Green Pond Mountain.
18.2	Cross upper branch of Old Arden Road.
18.3	Turn right onto lower branch of Old Arden Road.
18.35	Turn left onto Arden Valley Road.
18.55	Cross New York State Thruway.
18.75	Route 17.

From the tollgate at the west end of the Bear Mountain Bridge, the Appalachian Trail (AT) turns left through a gate into the area of the Trailside Museum and Zoo. (If the gate is locked — after about 5:00 p.m. — go to the traffic circle and turn left to Hessian Lake). Along the path is a nine-foot-high statue of Walt

Whitman. It was made by sculptor Jo Davidson for the 1939 World's Fair, and in 1940 it was given to the Palisades Interstate Park by W. Averell Harriman. Further along is a redoubt of old Fort Clinton, seized by the British on October 6, 1777. At 0.4 mile, the trail goes through an underpass beneath Route 9W, then follows a paved path around the south end of Hessian Lake. At 0.75 mile, it reaches a junction of paved paths behind the Bear Mountain Inn. Here the Cornell Mine (blue), Major Welch (red dot on white) and Suffern-Bear Mountain (S-BM) (yellow) Trails begin.

The S-BM Trail runs jointly with the AT, and both trails climb up a park service road, passing the ski jump. Soon S-BM leaves to the left. The AT continues to climb until it turns right onto the Scenic Drive at 1.8 miles. There are fine views from this road. The trail then continues uphill, crossing the Scenic Drive twice more before reaching the 1,305-foot summit of Bear Mountain at 2.6 miles. The stone tower on the summit is a memorial to George W. Perkins, Sr., first president of the Palisades Interstate Park Commission (from 1900 to 1920). Here also, fixed on a stone just below the summit, is a plaque in honor of Joseph Bartha, Trails Committee Chairman of the NY-NJ Trail Conference from 1940 to 1955. The Major Welch Trail crosses here. The AT and the Major Welch Trail go separately down the west slope of the mountain, meeting again at the Perkins Drive at 3.15 miles.

The AT follows the Drive down left for 0.5 mile, then leaves to the right (the end of the abandoned section of the Drive, once called Bear Mountain Bypass, is on the left). The trail crosses the Seven Lakes Drive and briefly joins old Doodletown Road, which also carries the historic 1777W Trail. At 4.45 miles, the Fawn Trail (red F on pink) departs right, to go over a low shoulder of West Mountain. The AT soon starts steeply up the mountain and reaches a viewpoint to the east at 4.9 miles. In another 500 feet, the Timp-Torne Trail (T-T) (blue) joins from the right. The joint trail passes another viewpoint to the east, then crosses to the western side of the ridge, with a number of striking views. The Anthony Wayne Recreation Area is in the valley to the west. At 5.8 miles, T-T departs to the left, while the AT begins its descent.

The first section of the Appalachian Trail was marked in 1922 through Harriman Park from the Elk Pen at Arden to Tiorati Circle. The entire trail from Arden to the Bear Mountain Bridge was officially opened on Sunday, October 7, 1923. The Bridge itself was opened on Thanksgiving Day, November 27, 1924. The new Appalachian Trail came across it, and for 0.5 mile followed the old Queensboro Trail high above Popolopen Brook. It then started steeply up Bear Mountain. This part of the trail was cut off in 1927 by the Popolopen Drive, and a new route was marked to the left of the road. The steep way up the north side of Bear Mountain was used as the route of the AT until 1931. Then, at the request of Major Welch, the AT was marked from the south end of Hessian Lake up past the ski chute to the firetower on the mountaintop. The firetower was replaced in 1934 by the Perkins Memorial Tower, and the older tower was rebuilt on Diamond Mountain in 1935. The old AT route up Bear Mountain was still maintained as an alternate approach to the AT, and it later became the Major Welch Trail. In 1939, the AT blazes were changed from yellow to white, to match the color used south of the Delaware River (the AT in Connecticut was blue until 1949). During the following years, the route up Bear Mountain was moved twice to avoid eroded sections. In 1976, the route down the west side was changed, to eliminate a dangerous sandy slope. It was given its present course down Perkins Drive to the point where the earlier trail had crossed. That older route, down to Seven Lakes Drive and up to West Mountain, had been joint with the Timp-Torne Trail, first blazed in 1921. T-T was rerouted away from Bear Mountain in 1960.

In 1988 and 1989, the trail from the ski jump up the east side of Bear Mountain was rerouted once more to avoid an eroded route and add new views. The relocated trail now follows a paved road (the Scenic Drive) for 0.3 mile, but beautiful views help compensate for the roadwalk.

After going down off West Mountain, the AT at 6.35 miles reaches Beechy Bottom East Road, an old woods road that was improved in 1933 by the Civilian Conservation Corps. Until 1997, the AT turned left and followed the grassy Beechy Bottom East Road for 0.1 mile, but now it crosses the road and parallels it on a footpath. It then drops down to cross the Anthony Wayne South Ski Trail (now marked with blue-on-white blazes as a bike path) and, at 6.65 miles, it crosses Beechy Bottom Brook on a wooden bridge. The AT then goes up and turns sharply right as the Ramapo-Dunderberg Trail (R-D) (red on white) joins from the left. At 6.9 miles, the joint trail goes across the Palisades Interstate Parkway. Immediately afterward, a faint old road, known as the Owl Lake Road, is crossed. Soon the 1779 Trail crosses, and AT/R-D goes up and over a low ridge. It then begins a steep climb to the 1,200-foot summit of Black Mountain, from which there are good views to the south and east. The line between Orange and Rockland Counties crosses the trail here, and runs northeast to Bear Mountain and the bridge. AT/R-D then descends, and at 8.2 miles it crosses a wide gravel path, the Silvermine Ski Road. This fire road was built in 1934 by the Temporary Emergency Relief Administration. AT/R-D then climbs gently to the level top of Letterrock Mountain, and at 9.1 miles reaches the William Brien Memorial Shelter. To the left of the shelter, a blue-blazed side trail goes to a spring-fed well nearby, and the unmarked Dean Trail leads to the Red Cross Trail. To the right is the start of the Menomine Trail (yellow), which goes down to the Silvermine Ski Area on Seven Lakes Drive in 1.35 miles.

This shelter is named after William Brien, the first president of the New York Ramblers. In 1954, he bequeathed $4,000 for a shelter, which was built in 1957 at Island Pond. Because of vandalism, that shelter was demolished in 1973 and the name transferred to the former Letterrock Shelter, which was built in 1933 (*N.Y. Post*, 6/23/33).

At 9.9 miles, AT/R-D comes down to a wooden bridge at the foot of Goshen Mountain. Here the unmarked Bockey Swamp Trail crosses. To the right, the Bockey Swamp Trail follows the little brook down towards Silvermine Lake. The R-D departs to the left, and begins to climb Goshen Mountain, while the AT goes right on a woods road. AT soon turns right, leaving this road. It goes down to another woods road, which it follows for a short distance, reaching the Seven Lakes Drive at 11.1 miles. The trail crosses the Drive, then a region with two brooks, and goes up Stevens Mountain. It then turns south, following an old woods road, known as the Youmans Trail. After leaving this road, the AT crosses a descending dirt road (the original Arden Valley Road) and, at 13.25 miles, rejoins the R-D Trail at the present-day paved Arden Valley Road on Fingerboard Mountain. Downhill, to the left, is Tiorati Circle, where there is a convenient parking area and restroom facilities.

The original route of the AT was *over* Goshen Mountain, joint with R-D. It came down west to cross an old woods road, where it parted from R-D, and continued over two knolls to the Seven Lakes Drive, 100 yards north of Tiorati Circle. It then climbed up to the Fingerboard Fire Tower (built 1922) and turned south to the R-D (*N.Y. Post*, 1/4/24). In November 1931, the AT was diverted through a tent camp on the knoll northeast of Tiorati Circle,

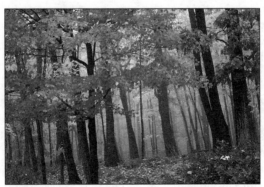
Red maple leaves and mist on Fingerboard Mountain

and then went jointly with R-D up Arden Valley Road (*N.Y. Post*, 11/13/31). In 1934, the AT was made to coincide with R-D from Goshen Mountain to Tiorati Brook Road, which it followed for 0.35 mile to Tiorati Circle. The present route up Stevens Mountain was devised in 1978 by Chief Ranger Tim Sullivan.

Proceeding now along the ridge of Fingerboard Mountain, AT/R-D passes a telephone line and a concrete water tank. This reservoir was built in 1927 to supply water to the facilities at Lake Tiorati and the camps at Lake Cohasset. At 13.75 miles, a half-mile from Arden Valley Road, the trail comes to a stone fireplace. Here was the beginning of the Fingerboard-Storm King Trail (FB-SK), which was blazed north to Storm King Mountain in 1922 by J. Ashton Allis and Raymond H. Torrey.

At 14.35 miles, the blue Hurst Trail begins to the left. It passes the Fingerboard Shelter (built in 1928) and goes down to the Seven Lakes Drive. In another 500 feet, R-D continues straight ahead, while the AT turns right and begins to descend. After 0.5 mile, the AT reaches Surebridge Mine Road, where it turns sharp left, passing the shafts of the Greenwood Mine to the left of the trail. During the Civil War, the ore from this mine was brought to the Greenwood Furnace at Arden. At 15.05 miles, the AT crosses Surebridge Brook and climbs the 1,240-foot Surebridge Mountain. It then goes down into a swampy region where the Long Path (turquoise) crosses. The AT continues up the northeast side of 1,303-foot Island Pond Mountain. At the summit, the remains of Edward Harriman's summer shelter are visible. When the new AT was described by

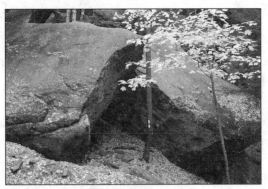
Entrance to the Lemon Squeezer

Raymond Torrey in 1924 *(N.Y. Post,* 1/4/24), he mentioned a wooden fire tower on the summit of Island Pond Mountain.

Now the AT goes downhill to the Lemon Squeezer, a narrow passage formed when a great piece of rock broke off the side of the cliff. There is a by-pass around the crevice.

Coming out of the crevice, at 16.55 miles, the AT briefly joins the Arden-Surebridge Trail, which comes in from the left, and soon departs to the left. After going over a little rise, the AT turns right, at 16.7 miles, onto the Crooked Road, an old miners' road which once marked the boundary of Harriman Park. The AT passes the north end of Island Pond, then turns left and ascends a hill, which affords a view of Island Pond to the south. Now descending, the trail passes, to the left, the rusted remains of a rotary gravel classifier, and then crosses a stone spillway, which carries water from the pond to Echo Lake in the Harriman estate (see pp.

358-59). After crossing a gravel road (built in 1963) that leads to Island Pond, the AT, at 17.15 miles, turns left onto Island Pond Road. In another 450 feet, the trail leaves the road to the right and begins its climb of Green Pond Mountain, reaching the summit at 17.65 miles.

At 18.2 miles, the AT crosses the upper branch of the Old Arden Road (built in 1894, and also known as "Harriman's level road"), then turns right on the lower branch of the road (the Arden-Surebridge Trail starts here). The AT bears left and joins paved Arden Valley Road at 18.35 miles, and soon passes the entrance to the hikers' parking area known as the Elk Pen. The AT now crosses a bridge over the New York Thruway, the Ramapo River and the Norfolk Southern Railway (formerly Conrail; previously the Erie Railroad), arriving at Route 17 at 18.75 miles. Agony Grind is just ahead.

The AT originally followed the northern shore of Island Pond, went over Green Pond Mountain and continued down to the Elk Pen. This pretty route gave great views to the south across Island Pond. However, after a fishermen's access road was built from Arden Valley Road to the lake in 1963, the area at the north end of the lake became littered and unsightly. To avoid that messy place, the trail was rerouted in 1980 around the southern end of the lake. However, conditions at the northern end of the lake subsequently improved, and the reroute around the southern end, which lengthened the trail and eliminated all views of the lake, was unpopular with hikers. In 1993, the original route along the northern end of the lake was restored (except that the AT now runs a short distance inland, rather than along the shore of the lake). Another relocation, which restored the original route over Green Pond Mountain, was completed in 1994.

Until 1947, Island Pond Mountain was called Echo Mountain. It has two 1,300-foot summits, connected across a half-mile by a saddle about 200 feet lower. There was confusion about names in this region until the Trail Conference decided that the northern summit, overlooking Echo Lake, was Echo Mountain. The southern summit was named Island Pond Mountain, and the ridge west of Island Pond became Green Pond Mountain (Trail Conference Minutes, 2/5/47).

The first section of the Appalachian Trail was blazed in 1922 from Route 17 over Green Pond Mountain, across the north end of Island Pond to the Crooked Road, and through the Lemon Squeezer. There it joined the A-SB up to the old firetower. The entire trail through the Park, from Arden to Bear Mountain, was officially opened on Sunday, October 7, 1923.

In those days, there were about 60 elk in a great enclosure between Southfields and Arden, known as the Elk Range. They had been brought from Yellowstone Park in December 1919. They did not thrive, and their num-

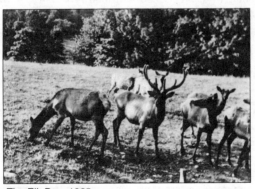

The Elk Pen–1925

ber gradually decreased until 1942, when the remainder of the herd was sold to a dealer from Hoosick Falls (Commission Minutes, 12/10/42).

How to cross the Ramapo River at Arden was a problem for the trail blazers. Arden Valley Road was a 16-foot-wide gravel road that came down to the old iron furnace at Arden, nearly a mile north of the present AT crossing. Prior to 1929, hikers on the AT had to cross the Ramapo River at the Arden railroad station and take the Old Arden Road to the Elk Pen — a detour of 1.25 miles. In 1929, a footbridge was built over the Ramapo River at the Elk Range by Raymond Adolph, Park Forester, and in 1934, the Park opened a new paved Arden Valley Road from the Elk Range to Lake Cohasset. From Route 17, the new road went 0.2 mile north down to the river level, where it went *under* the railroad tracks through an underpass. The Ramapo River went through the underpass, too, and met Arden Brook. The river bottom there was paved with concrete so that cars could ford the river. Stepping stones were provided for walkers. Naturally, hikers on the AT cut up over the bank to cross Route 17. The present bridge, which carries Arden Valley Road over the Thruway, the railroad and the river, was built in 1954.

ARDEN-SUREBRIDGE TRAIL

Length: 6.25 miles
Blazes: red triangle on white

Miles

0.0   Begin where dirt road from Elk Pen joins Arden Road.
0.03 AT leaves to left.
0.35 Turn left, leaving Arden Road.
0.5   Cross stream.
0.8   Turn left (leaving old AT route) and ascend steeply.
0.9   Pass cave.
1.0   Reach top of ascent and turn left.
1.25 Turn right onto Island Pond Road.
1.3   Cross outlet of Island Pond.
1.45 Bear right; road ahead leads to Island Pond.
1.5   Turn left, leaving Island Pond Road.
1.85 Turn left and descend.
3.05 Turn left onto Crooked Road.
3.2   Cross stream.
3.25 Turn right, leaving Crooked Road.
3.45 Briefly join AT at base of Lemon Squeezer.
3.7   LP joins from left; White Bar Trail starts to right.
3.75 Bottle Cap Trail starts; turn right.
4.0   Lichen Trail starts to right.
4.45 Turn right on Surebridge Mine Road.
4.55 "Times Square": R-D crosses; LP departs to right.
5.0   Cross brook; Dunning Trail starts to right.
5.1   Go right, leaving fire road.
6.0   Red Cross Trail starts to left.
6.25 Trail ends at Lake Skannatati.

To reach the start of the Arden-Surebridge Trail (A-SB), take Arden Valley Road east for 0.3 mile from Route 17, and park in the Elk Pen parking area. You will see a dirt road leading east across the meadow; follow this road for 0.1 mile until you reach the Arden Road (also known as "Harriman's level road") at the other side of the meadow. Here, a triple blaze on a tree marks the start of the A-SB Trail. Turn right and follow the Arden Road southward. The Appalachian Trail (AT) leaves to the left in 150 feet, but A-SB continues ahead on the road. At 0.35 mile, A-SB turns left, leaving the road, and begins to climb gradually up Green Pond Mountain. After another half mile, the trail turns left and climbs steeply up the mountain, following the route of the former Green Trail, and passing an interesting cave under a ledge. After reaching the top, A-SB goes down through laurels and, at 1.25 miles, turns right onto Island Pond Road.

A-SB crosses the outlet of the pond and then bears right at a road junction. (The road straight ahead leads to an abandoned ranger cabin at the south end of Island Pond.) Shortly after this junction, A-SB turns left, leaving the road, and goes around the south and east sides of Island Pond, passing through gullies and over knobs. After going down a long hill, the trail turns left, at 3.05 miles, onto the "Crooked Road," an old miners' road which once marked the boundary of Harriman State Park. A-SB crosses a stream and soon turns right, leaving the road, and climbs to the base of the Lemon Squeezer, where it briefly joins the AT.

A-SB does not go up through the Lemon Squeezer, but instead turns right, goes south along a rocky hillside, and soon joins a woods road. At 3.7 miles, at a large boulder, the Long Path joins from the left. Immediately afterward, the White Bar Trail starts to the right, while the joint A-SB/LP turns left, passes the end of a swamp, and starts to climb. In another 300 feet, the A-SB/LP turns right, while the Bottle Cap Trail (see pp. 31-32) continues straight ahead.

A-SB/LP now begins to climb more steeply. At 4.0 miles, after A-SB/LP passes a swamp on the left, the Lichen Trail (blue "L" on white) starts to the right. After passing through laurels and rhododendrons, the A-SB/LP descends a ledge, climbs briefly, goes down through a hemlock grove, and emerges on the Surebridge Mine Road. The section of A-SB from the Bottle Cap Trail up to the hemlock grove was named the "Lost Road" in 1921 by J. Ashton Allis (*N.Y. Post*, 11/11/21).

A-SB/LP turns right (east) on the Surebridge Mine Road and in about 500 feet reaches a junction known as "Times Square," marked by a stone fireplace beside a large boulder. Here, the red-blazed Ramapo-Dunderberg Trail crosses, and in another 75 feet the Long Path departs to the right. A-SB continues along the road and begins to descend. At 5.0 miles, it reaches a brook where the Dunning Trail (yellow) starts to the right. On the other side of the brook, there is a large mine opening to the left of the trail. After passing three smaller mine openings, A-SB bears right, leaving the wide path, and drops down a bank. It soon passes several stone foundations to the left. After going by the edge of Pine Swamp, the trail goes up Pine Swamp Mountain. There are limited views from the summit, but on the way down A-SB passes an excellent viewpoint over Lakes

Skannatati and Kanawauke. At 6.0 miles, the Red Cross Trail begins to the left. A-SB then descends steeply and, at 6.25 miles, ends at the parking area for Lake Skannatati. Here the Long Path comes in from the right, crosses Seven Lakes Drive and continues over a shoulder of Rockhouse Mountain.

The Arden-Surebridge Trail was first blazed during the summer of 1921 by J. Ashton Allis. He was a leader of the Fresh Air Club and the AMC and was a founder of the new Palisades Park Trail Conference. In preparation for his AMC hike the following weekend, he marked the route as a short-cut from Arden station to the R-D Trail on Hogencamp Mountain. It is shown as the "Allis Short Trail" on a map in the *N.Y. Post* (10/14/21). By December 1922, it had been extended by members of the Green Mountain Club from the R-D Trail to Camp Thendara on Lake Tiorati, and was marked with white wooden arrows and red metal triangles inscribed "A-SB."

From the Erie Station at Arden (located about 0.7 mile north of the present-day Arden Valley Road), the trail crossed Arden Brook at the Harriman Dairy bottling house and went up the wooden steps beside the old Greenwood Furnace. From the upper terrace, it followed the Echo Lake Road, which proceeded to the east on the south side of Arden Brook. At a fork, the trail turned right and went through the chicken farm and pastures. Then, at another fork, it turned left onto an old grass-grown road that led to the west side of Island Pond. After leaving the grassy road, A-SB went over a rise, crossed the outlet brook from Island Pond, and climbed to the top of Island Pond Mountain (then known as Echo Mountain).

It was there, on Echo Mountain, that the new Appalachian Trail, built in 1922, met the A-SB which J. Ashton Allis had built in 1921. Both trails followed the same route down through the Lemon Squeezer, which had been discovered and named by Allis. From the Lemon Squeezer to "Times Square," A-SB followed the same route that it still does today.

From "Times Square" to Lake Tiorati the trail was just a footpath in 1922. It was widened by the Park in 1936 as a fire road, from the Hurst Trail up to Pine Swamp Mine (Dunning Trail). In 1966 it was widened further, up to the Surebridge Mine Road (which also was widened to Lake Cohasset).

In 1924, because of a hunting incident, Roland Harriman closed the Echo Lake Road to hikers. They then used the Harriman Level Road south to the Elk Range. This route, too, was closed in 1953 when the new Thruway sliced into the hillside. After that, hikers went south from the Arden station along the west side of the Erie tracks, joining the original Arden Valley Road where it came down to the river level (see p. 17). They followed that old road up to the new entrance road and the bridge that was built across the Thruway in 1954. That route, too, was abandoned after rail service to Arden ceased about 1970.

In June 1978, A-SB was rerouted south over Pine Swamp Mountain. This change was made in order to divert the trail away from the entrance to Camp Thendara on the Seven Lakes Drive, near Lake Tiorati, where there had been parking problems and complaints of vandalism.

In the spring of 1995, the western end of A-SB was relocated. This reroute eliminated the roadwalk on Arden Valley Road and the steep climb up Island Pond Mountain, which was often icy in the winter. From its start near the Elk Pen, A-SB now follows a route around the southern end of Island Pond which was used by the AT from 1980 to 1993. However, A-SB uses the route of the old Green Trail to climb Green Pond Mountain, shortening the old AT route by nearly half a mile and passing by an interesting cave.

Beech Trail

Length: 3.85 miles
Blazes: blue

Miles

0.0	Start on LP near St. John's Church.
0.6	Cross Route 106.
0.75	Town line.
1.2	Rockhouse Mountain Trail, left.
1.6	Cemetery.
2.05	Hasenclever Fire Road.
2.8	Tiorati Brook Road.
2.95	Cross Tiorati Brook and go left from road.
3.4	Turn right onto older route of Beech Trail.
3.85	Red Cross Trail.

The Beech Trail begins at its intersection with the Long Path, 0.55 mile north of Lake Welch Drive. To reach this point, park at St. John's Church and proceed along St. John's Road a short distance to Lake Welch Drive. Follow the turquoise blazes of the Long Path to the north, proceeding up Polebrook Mountain through an area of old farms and cellar holes. After descending from an old farm field and crossing a small swampy area, you will find the blue blazes of the Beech Trail, which begins on the right. The trail goes northeast on a woods road (the old Green Swamp Trail). Near the start of this woods road is the foundation of a cabin, the home of Martin and Maybelle Youmans until 1928. The Beech Trail passes Green Swamp on the right. At 0.6

mile, it crosses Route 106 and continues northeast on another woods road (the old Rockhouse Mountain Trail), passing impressive boulders and cliffs. The town line between Haverstraw (to the south) and Stony Point (to the north) is crossed at 0.75 mile.

At 1.2 miles, the faint Rockhouse Mountain Trail goes off to the left (the junction is marked by a cairn), while the Beech Trail continues straight ahead. It reaches an old cemetery at 1.6 miles. (You will note Youmans' grave on one side of a stone wall, and several Jones graves on the other side.) A bit further along, the trail passes an old farm where there are remains of stone foundations, a root cellar and a huge Norway spruce. (From the farm, a rather vague road goes down easterly to a swampy area. It crosses a brook and climbs up to the Hasenclever Fire Road which once led to the village of Sandyfield, now covered by Lake Welch.)

Continuing to the northeast, at 2.05 miles the Beech Trail crosses the Hasenclever Fire Road. It gradually ascends Nat House Mountain, and then descends along a pretty brook, a tributary of Tiorati Brook, passing a fine cascade at 2.5 miles which the trail blazers named "Arthur's Falls." Tiorati Brook Road is reached at 2.8 miles. Here, to the left, there is a large filled area where parking is permitted (in winter, Tiorati Brook Road is closed, so this parking lot cannot be used.) The trail turns right onto Tiorati Brook Road and crosses a bridge over a tributary of Tiorati Brook. It re-enters the woods and follows the brook for 0.15 mile, and then rejoins the road and crosses a bridge over Tiorati Brook. Immediately after crossing the brook, the Beech Trail

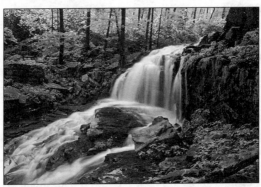
Arthur's Falls

turns left and heads up a flank of Flaggy Meadow Mountain through open woods, following an old woods road. It ends at the Red Cross Trail, 3.85 miles from the beginning. From this point, Tiorati Brook Road is 0.75 mile to the left on the Red Cross Trail.

This is one of the newer trails, blazed in 1972 after discussion by the NY/NJ Trail Conference (Trail Conference Minutes, 10/4/72). The work was done by members of Westchester Trails Association, who named the trail in honor of Art Beach. At that time, Art Beach was the representative of the Trail Conference to the Park administration. Due to a Park policy against naming trails for living persons, the name was spelled Beech (the 1984 Park map spells it Beach). It was during the construction of this trail that the device of using offset double blazes to show the direction in which the trail turns was invented.

The little cemetery on the trail has caused much speculation. Fifty acres on the south side of the stone wall were the farm of John Rose, which was acquired by the Park through condemnation in 1930. The grave is that of Timothy Youmans, who died on April 7, 1865 while serving in Company K of the 56th New York regiment. (The Civil War ended on April 9, 1865.) Samson Youmans, who served in that same Company, died in 1897 and was buried in St. John's Cemetery.

Twenty acres on the other side of the stone wall, including the farm with the root cellar, were owned until July 11, 1928 by Isaiah Charleston. He bought the farm in 1902 from William and Rebecca Jones. The graves are those of John R. Jones (1817-1896); his wife, Highlyann Babcock (1821-1886); and their little son Hiram Jones (1856-1859). Also buried there is John Strickland, who married Ruth Youmans (she died in 1897).

On the other side of the Cedar Ponds Road (Hasenclever Fire Road), about where Lake Welch Drive is now, was the 25-acre farm of John R. Jones, Jr. His father's grave is the one on our trail.

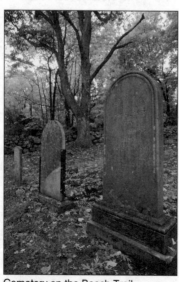

Cemetery on the Beech Trail

BLUE DISC TRAIL

Length: 2.8 miles
Blazes: blue dot on white

Miles

0.0	Johnsontown Road Circle.
0.15	Left, onto woods road.
0.45	Kakiat Trail joins briefly.
1.35	Gas line crosses.
1.5	Cross stream and turn right.
1.65	Elbow Brush.
2.0	T-MI Trail crosses.
2.05	Claudius Smith Rock.
2.8	End at Tri-Trail Corner.

The Blue Disc Trail formerly started from Seven Lakes Drive in Sloatsburg (at the second entrance to Johnsontown Road), but it now begins just west of the circle at the end of Johnsontown Road, where parking is available.

From 100 feet west of the bridge over the stream just west of the circle, the trail follows an unpaved road (the route of a gas pipeline) which goes up to a station of the Columbia Gas Transmission Co. This pipeline, which later again crosses our trail, was built in 1949. It goes across the Park in a southeast direction, from north of Tuxedo to Wesley Chapel (now Wesley Hills), and transports gas from Pittsburgh to Piermont, N.Y.

Beyond the gas pipeline station, the Blue Disc Trail turns left onto a woods road (until 1991, the blazes followed the gas pipeline road for another 0.15 mile to join the Kakiat Trail). After 0.3 mile on the woods road, the Kakiat Trail joins briefly, and Blue Disc starts a steep climb to the top of "Almost Perpendicular," a name given to the cliff in the early years by the Fresh Air Club (*N.Y. Post*, 4/21/36). At first, the trail goes up an eroded road. Leaving that about halfway up the cliff, the trail continues to the top where there is a good view to the south. After another 0.6 mile, the trail crosses the gas pipeline. Here the faint Fox Trail goes off to the right and descends to Spring Brook in the valley below.

In another 0.15 mile, Blue Disc crosses a stream and turns right along the foot of a ledge. A bit further, below the ledge, the trail is blazed through a crevice known as "Elbow Brush." The trail begins to parallel a stream and then runs along a swamp. At 2.0 miles, Blue Disc crosses the Tuxedo-Mt. Ivy Trail (T-MI) and climbs to the top of Claudius Smith Rock (see pp. 166-67). The Blue Disc Trail continues north over Big Pine Hill, with good views, and descends over bare, sloping rocks, often slippery in winter. The White Cross Trail (which begins from the T-MI Trail, 250 feet to the right of the Blue Disc crossing, and can be used as an alternate route) is less slippery. At the foot of the hill, Blue Disc crosses a rock dam (that retains the water in Black Ash Swamp) and ends at Tri-Trail Corner where it meets the Ramapo-Dunderberg and Victory Trails, 2.8 miles from the Johnsontown Road Circle.

In the '20s and early '30s, the Tuxedo Trail went from Tuxedo to Reeves Farm on Johnsontown Road, approximately following the route of the present-day Kakiat/Blue Disc trails. Hikers liked to climb the cliff which had been named "Almost Perpendicular." From the cliff top a trail, marked with green cairns, went to Claudius Smith Rock. In 1931, the New York Mountain Club scheduled a hike on the Green Cairn Trail (*N.Y. Post,* 1/9/31). Then, in the spring of 1932, Paul H. Schubert of Ridgewood (Queens) blazed a trail (marked with red discs with white centers) from Sloatsburg to the R-D Trail at the foot of Black Ash Mountain, using the Green Cairn Trail for part of the route.

Schubert had come from Germany in 1891 and worked as a printer for the *New York Staats-Zeitung.* A member of the Paterson Ramblers, the Woodland Trail Walkers, the Wanderbirds, and the NY/NJ Trail Conference, he also blazed the Trail of the Raccoon Hills. He died on October 8, 1961 at the age of 84 (*Walking News,* Dec. 1961).

From Sloatsburg, Schubert's Red Disc Trail went directly up Sleater Hill and continued along the ridge on the property of Miss Julia Siedler of Montclair, N.J. to Almost Perpendicular. That cliff and the land to the north, up to Black Ash Mountain, were the property of Tuxedo Park Association. At various times, both Miss Siedler and the Association closed their lands to ensure that these trails did not become public thoroughfares.

The Red Disc Trail went up the cliff with the help of a leaning dead tree on which Schubert had nailed slats as a ladder. A rope at the top helped climbers up the last stretch, where a sign read "Danger." By March 1938, the tree had fallen down, so he relocated the approach about 0.2 mile to the west, using a steep road toward Daters Mine. Just before the mine, the trail reached a level region and then turned right onto an old road that is part of the present route (which was chosen in 1970). After 1938, the blaze on this trail was changed to a half-and-half red/white disc, and the C.C.N.Y. Hiking Club took over the trail. In 1940, Miss Siedler closed the portion of the trail which was on her property, so it was rerouted to come up from Johnsontown Road. Then, in October 1943, the blazes were replaced by blue metal discs supplied by Alexander Jessup.

North of Almost Perpendicular, the trail goes over Pound Mountain. About 0.15 mile from the cliff, a side trail went left to a large rock, called Bonora's Rock. In 1928, John Bonora of 99 Varet Street, Brooklyn, a young member of the Paterson Ramblers Club, built a cabin against this rock. It had windows, a fireplace, double deck bunks, and a spring nearby. Known as Rockneath, it was a favored stopping place for those who knew the way.

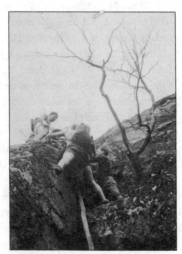

Coming down Almost Perpendicular – 1936

BOTTLE CAP TRAIL

Length: 1.9 miles
Blazes: bottle caps

Miles

0.0	Start from A-SB/LP.
0.05	Double caps; go up right.
0.4	Reach crest of ridge.
0.55	Descend steeply.
0.7	Cross brook and Surebridge Mine Road.
0.95	Cross R-D Trail.
1.25	Go up left from stream.
1.3	Go along hill, overlooking swamp.
1.5	Cross brook and ascend.
1.75	Top of hill.
1.9	End at fire road (old A-SB).

The Bottle Cap Trail, although marked, is not a Conference trail. Its origin has not been recorded, but it seems likely that the trail was made back in the '30s when members of the Green Mountain Club wanted an alternate route from the railroad station at Arden. The trail was marked with bottle caps nailed to the trees. The caps were renewed about 1945 by GMC members, and again in 1985 by the "Wednesday Hikers" led by Frank Haines. The latter group also marked the trail with many cairns.

The trail starts at a junction with the Arden-Surebridge Trail/Long Path (A-SB/LP) near the foot of Surebridge Mountain, 300 feet east of the end of the

White Bar Trail. (It is shown as a dashed red line on Trail Conference Map No. 4.) Here, A-SB/LP turns right, while the Bottle Cap Trail proceeds uphill along a broad path made by bulldozers during the 1988 fire season. In 350 feet, it turns right, leaving the bulldozer path, and continues up Surebridge Mountain.

After reaching the ridge of Surebridge Mountain at 0.4 mile, the Bottle Cap Trail continues north, along the ridge, for 0.15 mile. It then curves to the right and drops down several steep places. At 0.7 mile, it joins a bulldozer track which comes in from the left, crosses the brook which drains Surebridge Swamp, and crosses the Surebridge Mine Road. The trail then continues on an old mine road (the Surebridge Mine is in the trees to the right). It goes up a hill and, at 0.95 mile, crosses the Ramapo-Dunderberg Trail.

From here, the Bottle Cap Trail descends a gully, crosses a little brook, and follows along the north side of the brook for about 0.15 mile. It then veers left, away from the brook, and traverses the hillside overlooking a large swamp. It descends to another stream (the inlet of the swamp), which it soon crosses, and then proceeds uphill. At 1.75 miles, it reaches the top of a hill and descends to end at a fire road (the former route of the A-SB Trail) at 1.9 miles. From here, the hiker should turn left on the fire road and, in 60 feet, bear right on an old road which leads downhill for 400 feet to Seven Lakes Drive, opposite the entrance to Camp Thendara.

BREAKNECK MOUNTAIN TRAIL

Length: 1.5 miles
Blazes: white

Miles

0.0	Start on T-MI Trail.
0.15	West Pointing Rock.
0.8	Viewpoint, left, to lake.
1.0	Viewpoint to north and east.
1.2	Viewpoint to lake; turn left and descend.
1.5	End at S-BM Trail.

The Breakneck Mountain Trail starts from the Tuxedo-Mt. Ivy Trail, about 400 feet north of Pine Meadow Road East. It proceeds to the northeast along the ridge of Breakneck Mountain, passing (at 0.15 mile) "West Pointing Rock," a 10x14-foot boulder, with a sharp projection on its west side. At 0.8 mile, there is a limited view to the left over Breakneck Pond. After turning right and descending, the trail continues in a northeast direction. At 1.0 mile, the trail comes out on open rocks, with views to the north and east. The towers on Jackie Jones Mountain are visible straight ahead. Another viewpoint over the lake is reached at 1.2 miles; from here, an unmarked trail departs to the left and descends to the lake. The Breakneck Mountain Trail now turns left and goes down. It proceeds through a hollow and then turns left and ascends. At 1.5 miles from the start, it ends at the Suffern-Bear Mountain Trail (S-BM). Here, the (abandoned) Red Arrow Trail departs from the S-BM to go down to the camp on Breakneck Pond.

The Breakneck Mountain Trail was first blazed in the fall and winter of 1927 at the suggestion of Major Welch, General Manager of the Park (*N.Y. Post*, 9/2/27). It was built to connect the T-MI Trail with the S-BM Trail. Breakneck Mountain itself (known among local people as Knapp Mountain) had been acquired by the Park from Emma Louisa Knapp on June 27, 1917. Breakneck Pond had been the property of Rockland Finishing Company of Haverstraw (*N.Y. Times*, 4/8/28), while Cranberry Mountain, on the west side of the lake, belonged to William Huffman. Both of these properties were acquired by the Park in 1928.

In January 1924, George F. Parmelee of the Fresh Air Club cleared a trail along the east side of Breakneck Pond. There were no camps then, and the lake shore was quite wild. The trail ran from the old earth dam at the north end of the pond (built about 1890) through the laurels beyond the south end, and terminated at the woods road which carried the T-MI Trail across the north end of Big Green Swamp. (This road continued northwest to a junction with the Cranberry Mountain Trail and is now known as Pine Meadow Road.) The old trail through the laurels can still be followed by curious hikers.

CONKLINS CROSSING TRAIL

Length: 0.6 mile
Blazes: white

This trail is a short-cut between the Suffern-Bear Mountain (S-BM) and Pine Meadow Trails. It starts from the Pine Meadow Trail at the east end of Pine Meadow Lake, about 0.1 mile from the site of Conklin's Cabin, and crosses a rocky gully. On the right, an unmarked trail leads around the south side of the lake. The trail ends, 0.6 mile from the start, at the S-BM Trail on the Ramapo Rampart (a name coined by Frank Place). A very large boulder, known as "The Egg," is 0.15 mile to the left on the S-BM Trail, and another 0.2 mile further is the Stone Memorial Shelter.

Prior to 1935, when Ramsey Conklin and his family were still living at Pine Meadow, this trail started at their farm and crossed over the Rampart. It continued down into the valley, and followed Sky Meadow Road to Route 202 at Wesley Chapel (now Wesley Hills). In 1942, the owner of the land at the upper end of Sky Meadow Road closed the trail to hikers. The section down from the S-BM Trail was abandoned, as was another trail to Horse Stable Rock. From Pine Meadow to S-BM the trail was maintained by Jim Stankard of Westchester Trails Association from 1962 to 1973. As late as 1973, the abandoned section could still be followed. (Since then, it has become overgrown.)

CORNELL MINE TRAIL

Length: 2.5 miles
Blazes: blue

Miles
0.0	Trail begins at Bear Mountain.
0.75	Make sharp left off Bridle Path.
1.05	Reach Route 9W.
1.65	Cross old dirt road.
2.5	End at R-D Trail.

The Cornell Mine Trail (often known simply as the Cornell Trail) begins at a junction with the Appalachian Trail, the Suffern-Bear Mountain Trail and the Major Welch Trail, near a playground just west of the Bear Mountain Inn. It proceeds south along a paved path, and soon passes a skating rink to the right. After following the edge of the south parking area, the trail goes through a tunnel under Seven Lakes Drive. It then turns right from the paved path and goes through another tunnel under the South Entrance Road. This portion of the Cornell Mine Trail coincides with the Doodletown Bridle Path (see pp. 337-39), now a ski trail (red markers), and the 1777E Trail.

At 0.75 mile, the Cornell Mine Trail makes a sharp left and leaves the Bridle Path. It descends to the abandoned Doodletown Road and follows it to Route 9W, just north of where Doodletown Brook goes under the highway. From this point (elevation 20 feet) the trail climbs nearly 1,000 feet in the next 1.45 miles. It re-enters the woods and follows the brook uphill, using the route of the Iona Island Aqueduct for a short distance. On the way, there are views of the reservoir and water treatment plant built in 1974 to serve Iona Island, which had been acquired by the Park in 1965.

At 1.65 miles, the trail crosses an old dirt road. In another 0.45 mile, after briefly following a second dirt road, the trail begins to go steeply uphill along a ravine. Small mine openings may be seen on the way up. The Cornell Mine Trail ends at the Ramapo-Dunderberg Trail, 2.5 miles from the start, where another small mine opening is visible. On the hillside west of that point there are two larger horizontal shaft openings.

Bill Hoeferlin's Hikers Region Map #16 of August 1943 shows the original route of the Cornell Mine Trail. It began where the old (1809) Dunderberg Road crossed Timp Brook (this point has been covered by the reservoir which was built in 1974). The trail climbed towards Bald Mountain where it crossed a little brook on the 400-foot contour. The present-day route, which comes up somewhat to the east of the older route, joins the latter at the brook, and continues up the ravine, following approximately the original line.

At its meeting of December 1, 1971, the Trail Conference decided to make a new Cornell Mine Trail starting from the Bear Mountain Headquarters. By the end of February 1972, the new route had been cleared and blazed by the AMC. The steep route up the ravine, which had become badly eroded, was relocated in part by the West Hudson Trail Crew during 1998 and 1999.

The present Cornell Mine Trail goes up through a parcel of land on the side of Bald Mountain which was acquired by Thomas A. Edison in 1890. His 194-acre lot started at the old Dunderberg Road and went to the 1,080-foot level (the knob which the R-D Trail crosses, east of its junction with the Cornell Mine Trail). Edison's property line crossed the Cornell Mine Trail at the 810-foot level, so his land did not include the larger mine openings near the top of the mountain. (The history of these mine openings is given in our discussion of the Cornell Mine, pp. 451-53.)

The land on the north side of Bald Mountain was part of a grant made on October 30, 1749 by King George II to four children of Richard Bradley, who was the Attorney General of New York. In 1849, it was bought by Caleb June of Doodletown from three Sheldon brothers for $48.88. Thereafter, it was known as the Sheldon Lot.

In 1885, the parcel was sold by Andrew June to Thomas Nelson of Brooklyn, who sold it five years later to Thomas Edison.

At that time, Edison was deeply involved in a project to concentrate iron ore with magnets. He had extensive works in Ogdensburg, New Jersey, and another in Putnam County, New York. There is little evidence of mining activity on Edison's property. At the 610-foot level, there is a large trench near the trail. Another test hole is at the 810-foot level, the upper edge of the parcel.

In 1891, Edison transferred title to the Bald Mountain lot to his New York Concentrating Works, but he abandoned all of his iron projects soon afterwards, because the price of iron had dropped after the opening of the Mesabi Range mines in Minnesota in 1892. Edison sold his lot to the Park in 1928.

DIAMOND MOUNTAIN-TOWER TRAIL

Length: 0.8 mile
Blazes: yellow

Miles
West Branch (former Diamond Mtn. Trail)

0.0   Start from Pine Meadow Trail.
0.03 Bear left at junction.
0.25 End at Seven Hills/Hillburn-Torne-Sebago Trail.

East Branch (former Tower Trail)

0.0   Start from Pine Meadow Trail.
0.03 Bear right at junction.
0.05 Pass septic tank.
0.25 Climb over ledges, with views.
0.5   Site of fire tower.
0.55 End at Seven Hills Trail.

The Diamond Mountain-Tower Trail starts uphill from the Pine Meadow Trail (red square on white) about 100 feet west of where the latter crosses Christie Brook, 0.15 mile west of Pine Meadow Road. In about 150 feet, it reaches a junction. Here one branch of the trail (the former Tower Trail) goes off to the right, while the other branch (the former Diamond Mountain Trail) turns left.

The west (left) branch of the trail climbs steeply up Diamond Mountain. After crossing open ledges, it ends, 0.25 mile from the start, at the Seven Hills/

Hillburn-Torne-Sebago Trail. There is a good view at this point toward New York City.

The east (right) branch of trail goes up on a wide path. In another 100 feet, it passes a large concrete septic tank, built in 1934 to collect the sewage from the camps that were to be built on the four new lakes. The camps were not built, and the sewage system was never used. Upstream from the tank is an incomplete dam that was intended to create Lake Oonotookwa ("place of cattails") on Christie Brook.

The trail then turns left and goes steeply up over ledges, reaching one at 0.25 mile with a good view of Lake Wanoksink and Pine Meadow Lake. At 0.5 mile, the trail passes the site of the fire tower which was removed in 1986. Just beyond, the Diamond Mountain-Tower Trail ends at the Seven Hills Trail (blue on white).

On April 14, 1937, Raymond Torrey wrote to Major Welch: "Someone has made a new trail from the firetower on Diamond Mountain down to Christie Brook without asking anyone. . . . It is a handy short trail. I think we have enough trails." The new trail, known as the Tower Trail, was marked with a red T. Years later it was learned that it had been made by Kurt Stettner, a member of the Wanderlusters Club. His trail actually ended at the Stone Giants (Ga-Nus-Quah), 0.4 mile down the Pine Meadow Trail. In 1944, the color was changed to yellow, and in 1974 a black T was added at the beginning and end. Stettner died in February 1945 (Trail Committee Minutes, 3/21/45). In 1981, the trail was made to start from the Pine Meadow Trail near the old CCC ruin.

The Diamond Mountain Trail was first marked about

1939, but the name of its builder is not recorded. Until 1993, it was blazed white. In 1993, it was consolidated with the Tower Trail, and the joint trail—now officially known as the Diamond Mountain-Tower Trail—was reblazed yellow.

DUNNING TRAIL

Length: 3.75 miles
Blazes: yellow

Miles

0.0 Start from Nurian Trail.
0.15 Overhanging rock at edge of Green Pond.
0.4 Cross Nurian Trail.
0.45 Left on Island Pond Road.
0.55 Boston Mine.
1.1 Left on White Bar Trail.
1.35 Right on Crooked Road.
1.7 Cross R-D Trail.
2.1 Bowling Rocks.
2.25 Abandoned Dunning Trail leaves, left.
2.65 Crooked Road leaves, right.
2.85 Hogencamp Mine, up on left.
3.05 LP comes in from left.
3.1 LP leaves, right.
3.6 Pine Swamp Mine, left.
3.75 End at A-SB Trail.

This beautiful trail starts from the Nurian Trail (white) where the latter reaches the hilltop from the Valley of Boulders. Dunning proceeds south over a little rise, then goes left along the rocky edge of Green Pond, passing under an overhanging rock. It parallels the Nurian Trail which, at places, is only a few yards away. Although it provides a sheltered route in cold, windy weather, it is rather slippery when there is ice on the rocks. The Nurian Trail soon comes in from the left and, in 75 feet, leaves to the right. At 0.45 mile, Dunning reaches Island Pond Road. It turns left on this road for a short distance, and then turns right and passes by the Boston Mine. This mine, which was last worked in 1880, is a large cut in the hillside, with a water-filled shaft. The ore was sent to the Clove Furnace at Arden (see p. 448).

Dunning goes over the hill to the right of the mine (it went to the left until 1972) and continues eastward. At 1.1 miles from the start, Dunning turns left and joins the White Bar Trail. Both trails run together for 0.25 mile. Dunning then turns abruptly to the right and soon starts uphill, following the old "Crooked Road." On the ridge of Black Rock Mountain, 1.7 miles from the start, the Ramapo-Dunderberg Trail (R-D) (red on white) crosses. (The Bald Rocks Shelter is 0.15 mile to the south on the R-D Trail.) From here, Dunning proceeds downhill and eastward, crossing a little stream

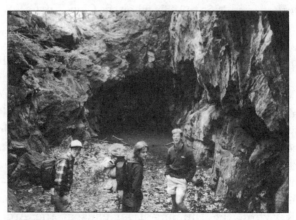

Hikers at the Boston Mine

and then a bare, rocky area. The boulders that dot the bare rock gave rise to the name "Bowling Rocks."

About 0.15 mile downhill from Bowling Rocks, the original route of the Dunning Trail goes left into the laurels. Brown paint covers the old yellow blazes on this path, which leads in 0.3 mile to the Long Path. Dunning continues downhill, following the Crooked Road. At 2.65 miles, the Crooked Road turns sharply down right, while Dunning continues straight ahead. (The Crooked Road, a lovely old grassy road, descends 0.5 mile to Little Long Pond, passing through the abandoned Girl Scout Camp Quid Nunc, which means "what now.")

In another 0.2 mile, the trail passes the extensive cuts of the Hogencamp Mine on the hillside to the left. A short distance beyond, as the trail passes a swamp on the right, the tailings from another shaft of the Hogencamp Mine can be seen on the left. This mine was worked from 1865 to 1885, when the Clove Furnace was finally shut down (see pp. 458-60).

At 3.05 miles, the Long Path (turquoise) joins from the left. It runs jointly with Dunning for a short distance, and then departs to the right and goes to Lake Skannatati. Dunning continues to the northeast on fairly level ground. It runs along the west side of Pine Swamp and passes the Pine Swamp Mine to the left (see pp. 462-63). A high pile of tailings can be seen from the trail, and the 25-foot cut — which leads into an interesting passageway tunnelled into the hillside — is visible if one climbs up beyond the pile of tailings. Soon afterward, the Dunning Trail ends at the Arden-Surebridge Trail, 3.75 miles from the start.

In 1934, Dr. James M. Dunning, chairman of the AMC Trails Committee, personally maintained the AT from the Bear Mountain Bridge to the Connecticut line. In April 1933, he proposed a new trail, to be a short-cut to the R-D Trail for hikers from Southfields. The proposal was endorsed by Major Welch, General Manager of the Park. Dunning, Ridsdale Ellis and other AMC members cut the new trail from Nurian's trail to the Crooked Road and thence to the R-D on the ridge. By June 1933, the red-blazed trail was complete. Unfortunately, Dunning had used Nurian's route from Stahahe Dam to Island Pond Road, and this led to a historic dispute. Kerson Nurian would not tolerate the new red markers, and he painted them out. Dunning then started his trail on the top of the ridge and relocated it along nearby Green Pond, and the dispute subsided.

The Dunning Trail was blazed red until 1943, when Joseph Bartha repainted it yellow and extended it from the R-D Trail past Hogencamp and Pine Swamp Mines to end at the A-SB Trail. In 1979, the Dunning Trail was rerouted to avoid passing an open cut of the Hogencamp Mine at the edge of the trail (the Long Path now uses that route, however).

FAWN TRAIL

Length: 1.0 mile
Blazes: red F on pink

Miles

0.0	Begin on AT, 0.25 mile from Seven Lakes Drive.
0.1	County line.
0.75	Cross T-T Trail.
1.0	End at Beechy Bottom East Road.

The Fawn Trail provides an easy route from the Appalachian Trail (AT) and Doodletown Road to the Anthony Wayne Recreation Area on the other side of West Mountain. It is a fairly level trail, and in June it passes through masses of laurels in bloom.

The Fawn Trail begins on the AT, 0.25 mile south of Seven Lakes Drive, where it goes off to the right. At 0.75 mile, on a low ridge, it crosses the Timp-Torne Trail (blue on white). At 1.0 mile, it ends at the Beechy Bottom East Road. Just a short distance to the right, a park path goes downhill to the Anthony Wayne Recreation Area.

The Fawn Trail was shown on the first Park trail map (1920). It started from the junction of Doodletown Road with Seven Lakes Drive. That Drive, built in 1913, used an already existing road (built in 1809) from Queensboro through Doodletown to Jones Point. Later, the AT was built (1922) and then a Bridle Path (1935).

In 1971, the Tramp and Trail Club asked permission from the Conference to mark and maintain the Fawn Trail, from the old fireplace on the AT to the Timp-Torne Trail. They marked it orange. In later years it was marked by the Park with red plaques as a ski trail, but in 1984 it was reinstated as a Conference Trail and reblazed red by Dick Warner. In 1987, Paul Leikin marked it in its present color.

During the 1988 forest fire season, bulldozers were used to make a fire lane which included parts of the Fawn Trail. It is hoped that, in time, the bulldozer scars will fade.

HILLBURN-TORNE-SEBAGO TRAIL

Length: 4.8 miles
Blazes: orange

Miles

0.0	Start at foot of Sebago Dam.
0.15	Cross T-MI Trail.
0.25	Turn left, uphill.
0.35	Cross Diamond Creek.
0.75	Join Seven Hills Trail.
1.0	Diamond Mountain Trail leaves, left.
1.05	Seven Hills Trail leaves, left.
1.95	Cross Pine Meadow Brook.
2.0	Briefly join Pine Meadow Trail.
2.4	Briefly join Seven Hills Trail.
2.8	Cross gas pipeline.
3.2	Raccoon Brook Hills Trail crosses.
3.45	Top of "Russian Bear."
4.3	Join Seven Hills Trail.
4.5	Turn left, off Seven Hills Trail.
4.8	End at Ramapo Torne.

When the Hillburn-Torne-Sebago Trail (HTS) was first blazed, it went from Lake Sebago dam, over Ramapo Torne, and down to Route 17 (now Route 59) in Hillburn, a distance of 5.9 miles. This accounts for the name of this trail, which now ends at the Torne.

From the foot of Sebago Dam, 0.65 mile south of the Sebago hikers' parking area, the trail follows Woodtown Road (West). It soon turns right and runs along Stony

Brook. At 0.15 mile, the Tuxedo-Mt. Ivy Trail (red on white) crosses, and in another 400 feet HTS turns left, uphill. After crossing Diamond Creek, a tributary of Stony Brook, the trail goes steeply up Diamond Mountain. On the way up, there are several limited viewpoints over Lake Sebago. At the top of the ridge, the Seven Hills Trail (blue on white) joins from the left, and both trails continue southwest along the crest of the ridge. The Diamond Mountain-Tower Trail (yellow) goes off to the left at 1.0 mile, after which HTS reaches an excellent viewpoint at the summit of the mountain. Soon afterwards, the Seven Hills Trail diverges left, while HTS turns right and descends over Halfway Mountain. At 1.95 miles, HTS reaches Pine Meadow Brook.

This point on the brook, where the water tumbles down over boulders, is called the Cascade of Slid, a name given by Frank Place. HTS turns left onto the Kakiat Trail (white), which follows the north side of the brook. A few yards upstream, HTS turns right and crosses the brook on a wooden bridge (which occasionally is washed away). The trail climbs up from the brook, turns left briefly on the Pine Meadow Trail (red on white), and then goes right, up Chipmunk Mountain. At 2.4 miles, the Seven Hills Trail (blue on white) joins from the left, then soon departs again to the right. HTS climbs to the hilltop and crosses the pipeline of the Columbia Gas Transmission Company, built in 1949. Downhill to the right, the gas line (which is walkable) crosses the Pine Meadow Trail 0.5 mile from Reeves Meadow.

At 3.2 miles, the Raccoon Brook Hills Trail (black on white) crosses, and at 3.45 miles HTS arrives at the top of the "Russian Bear." This cliff provides a good view of the Torne Valley and the Ramapo Rampart beyond, with the Ramapo Torne visible to the southwest. The trail then descends, climbs again, crosses a hollow and then climbs the opposite slope to meet the Seven Hills Trail once more. After running together for 0.2 mile, Seven Hills bears down to the right, while HTS turns left and continues gently upward to end at the top of Ramapo Torne, 4.8 miles from Sebago Dam.

HTS was first blazed in 1928 by Kerson Nurian. Nurian made the trail without asking permission of the landowner, of the Park or of the Trail Conference. He started the trail on Route 17 (now Route 59) in Hillburn, 0.3 mile north of the Hillburn Erie R.R. station (where a brook crosses the road). It went up over the side of Hillburn Mountain, then down across Torne Valley (where the Orange and Rockland Power substation is now) on an old route first blazed in 1922 by J. Ashton Allis. There was no landfill there then. The trail then climbed steeply to the top of Ramapo Torne. Today, one can still follow the white blazes from the Torne down to the service road under the power line.

Going north from the Torne, HTS used the older (1922) route of the Seven Hills Trail (white blazes) for 0.2 mile, then turned right toward Little Torne (later named Russian Bear). It was Dr. Myrtle Lothrop Massey of the Interstate Hiking Club who, in 1929, saw on the cliff the profile of a performing bear (*N.Y. Post*, 1/10/30). Dr. Massey often invented fanciful names for rock formations, but this is the only one still remembered. She died on September 30, 1945, at the age of 69.

In 1931, Paul Schubert of the Paterson Ramblers marked the Trail of Raccoon Hills. His trail, which started from the Ramapo Torne and followed the route of HTS for some distance, was marked with a red half disc with a white center. In the fall of 1936, Jack Spivack of the New York Ramblers extended the Seven Hills Trail to Suffern. Going south from the Torne, he used the route first marked by Allis, and his extension joined the S-BM Trail just south of the Kitchen Stairs. Spivack also reblazed the entire Seven Hills Trail, using blue blazes instead of white.

In 1937, there were three sets of blazes leading north from the Torne, and hikers became aware of the "Great Ramapo Trail War" (*N.Y. Post*, 12/3/37). One day, Schubert found that his Raccoon Hills blazes had been painted black. Spivack's Seven Hills extension to Suffern was painted black, too, while the blue blazes north from the Torne were painted yellow. A sign was put up at the junction of the Seven Hills extension and S-BM which read: "Tie-trail to HTS." The extension itself was reblazed with a T. In January 1938, Torrey discovered that the "painter-outer" was Kerson Nurian. He was single-handedly eliminating the joint markings (although he himself, ten years earlier, had used a portion of the Seven Hills Trail for his HTS Trail). Because all these trails were on private land, neither the Trail Conference nor the Park had jurisdiction over them.

Schubert angrily removed his blazes north from the Torne, and started his trail from Torne View instead. Spivack repainted his Seven Hills blue blazes, and after Nurian's identity became known, the Trail War subsided. In 1933, Nurian had a dispute with Jim Dunning (see p. 45), and he would have another dispute with the Conference in 1948 about the Triangle Trail (see p. 163). Nurian maintained the HTS Trail until 1939, when he turned it over to Charles Wolfman.

In 1940, the trails south of Pine Meadow Brook were officially closed to hikers by the landowner, the Ramapo Land Company (Pierson Estate). It was only after 1963, when the Park acquired a large parcel of Pierson land (including the Torne), that these trails were restored to their present length. Since the land immediately south of the Torne remains in private ownership, the trails in this area have not been reopened.

Hurst Trail

Length: 0.5 mile
Blazes: blue

The Hurst Trail starts from Seven Lakes Drive near the south end of Lake Tiorati, about 0.1 mile north of the entrance to Camp Thendara. At the edge of the road there is a cable barrier across the trail (the bar closes the fire road which also starts at this point). The Hurst Trail follows the fire road for 125 feet, then goes up to the right. After passing under telephone wires, it bends left and climbs Fingerboard Mountain. It passes around the left side of Fingerboard Shelter and shortly afterward ends at the Ramapo-Dunderberg/Appalachian Trail.

The Hurst Trail was first blazed in November 1922 by Haven C. Hurst, a member of the Green Mountain and Sierra Clubs. After his accidental drowning in the Hudson River off 119th Street on June 5, 1923, the trail became known as the Hurst Memorial Trail (*N.Y. Post*, 6/15/23). When first made, the Hurst Trail crossed the R-D/AT on the ridge of Fingerboard Mountain about 125 yards north of the shelter, on the north side of a knob. This point is a few hundred feet north of the present end of the trail. From here, the trail went west and northwest down the slope. Passing around the north end of a swamp (where the Long Path meets it today), it joined the Surebridge Mine Road, which it followed out to Upper Cohasset Lake.

The Hurst Trail was a favorite way to Paradise Rock, on a rocky hilltop overlooking Upper Cohasset Lake. A short bushwhack uphill from the trail where it followed the road around the swamp led to the rock. Traces (a trash basket and water pipes) can still be found there of a shelter which was built about 1937, with private funds, for the use of the girls' camps on the Cohasset Lakes below.

Before 1949, the Hurst Trail was blazed with a black H on a white square. The trail was then regarded as unauthorized. In 1949, the blazes were changed to blue, and on October 5, 1955 the Conference voted it an official trail. By this time, the trail appears to have been abandoned west of AT/R-D. The first Conference Map #4 (1975) shows the Hurst Trail ending at AT/R-D.

Kakiat Trail

Length: 7.4 miles
Blazes: white (at junctions, a black "K" on white)

Miles

0.0	Tuxedo (Grove Drive).
0.25	Level off on abandoned telephone line.
0.5	Descend steeply to cross stream.
1.0	County line crosses.
1.35	Path goes up left towards Daters Mine.
1.5	Blue Disc Trail joins briefly.
1.8	Gas pipeline crosses.
2.05	Cross Spring Brook.
2.2	Briefly join White Bar Trail.
2.3	Cross Seven Lakes Drive.
2.6	Hilltop.
3.05	Bridge over Stony Brook.
3.15	Bridge over Pine Meadow Brook.
3.4	Cascade of Slid; HTS Trail crosses.
3.75	Seven Hills Trail joins.
3.8	Cross Pine Meadow Brook.
4.1	Raccoon Brook Hills Trail starts.
4.6	RBH Trail loop crosses.
4.85	Torne Valley Road crosses.
5.0	Cross Torne Brook.
6.0	S-BM Trail crosses.
6.4	Power line; sharp left.
6.65	Gas line crosses.
7.15	Turn right, near river.
7.4	Trail ends; parking area is 0.1 mile to left.

The Kakiat Trail starts in Tuxedo. To reach the trailhead, follow the Ramapo-Dunderberg Trail (R-D) (red on white) from the railroad station a bit south along the tracks and down to the footbridge over the Ramapo River. (Or follow East Village Road, north of the station.) After going under the Thruway, turn left on Grove Drive, then follow the R-D when it turns right, into the woods. Forty feet from where R-D leaves the paved road, Kakiat goes up to the right, on a woods road. The trail climbs Pine Hill, leveling off on an abandoned telephone line. Then, at 0.5 mile, it goes steeply down to cross a stream. Soon it joins a woods road which curves to the east, around the foot of Daters Mountain. A concrete monument to the right at 1.0 mile marks the boundary between Orange and Rockland counties.

At 1.35 miles, as Kakiat bends sharply to the right, a path goes up left toward Daters Mine. This once was the start of the Blue Disc Trail (see pp. 29-30). Now, however, Blue Disc joins briefly at 1.5 miles. In another 0.3 mile, Kakiat crosses a gas pipeline and goes down to cross Spring Brook on stepping stones. At 2.2 miles, Kakiat briefly joins the White Bar Trail, which follows abandoned Johnsontown Road, and, in another 500 feet, it crosses Seven Lakes Drive. Kakiat climbs a bank into the woods again and goes uphill on a woods road, then down through an evergreen grove past an old farm site. At 3.05 miles, Kakiat crosses Stony Brook on a log bridge. It goes left on the unmarked Stony Brook Trail and, after 500 feet, crosses to the north side of Pine Meadow Brook on another log bridge.

The hemlock grove and cellar hole on the hillside above Stony Brook are the site of a farm known as "the old Bentley place." In 1855, Henry C. Wanamaker sold the 75-acre farm on the ridge to John and Cornelia Becraft. At the same time, he sold the adjacent 62 acres along Johnsontown Road to Jacob Waldron, retaining a right of way to the ridge farm. That right of way is now the route of our Kakiat Trail. John and Cornelia immediately sold 50 acres on the ridge to Andrews and Susan Hill. In 1864, the Hills sold the place to Joel Becraft. Joel kept it until 1904, when he was 75 years old. Then he sold the ridge farm to Fred and Sarah Bentley of Tuxedo Park. Bentley sold the farm in 1906 to Robert Prentice of New York City, but continued to use it for a number of years. Prentice sold the farm to the Park in 1916. In 1919, the old farmhouse was demolished and the evergreens planted.

Although they lived in Tuxedo Park, Fred and Sa-rah Bentley were not rich people. They arrived in New York City from England in 1888. Their friend Pierre Lorillard met them at the boat, and made them welcome at his new country place, Tuxedo Park. Fred Bentley became the head gardener at Tuxedo, and developed quite a good business working for the well-to-do residents there. Lorillard gave him the use of a farm, east of the river, where the Italian Village was later built. Bentley had twelve teams of horses for his gardening/hauling business, and to get more hay for his horses he bought the Becraft farm above Stony Brook. He died in 1934.

The Kakiat Trail originally started where Pine Meadow Brook joined Stony Brook. There it met the (unmarked) Stony Brook Trail. In October 1935, Frank Place and Park Ranger William Gee extended the trail from Stony Brook to Tuxedo. They used the older Tuxedo Trail (Hikers Region Map #5, 1935) which went to Tuxedo from

Robert Reeves' farm on Johnsontown Road. To avoid crossing Reeves' land, they built a bridge over Stony Brook. By March 1936, the new bridge had been washed away, but it was rebuilt a month later. It has been washed away and rebuilt many times since then.

After crossing Johnsontown Road and going around Daters Mountain, the new extension headed north and downhill towards Tuxedo. It joined a woods road along the Ramapo River that led to the Italian Village and the footbridge over the river. When the Thruway was built in 1954, the Kakiat Trail went down along the Thruway fence to the Village. The residents of the Village objected to the trail and, in December 1974, Art Paul of the Tramp and Trail Club relocated the Kakiat Trail to follow an abandoned power line on the hillside and then go down to Grove Drive at the end of the Ramapo-Dunderberg Trail.

The trail goes over boulders up along the north side of Pine Meadow Brook. At 3.4 miles, it passes the Cascade of Slid. This cascade is quite impressive during the spring. Here, the Hillburn-Torne-Sebago Trail (orange) comes down from Halfway Mountain and crosses the brook on a log bridge. Before 1946, Kakiat also crossed the brook on this bridge.

In the early 1920s, Frank Place had been reading the fanciful works of Edward Plunkett, Lord Dunsany. One of Dunsany's first books was *The Gods of Pegāna* (London, 1911), a tale about a mysterious kingdom where geography ends and fairyland begins. One of those gods was Slid, "the Lord of gliding waters and of still, Lord of all the waters of the world, and all that long streams garner in the hills; but the soul of Slid is in the sea." About 1920, Frank Place decided to name the cascade for this Dunsany character. Lord Dunsany died in Dublin on October 25, 1957, while Frank Place died on September 8, 1959. In April 1962, his Tramp and Trail Club placed a tablet in Frank Place's memory on a tree near the Cascade. The tablet disappeared about 1970.

The Kakiat Trail continues up the north side of the brook, meeting the Seven Hills Trail (blue on white) at 3.75 miles. The Pine Meadow Trail comes in here, too, and all three trails cross Pine Meadow Brook on a log bridge (once called "Hauptman's Bridge," after its first builder, Adolph Hauptman, a member of the Nature Friends Club). Kakiat then turns left and goes up Raccoon Brook, a tributary stream. At 4.1 miles, the Raccoon Brook Hills Trail (RBH) (black on white) starts from the left.

Until 1963, the area to the south of this point was owned by the Ramapo Land Company, controlled by the Pierson family. The Kakiat, HTS, Seven Hills and RBH Trails, as well as the Quartz Brook and Reeves Brook Trails, ran through the Pierson land. The Boundary Trail also started here, at the junction of Kakiat and RBH. It was marked in 1942 with a black B on white, as well as with the yellow blazes that designated the Park boundary. Little used, the Boundary Trail was abandoned in 1954.

Kakiat now climbs over a ridge and, at 4.6 miles, the RBH Trail joins from the right. The two trails run together for 125 feet, after which RBH turns left, while Kakiat continues straight ahead. At 4.85 miles, Torne Valley Road is crossed, and shortly afterward Kakiat crosses Torne Brook. Soon Kakiat begins to parallel the Columbia Gas Transmission Company pipeline, constructed in 1949. The trail then climbs to the Ramapo Rampart (a name invented by Frank Place) at Cobus Mountain. (A rather poetic tale about Claudius Smith, "Cowboy of the Ramapos," said that he had a brother named Jacobus (he didn't) — hence the name Cobus.)

At 6.0 miles, the Suffern-Bear Mountain Trail (S-BM) (yellow) crosses. On the S-BM just south of this junction are two huge boulders (many others are nearby) which were named "Grandma and Grandpa Rocks" by Place and Torrey when they scouted the S-BM in 1926 (*N.Y. Post*, 4/21/36).

Descending Cobus Mountain partly on woods roads, Kakiat reaches the power line of Orange and Rockland Utilities at 6.4 miles. Here it makes a sharp left turn. At 6.65 miles, the trail crosses a wide gas pipeline (look carefully here for the blazes). Further down it again uses wide woods roads. Some of these roads are also marked with a green stripe on white by the Kakiat County Park. This county park was created in 1963 when Rockland County acquired 239 acres owned by Anthony Cuccolo (he also owned Kakiat Farm) and the adjoining 105 acres owned by Baillie. At 7.15 miles, the trail approaches the Mahwah River. The old Kakiat Lodge was across the river here. The Kakiat Trail now turns right on a park road, and ends 0.25 mile further, 7.4 miles from the start. A parking area is across the Mahwah River, 0.1 mile to the left.

In the 1920s, the Tramp and Trail Club of New York City rented a lodge at the corner of Route 202 (it was then known as Route 122) and Grandview Avenue. It was called the Kakiat Lodge, probably because it was across the road from the Kakiat Farm. In 1926 that club, led by Frank Place and Raymond Torrey, marked a trail (white K blazes) from the Kakiat Lodge to Stony Brook. They often referred to it as the Tatcony Trail (the initials of Tramp And Trail Club Of New York).

The name Kakiat is derived from a grant of land made in 1696 by Governor Benjamin Fletcher, in the name of King William III, to Daniel Honan and Michael Hawdon. The grant included the land from Sloatsburg to Monsey and Pomona. The Minsi Indians called it Kackyachtaweke. This region, once known as Kakiat, was later named New Hempstead by settlers from Long Island. Eventually it became the Town of Ramapo.

The curious hiker who visits the junction of Route 202 and Grandview Avenue, 0.5 mile northeast of the entrance to Kakiat Park, will find there (just north of the intersection) a marker which reads:

KAKIAT LODGE
Aaron (Aurie) Blauvelt (1738-1801), French & Indian War veteran and Orangetown Militia captain in the Revolution, occupied a stone house here and ran a saw and grist mill on the Mahwah River nearby. Son, Cornelius Blauvelt (1766-1843), a colonel in the War of 1812, inherited the farm. His son, Richard, added a foundry to the mill and probably built this homestead c. 1830. It served as an inn in recent decades.

LICHEN TRAIL

Length: 0.45 mile
Blazes: blue "L" on white

The northern end of the Lichen Trail is on the Arden-Surebridge Trail, about 0.5 mile from the Lemon Squeezer. The trail starts uphill from a rhododendron grove, climbs about 100 feet through a hemlock grove, and then levels out over rocky ledges in a burned-out area, soon passing a beautiful view to the west, over Island Pond. The Lichen Trail ends at the Ramapo-Dunderberg Trail, 0.45 mile north of the Dunning Trail and just south of a large boulder known as "Ship Rock."

"Frank Place of Tramp and Trail Club, with permission of W.A. Welch, is locating a new shortcut trail from A-SB to RD. To be painted white. He strung it last Saturday." (*N.Y. Post*, 4/22/33).

By mid-June, the trail was ready, painted blue. Frank Place called it the Surebridge Shortcut. By mid-September, R.H. Torrey had found the new trail to be rich in common and unusual lichens, especially the one known as "Iceland Moss." The scientific name for this species, which grows in brown clumps, is Cetraria Islandica. Torrey also found several varieties of Cladonia. He decided to name the new trail the Lichen Trail (*Torreya, Journal of Torrey Botanical Club*, May 1934; *N.Y. Post*, 9/15/33).

An amusing anecdote relates that Torrey, in his enthusiasm for the new trail, persuaded Major Welch to come with him to hike it. He was greatly embarrassed when he realized that he could not find it.

LONG PATH

Length: 25.15 miles (Mt. Ivy to Florence Mountain)
Blazes: turquoise

Miles

0.0	Intersection of Routes 202 & 45 at Mt. Ivy.
0.2	Turn right onto Parkway ramp.
0.4	Leave paved road and enter woods.
1.45	Cross bridge over Minisceongo Creek.
2.35	Knob of Cheesecote Mountain.
2.45	Cheesecote Pond.
3.3	Turn left at Letchworth Village Cemetery.
3.5	Turn left onto Calls Hollow Road.
4.55	Cross Old Turnpike.
5.45	S-BM Trail (yellow) joins from right.
5.6	Big Hill Shelter.
5.75	Cross Old Turnpike.
6.25	Cross stream on rocks.
6.35	Site of plane crash.
6.5	Turn right, onto woods road.
6.65	Footbridge over Beaver Pond Brook.
7.05	Bear left (right goes to St. John's).
7.55	Cross Lake Welch Drive.
8.1	Beech Trail (blue) goes right.
8.75	Cross Route 106 (Gate Hill Road).
9.2	Cross Seven Lakes Drive (to Lake Skannatati).
10.5	Join Dunning Trail (yellow).
10.55	Dunning Trail leaves, left.
11.3	"Times Square"; join A-SB.
11.85	Lichen Trail (blue), left.

12.15	White Bar Trail, left.
12.85	AT (white) crosses.
13.7	View of Upper Cohasset Lake.
13.85	Cross Surebridge Mine Road.
14.0	Old Hurst Trail goes right.
15.0	Cross Arden Valley Road.
16.15	View toward Arden House.
17.0	Hippo Rock.
17.15	Menomine Trail (yellow), right.
17.25	Stockbridge Shelter.
17.55	Stockbridge Cave Shelter.
18.75	Join park fire road.
19.25	Cross Route 6 (parking).
19.7	Junction with Popolopen Gorge Trail.
20.0	Long Mountain Summit; Torrey Memorial.
20.2	Go down left.
20.55	Cross Deep Hollow Brook.
21.05	Cross Deep Hollow Trail.
21.6	View from Howell Mountain.
22.0	Cross Brooks Hollow Brook.
23.15	Cross Route 293.
24.5	Join Route 6.
25.15	Go right, off Route 6, down Florence Mountain.

The Long Path (LP) starts at the George Washington Bridge and presently ends at John Boyd Thacher State Park in Albany County. The section described in this guide begins at the intersection of Routes 202 and 45 in Mt. Ivy, adjacent to Exit 13 of the Palisades Interstate Parkway.

Parking is permitted (weekends and holidays only) in the commuter lot at the junction of Routes 202 and 45. Phone your license plate numbers to the Haverstraw police (914-354-1500) on the day of the hike. You should have a Trail Conference decal visible in the rear driver-side window.

The Long Path goes west on Route 202 and crosses under the Parkway. It then turns right, up the Parkway entrance ramp and past the start of Quaker Road, and enters the woods in a small pine grove. The trail parallels the Parkway for about a mile. For the first 0.7 mile, the trail runs along a narrow strip, with the Parkway to the right and a chain-link fence (beyond which there is residential development) to the left. At 1.3 miles, after passing through a wet area, the trail turns right and continues along a grassy woods road. Shortly after crossing the south branch of the Minisceongo Creek on a wooden bridge (built by the PIPC's Summer Youth Work Program in 1984), the trail turns right, then goes left and continues uphill into the Cheesecote Town Park. This mountain — known variously as Cheesecote or Cheesecock Mountain — lies within the royal Cheesecock's Patent granted by Queen Anne to seven New Yorkers on March 25, 1707.

After reaching the crest of a knob, the trail descends and approaches the east side of Cheesecote Pond. It turns left onto the old Letchworth Village Road, which is "paved" with stones, and goes around the south side of the pond. At the southwest corner of the pond, there is a wide turnaround. (The parking here is for Haverstraw residents only.) The old Letchworth Village Road curves to the right and continues down to Willow Grove Road, while LP turns left, goes up over a rise, and then goes down along a gravel road to the northwest. After passing under a power line, it reaches Letchworth Village Cemetery (where most of the graves are marked only by numbers) and turns left. It soons turns left again and, at 3.5 miles, reaches Calls Hollow Road. From this point, Ladentown is 2.6 miles to the left, and the Palisades Interstate Parkway is 0.8 mile to the right (at Willow Grove Road). Parking at this trail crossing is not advisable.

In 1921, Major Welch, General Manager of the Palisades Interstate Park, proposed creating a hiking trail from Fort Lee to Bear Mountain via Piermont, Hook Mountain, High Tor and Mt. Ivy (*N.Y. Post*, 3/11/21). Nothing was done, however. In 1928, R.H. Torrey proposed a trail from Englewood landing to Mt. Ivy (*N.Y. Post,* 1/13/28). Again, the proposal was not acted on. In 1932, Vincent J. Schaefer of the Mohawk Valley Hiking Club of Schenectady suggested a new long trail from Bear Mountain to Lake Placid (*N.Y. Post*, 12/23/32). Schaefer laid out his trail in detail on topo maps. He intended that it be followed by map and compass, but did not want it to be blazed. Florence Puller of the New York Hiking Club brought this plan to the attention of W.W. Cady of New York City. In the fall of 1933, Cady began blazing a trail from the George Washington Bridge to Lake Placid (*N.Y. Post*, 11/7/33). Cady's route was described in great detail in R.H. Torrey's Tuesday *New York Post* columns from March 3, 1934 to September 14, 1934. It extended as far as the Adirondack Mountain Club's Johns Brook Lodge in the Adirondacks. It appears that Cady never blazed the trail further north than Route 23, near Windham High Peak, and for years after that, the trail was untended. In 1943, Alexander Jessup again marked the trail as far as Peekamoose Mountain in the Catskills. It included lots of road walking. Again it was left untended. Jessup died on March 11, 1944.

In the spring of 1961, Robert Jessen, Kurt Ramig and Michael Warren of New York City issued a booklet planning a 350-mile route from the George Washington Bridge to Whiteface Mountain. Jessen was a 21-year-old textile worker (*N.Y. Times*, 8/16/61) and president of the Ramapo Ramblers. By October 1961, the blazing and clearing north from the George Washington Bridge was started. In 1964, the Trail Conference decided on the route through Harriman Park, and in January 1965 it was adopted as a Conference trail. The route chosen was joint with T-MI from Mt. Ivy to Ladentown and across the Park to the Dutch Doctor Shelter. There the new Long Path joined the old Boy Scouts' White Bar Trail over the saddle of Parker Cabin Mountain, over Car Pond Mountain, and north to the

AT at Island Pond. Together with the AT, it went up to Fingerboard Mountain (here the R-D also joined) and continued north to a fireplace where it left AT/R-D and picked up the old route of the Fingerboard-Storm King Trail.

The history of the Long Path was recounted by George Zoebelein in the July 1966 *Trail Walker*.

On September 28, 1971, Secretary of the Interior Rogers C.B. Morton dedicated the Long Path in New Jersey and New York as a National Recreational Trail. Also present for the dedication ceremony were Palisades Interstate Park Commissioners Laurance Rockefeller and Donald Borg, and New York State Commissioner of Parks and Recreation, Alexander Alrich.

In 1981, the Long Path was extensively rerouted to approximately its present line. The purpose of this relocation was to eliminate the two-mile road walk from Mt. Ivy to Ladentown.

The Long Path goes left on Calls Hollow Road and after 500 feet turns right, into the woods. Soon it crosses Horse Chock Brook (which drains the three Letchworth Reservoirs) and climbs fairly steeply uphill. About half a mile above the brook the ruins of the Call family home are visible on the left. At 4.55 miles, the Long Path crosses a wide dirt road known as the Old Turnpike, which is now the route of a buried coaxial telephone cable. Until 1992, this road carried the Long Path for 1.5 miles, but the trail has now been rerouted through more sylvan glades. About 500 feet to the right along the Old Turnpike, a path leaves to the right and goes to the site of ORAK, an old mansion (see p. 143).

Soon the Long Path crosses a small brook and ascends a hill. At the top of the hill, at 5.0 miles, it passes a small swamp to the left. It then goes down and, after a short climb, joins the Suffern-Bear Mountain Trail (S-BM) (yellow) which comes in from the right. A moment later, the joint trails meet a faint woods road, known as the Second Reservoir Trail. To the left, this road goes to the Second Reservoir; to the right, it ends at the Old Turnpike nearby.

In another 250 feet, LP/S-BM goes steeply uphill to the Big Hill Shelter, which it reaches at 5.6 miles. Here, the Long Path turns right and goes down to cross the Old Turnpike again. It then goes over another small hill and descends to cross a stream. At 6.35 miles, the trail enters a clearing. This is the site of a 1974 crash of a jet plane which had been enroute to Buffalo to pick up the Baltimore Colts football team. The three crewmen were killed (*N.Y. Times,* 12/2/74).

Beyond the clearing, the trail crosses a boulder field, and at 6.5 miles it turns right, onto a woods road. Until 1981, this road was the route of the Skannatati Trail. Just 100 feet to the left of this junction, the woods road ends at the paved road to Breakneck Pond.

The Long Path now goes down to cross Beaver Pond Brook, which comes from the Breakneck Pond dam. There is a good footbridge across the brook now, but, in years past, hikers crossed on a beaver dam. The bridge was built in 1986 by Park ranger Andy Smith. He named it the Jake Gannon Memorial Bridge in memory of his grandfather, who served for many years as the caretaker of St. John's Church.

At 7.05 miles, a trail to the right leads to St. John's Church. LP bears left and soon crosses Lake Welch Drive at its intersection with St. John's Road. The trail goes northwest along a farm road, passing old cellar holes. This farm — part of the Sandyfield community — was the home of Charles Conklin until September 1938.

LP then goes down a slope and across a low area. At 8.1 miles, the Beech Trail (blue) starts, to the right. About 0.7 mile further, LP reaches Route 106 (Gate Hill Road). It turns right and follows the road for 250 feet, then turns left and goes up over the shoulder of Rockhouse Mountain (the "Rock House" is a cave to the right of the trail, *below* the highway). LP passes under a telephone line, rounds the end of Lake Askoti and, at 9.2 miles, crosses the Seven Lakes Drive and reaches Lake Skannatati. At the edge of the lake, LP passes the beginning of the Arden-Surebridge Trail (red triangle on white). LP follows the north shore of the lake, crosses Pine Swamp Brook, and then turns uphill to the right. At 10.5 miles, it joins the Dunning Trail (yellow).

Lake Askoti dam, which carries the Seven Lakes Drive, was built in 1935. Lake Skannatati dam was built three years later. The names of both lakes were chosen by Major Welch. In the Algonquin language, Askoti means "this side," and Skannatati means "the other side." Some time after Lake Skannatati was filled with water, perhaps in 1942, a trail was made by the Boy Scouts from there west to the Hogencamp Mine. On December 1, 1943, the Trail Conference planned a new trail, to be marked with a red cross. It started from the Dunning Trail near Hogencamp Mine, used the Boy Scout route to Lake Askoti, then went up Rockhouse Mountain to Hasenclever Road. After 1947, when the Red Cross Trail was rerouted, this trail route was unblazed. Then in 1961 it was marked as the Skannatati Trail (white) from the Dunning Trail to Lake Skannatati. In 1963, Bill Hoeferlin blazed it to St. John's Church, and in the spring of 1964 he extended it to Big Hill Shelter. In the fall of 1981, most of the Skannatati Trail was taken over by the Long Path.

The Long Path goes west with the Dunning Trail for about 250 feet. It then turns right and goes uphill. A shaft of the Hogencamp Mine is soon visible on the left (the main mine is near the Dunning Trail). LP then goes around a great boulder, called Cape Horn. In the rocks behind the boulder is a cave known as the Cat's Den.

A short distance beyond Cape Horn, LP goes right (here, the original route of the Dunning Trail went left; see p. 44). LP heads north along the side of a little valley and soon joins an old woods road — a continuation of the

Surebridge Mine Road — that goes to "Times Square." Here, at 11.3 miles, LP meets the Ramapo-Dunderberg (R-D) and Arden-Surebridge (A-SB) Trails. LP now joins A-SB. The joint trail briefly follows the Surebridge Mine Road and soon turns left into a hemlock grove. It then descends Surebridge Mountain through rhododendrons, passing the ends of two swamps. This part of the trail was named the "Lost Road" by the blazers of A-SB in 1921.

At 11.85 miles, LP/A-SB passes the end of the Lichen Trail (blue L on white). In another 0.3 mile, it reaches a junction. Here, the White Bar Trail starts to the left and A-SB goes straight ahead to the Lemon Squeezer, while LP bears right (north) and continues along the west side of Dismal Swamp. At 12.85 miles, the Appalachian Trail crosses. Winding now through groves of maple and hemlock, LP climbs the eastern side of Echo Mountain. At 13.7 miles, there is a view of Upper Cohasset Lake, and just below is a shelter that was built in 1937 for the girls' camps on the lake. From here, LP goes down to Surebridge Mine Road and joins a woods road that goes northeast around the end of a swamp. This road is part of the abandoned section of the Hurst Trail (see p. 53). A bushwhack left uphill away from the swamp will take you to Paradise Rock on the summit — a beautiful spot for lunch.

At 14.0 miles, the old Hurst Trail goes right. LP continues northeast along the western foot of Fingerboard Mountain to Arden Valley Road, which it reaches at 15.0 miles. LP crosses the road and follows a woods road to the north.

On the left as one starts up this woods road, a faint trail may be seen going northwest through the saddle between two summits of Bradley Mountain. That path — the Forest Lake Trail — was part of the first road, built in 1760, through the Highlands from Stony Point to Central Valley. It leads into the Harriman estate and should not be used without written permission. The woods road that carries the Long Path here for 0.2 mile was part of that old road, and of the Arden Valley Road before the Park built the present paved road down to Tiorati Circle about 1917.

After 0.4 mile on the woods road, LP diverges left and climbs gradually to the summit of Stockbridge Mountain (named for Elisha Stockbridge, 1826-1916, who owned a hotel near Summit Lake in 1893). From the ridge, Arden House can be seen to the west.

Arden House was the home of Edward Harriman. The plans were drawn by architects John Carrere and Thomas Hastings, who are best known for designing the New York Public Library. The house took three years to complete, and cost $2,000,000. Edward Harriman moved into his new home in August 1909 and, unfortunately, died of stomach cancer on September 9, 1909. Arden House is now used as a conference center for Columbia University.

At about 17.0 miles, a great boulder named Hippo Rock overhangs the trail. In another 0.15 mile, the Menomine Trail (yellow) leaves to the right. (The continuation of this trail, going west, is the unmarked Nawahunta Trail.) LP then climbs a ledge to reach Stockbridge Shelter (built in 1928) at 17.25 miles.

About 0.3 mile further north, the trail descends a ledge to the Stockbridge Cave Shelter.

The scouting of this trail, the old Fingerboard-Storm King Trail, began in the summer of 1922. In July, the cave was discovered by J. Ashton Allis, who was exploring this section of the trail with his two young sons. The Park improved the cave in 1928 so that it could be used as a second Stockbridge Shelter. Other trails that were first blazed by Allis are the Seven Hills Trail, the Arden-Surebridge Trail, and a long trail from Harrison Mountain in the Wyanokies over Sterling Ridge to Mombasha High Point (1913). A short section of that latter trail is still called the Allis Trail. J. Ashton Allis, a founder of our Trail Conference, died at age 89, on December 29, 1970.

Coming down from the ridge, LP at 18.75 miles joins a fire road that goes north from Lake Nawahunta. In another 0.5 mile, it crosses Route 6 (Long Mountain Parkway). The paved loop, where cars may be parked, is the older (1919) line of Route 6. LP turns left into the woods again and soon reaches a junction with the Popolopen Gorge Trail (red dot on white). The path which goes down left from here was the route of Long Path until September 1988. It is an "ankle breaker" road, paved with broken stones in 1934 by the Civilian Conservation Corps.

From its junction with the Popolopen Gorge Trail, LP turns up to the left and climbs to the summit of Long Mountain, which it reaches at 20.0 miles. This was the route of the older and much longer Fingerboard-Storm King Trail, and subsequently was designated the Long Mountain Trail. The 1,155-foot summit affords a fine view to the east, with Turkey Hill Lake below. This was

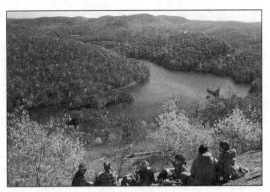

Hikers on Long Mountain overlooking Turkey Hill Lake

a favorite spot of Raymond Torrey, much loved leader of the Trail Conference who, with J. Ashton Allis, scouted this section of the trail in 1922. Torrey died on July 15, 1938. In his memory, his friends inscribed a memorial on the summit of Long Mountain:

**In Memory of
RAYMOND H. TORREY
A Great Disciple of the
"LONG BROWN PATH"
1880 - 1938**

The memorial was dedicated on Sunday, October 30, 1938, and Torrey's ashes were scattered there to the winds by his friend Frank Place.

0.2 mile north of the memorial, LP turns left and goes down off the ridge (the older markers, which head north into West Point land, can still be seen). The trail descends on switchbacks, following a 1992 relocation.

As it approaches Deep Hollow Brook the trail passes the site of the former Deep Hollow Shelter (1933-1975). The original path down from the ridge was cleared in 1929 by Alexander Jessup, who was at that time the maintainer of the entire Fingerboard-Storm King Trail.

The Long Path crosses Deep Hollow Brook (there *may* be stepping stones) and then a tributary stream, and goes up a wide firebreak, the boundary of West Point Military Reservation. About 0.4 mile beyond the second stream crossing, an old woods road crosses. This was named the Deep Hollow Trail because it starts at the north end of Deep Hollow, near Stillwell Lake, and goes southwest along the mountainside to end at Route 6, 0.5 mile west of the LP crossing (see pp. 292-93).

LP continues upward, reaching a fine viewpoint on Howell Mountain (named for William Thompson Howell, 1873-1916, a pioneer hiker in these Highlands). The trail descends steeply into Brooks Hollow,

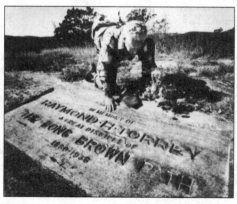

At the Torrey Memorial – October 26, 1986

and at 22.0 miles crosses the brook that drains Lake Massawippa. It climbs up Brooks Mountain, turns southwest along the ridge, and then turns right (west) and goes downhill to cross Route 293 (0.15 mile north of Barnes Lake). After going a short way up Blackcap Mountain, the trail turns southwest, down a long ridge, to reach Route 6 just west of its junction with Route 293.

When LP was first blazed in this area in 1962, it went on over Blackcap Mountain to join Lawn Road/Trout Brook Road/Pine Hill Road into Highland Mills. In 1974, it was relocated to approximately its present route to avoid West Point land. Now the trail follows the fence along Route 6 for 0.65 mile, and then, at 25.15 miles, turns right toward Central Valley, using the abandoned line of Route 6 down Florence Mountain.

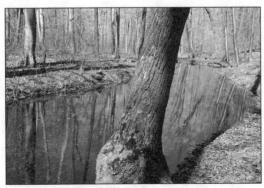

Deep Hollow Brook

Major Welch Trail

Length: 2.65 miles
Blazes: red dot on white

Miles

0.0	Bear Mountain Inn.
0.45	Go left, uphill.
0.95	Turn left and start steep climb.
1.2	Views.
1.4	Cross Perkins Drive.
1.8	Go right, onto Perkins Drive.
1.9	Perkins Tower.
2.65	End at Perkins Drive.

The Major Welch Trail, named in 1944 in memory of Major William A. Welch, the first General Manager of the Park, starts behind the Bear Mountain Inn, and follows the paved path along the west side of Hessian Lake. After 0.45 mile, near the north end of the lake, the trail turns left and goes uphill. It passes the Bear Mountain covered reservoir (see p. 340), on the hillside to the left, and goes above Overlook Lodge, which may be seen below to the right. Soon it levels off on the 400-foot contour on the northeast side of Bear Mountain. At 0.95 mile, the trail turns sharply left (the Appalachian Trail (AT) originally came from below to this point) and climbs steeply 900 feet to the summit. At about 1.2 miles, there are good views of the Hudson River and the hills beyond. The Major Welch Trail crosses Perkins Memorial Drive at 1.4 miles. It continues straight ahead and goes through a picnic area on the summit. At 1.8 miles, it turns right onto Perkins Drive, and soon passes the Perkins Memorial Tower. The trail then leaves the Drive and descends the south slope of Bear Mountain, following an old route of the AT. It bears right (still following the old AT route) and passes some excellent viewpoints. Soon the old AT route bears left (downhill), while the Major Welch Trail continues straight ahead (on the old route of the Timp-Torne Trail, abandoned in 1960), crossing many rock outcroppings with good views. At 2.65 miles, it ends at the Perkins Drive. Until 1991, the blazes continued another 0.6 mile up the Drive, to end at the ascending route.

This trail was first marked in 1922 as the route of the new Appalachian Trail up Bear Mountain. The trail builders were expecting a bridge to be erected across the Hudson here. In anticipation, they started the AT up the mountain about a half mile west of the bridge-to-be. There was no Popolopen Drive then, only an old woods road above the gorge. The new Popolopen Drive, started in 1925 (now the route of the Palisades Interstate Parkway), made a 20-foot cut where the AT had started uphill, so the trail was moved 50 yards to the east.

In the fall of 1931, the AT was relocated to pass by the ski jump at the south end of Hessian Lake. The old route was left as an alternative approach trail to the AT, joining the relocated AT on the summit of Bear Mountain (*N.Y. Post*, 1/29/33). In 1934, the old route was repainted white (the AT was blazed yellow, then). In 1940, the Cygian Society added a red ring to the white squares. (In 1991, the blazes were changed to a solid red circle on a white square.) Then, in 1944, Joseph Bartha, Trails Chairman of the Conference, suggested starting the trail from the Inn instead of the Bridge, and naming it for Major William A. Welch, who had died on May 4, 1941. The relocation was done by Charles Luscher in the spring of 1946.

At the top of the mountain, the trail originally ended at Perkins Tower. In June 1960, the Timp-Torne Trail was rerouted away from Bear Mountain, and the former route of that trail was used to make the upper end of the Major Welch Trail.

Where the Major Welch Trail comes up from below to cross the Perkins Memorial Drive, there is a point of interest. Uphill, 200 feet above the road and 50 feet east of the trail, a five-foot stone monument, with an iron spike sticking out of the top, may be seen. This is an old boundary marker. When the Park was formed in 1910, the West Point Military Academy retained ownership of a

pie-shaped parcel on Bear Mountain. From its apex near the summit, the West Point line went north to Popolopen Brook and west to a point on the old Fort Montgomery Road (a similar monument can be seen there). In 1939, West Point proposed a land exchange with the Park (*N.Y. Times*, 6/4/39). The deal was closed on April 20, 1942 (Commission Minutes, 5/13/42). The Park acquired 50 acres of West Point land on Bear Mountain and a 252-acre parcel north of the brook (which included the Popolopen Torne). In return, West Point acquired 108 acres of Park land northeast of Turkey Hill Lake and 718 acres in the hills northwest of Fort Montgomery (which the Park had bought in 1928 from the Fort Montgomery Iron Corporation). The Park also received a cash settlement of $14,526.19.

West Point was not the only "other" property owner on Bear Mountain. When the Commission acquired the prison site in 1910, their land extended up the mountain to within one-tenth of a mile of the summit. The 237 acres at the very top were the property of Addison Johnson of Port Chester, New York. He also owned the land on the north side of the mountain, down to Popolopen Brook. (The latter tract had, until 1817, been the property of Ithiel June, the first resident of Doodletown.) Johnson sold his land to the Commission on August 19, 1912.

A tenth of a mile west of Perkins Tower was the start of a 23-acre parcel owned by Harriet W. Graham of Queens Village, Long Island. This piece included the land through which the AT and Major Welch Trails were blazed, down to Perkins Drive. Mrs. Graham also had a right-of-way "from the above-described premises to the Dunderberg Turnpike" (now known as Doodletown Road). Except for West Point, she was the last of the "other" landowners on Bear Mountain, selling to the Commission on June 26, 1930.

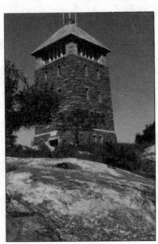

Perkins Memorial Tower

MENOMINE TRAIL

Length: 2.85 miles
Blazes: yellow

Miles

South to William Brien Memorial Shelter (AT/RD)

0.0   Start at south end of Silvermine parking area.
0.45 Join old road which comes out of lake.
0.65 Reach end of Silvermine Lake.
0.95 Turn left on grassy woods road.
1.35 Trail ends at William Brien Memorial Shelter.

North to Stockbridge Shelter (Long Path)

0.0   Start at south end of Silvermine parking area.
0.25 Cable barrier across road; turn up right.
0.35 Grave of "Scobie" Jim Lewis, right.
0.4   Cross Seven Lakes Drive.
0.55 Turn left off Nawahunta Fire Road.
0.65 Cross brook.
0.85 Begin to ascend.
1.1   Cairn; trail, right, leads to Cave Shelter.
1.35 Trail, left, to Stevens Mountain.
1.5   End at Long Path.

The Menomine Trail connects the Silvermine parking area with the Appalachian/Ramapo-Dunderberg Trails (AT/R-D) at the William Brien Memorial Shelter on Letterrock Mountain, and with the Long Path at the Stockbridge Shelter on Stockbridge Mountain. Since the Menomine Trail primarily serves as a means of accessing these two major trails from the parking area, we will describe the trail in two sections, beginning in each case from the parking area.

South to William Brien Memorial Shelter (AT/RD)

From the southern end of the Silvermine parking area, the Menomine Trail crosses a bridge and turns left. Just before it reaches the lake, it turns right, and then it turns left and follows along the shore of the lake, passing through a very rocky area. At 0.45 mile, the trail joins a woods road which comes up from the lake. Before the lake was built, this road went along the edge of what was then known as the Bockey Swamp. Since the creation of the lake, the northern section of the road has been submerged, and the remaining portion of the road (now followed in part by the Menomine Trail) became known to hikers as the Bockey Swamp Trail.

After reaching the end of the lake, the Menomine Trail goes up a valley along Bockey Swamp Brook. At 0.95 mile, it comes to an intersection with another woods road. (To the right, this road leads 0.8 mile to the Seven Lakes Drive.) The Menomine Trail turns left on the road, crosses a stream, and begins a steady ascent. At 1.35 miles, the trail ends at an intersection with the AT/RD at the William Brien Memorial Shelter.

North to Stockbridge Shelter (Long Path)

This part of the Menomine Trail begins just before the bridge at the southern end of the Silvermine parking area. It proceeds west along the guardrail at the edge of the parking area, then follows a dirt road leading through a picnic area. It turns right, uphill, at a cable barrier at the end of the picnic area, crosses a road which leads to an abandoned parking area, and enters an evergreen grove on a knoll above Seven Lakes Drive. Just to the right of the trail is the grave of "Scobie" Jim Lewis, whose farm was where Lake Nawahunta was created in 1915.

After crossing Seven Lakes Drive at 0.4 mile, the Menomine Trail briefly follows the Nawahunta Fire Road, passing to the left the cellar hole of the Lewis family home. At 0.55 mile, near the end of Lake Nawahunta, the Menomine Trail turns down left and crosses the inlet of the lake (Nawahunta Brook) on stepping stones. It passes through a pine grove, crosses a causeway across a swamp, and follows an old wagon road up Stockbridge Mountain. At 1.1 miles, just beyond a bend in the road, a cairn on the right marks the start of a trail which leads 0.3 mile to the Stockbridge Cave Shelter. This trail, once blazed red, has been painted out with black paint, and the black blazes can still be followed (with care). Now the Menomine Trail begins to level off. At 1.35 miles, a road forks left to Stevens Mountain, and the Menomine Trail again begins to climb. The yellow Menomine blazes end at 1.5 miles, where the Long Path (turquoise) crosses. The Stockbridge Shelter is about 0.1 mile up to the right.

The Menomine Trail was created on Labor Day, 1994, as a means of linking the AT/RD and the Long Path with the convenient Silvermine parking area. For the most part, it follows the routes of two old woods roads — the Bockey Swamp Trail and the Nawahunta Trail — which had long been used by knowledgeable hikers to access these marked trails from the Silvermine parking area.

The name of the trail, Menomine, was originally given by Major Welch to the lake south of Seven Lakes Drive that was created in 1934 by the Civilian Conservation Corps. Prior to then, the area was a large swamp, known as the Bockey Swamp. In an attempt to attract birds, the Park planted wild rice in the swamp. But, instead, the rice was eaten by deer. When the lake was built, it was named Lake Menomine, an Indian name for wild rice. It was renamed Silvermine Lake in 1951.

NURIAN TRAIL

Length: 3.4 miles
Blazes: white

Miles

0.0	Former Southfields railroad station.
0.1	Go down, right.
0.25	Cross Ramapo River.
0.35	Cross New York Thruway.
0.65	Turn right and start uphill.
1.1	Top of Green Pond Mountain.
1.4	Join paved road.
1.65	Begin steep climb.
2.05	Dunning Trail starts, right.
2.3	Dunning Trail crosses.
2.35	Briefly join Island Pond Road.
2.85	White Bar Trail joins from left.
2.95	Turn left and go down.
3.4	End at R-D Trail.

The Nurian Trail is named for its builder, Kerson Nurian. He called it "the Short Trail" to the R-D, making possible a hike from Southfields to Tuxedo.

The trail starts (for most hikers) at the Red Apple Rest, where the Short Line bus stops in Southfields. This warm meeting place is much appreciated in winter (cars should be parked at the rear of the lot). Cross the parking area to the northeast corner, near the tracks, and walk north along the tracks for about 0.25 mile. Watch for a triple white blaze on a utility pole on the right, just north of Railroad Avenue, at the site of the former station. The trail continues along the tracks for 0.1 mile, then goes down right, along an old woods road, toward the river, which is crossed on a steel bridge. At 0.35 mile (from the old station), the trail crosses the New York Thruway on the Nurian overpass.

In 1824, the old woods road from the railroad tracks to the river was part of the "Monroe and Haverstraw Turnpike," which we now know as Route 106/Gate Hill Road (the railroad did not come through until 1838). The old toll road turned up through the hills past Car Pond (Lake Stahahe), Little Long Pond, and Beaver Pond (Lake Welch).

In 1894, Edward Harriman built a road south from Arden which crossed the Ramapo River 0.25 mile north of the Turnpike bridge. About 1929, Nurian marked his trail to cross the river at a ford where Harriman's bridge had stood. Soon afterward, the Park built a wooden footbridge where the Turnpike had crossed, and Nurian's trail was rerouted to cross that bridge. The bridge was washed away in

April 1936 and rebuilt a month later. It was washed out again in December 1938 and replaced in January 1939. That bridge was washed out in 1946, and the present bridge of steel beams was built in 1950. From 1948 to 1950, hikers crossed the river on two steel cables.

During the construction of the Thruway in 1953, the western end of the Nurian Trail was closed. Indeed, it appeared that it would be permanently closed. Agitation for an overpass was started by the Trail Conference in 1954. Initially, Thruway officials rejected a proposed stone-faced bridge on the ground that it would cost $80,000 and serve only a small number of hikers.

William Burton, Conference Trails Chairman, who was a naval architect, then designed a steel-and-concrete bridge, which could be built for half the price. John Coggeshall, a former President of the Conference, who worked for the State, showed the new design to Thruway officials and persuasively argued the need for a bridge in this location. He was successful in convincing the officials to construct the bridge, which was opened with a ceremony on July 15, 1956.

From the overpass, the trail goes north along Harriman's Level Road (the Old Arden Road), turning right, uphill, at 0.65 mile from the railroad station. It climbs 320 feet to the summit of Green Pond Mountain and then descends. On the way down, at 1.2 miles, a cement box-like structure may be seen on the hillside to the right. That was once a latrine for a camp operated by Grace Church of New York City. The camp's mess hall burned on September 5, 1947, but its fireplace chimney is still standing.

At 1.4 miles, Nurian reaches a paved park road which serves the camps on both sides of the lake. Just before reaching the paved road, the trail crosses a woods road. To the left, this woods road follows Stahahe Brook for 0.65 mile down to Harriman's Level Road, which it reaches about 0.7 mile north of the Nurian junction, and 0.8 mile south of the hikers' parking area at Arden (the "Elk Pen"). Nurian turns left along the paved road and crosses the outlet brook of Lake Stahahe.

In 1929, Torrey described the original route of the Nurian Trail: "Cross the Ramapo River northeast of the station, and follow a trail along the telephone line to Lake Stahahe" (*N.Y. Post,* 6/14/29). That "telephone trail" turned uphill from Old Arden Road just a bit south of where the present-day trail starts up, and reached the road along Lake Stahahe about 0.4 mile south of the dam. The trail then followed the road north along the lake. At first, Nurian's trail crossed the Stahahe dam (*Paterson* *Morning Call*, 8/19/32), but by 1935 the present route over the mountain and on the paved park road was in use.

Nurian turns left off the paved road near a concrete septic tank, briefly follows a gravel road, passing filter beds to the left, and then continues straight ahead where the road turns right. It soon begins to ascend, steeply in places, following the south side of Island Pond Brook (Island Pond has two outlet brooks). The ravine of the brook is known as the Valley of Boulders.

After climbing further up, there are great boulders immediately to the left of the trail at 1.9 miles. The Nurian Trail then goes around the end of a long sloping rock, and continues by going up alongside the rock. Near the top of the rock there is a limited viewpoint to the northeast over Green Pond Mountain. At 2.05 miles, Nurian reaches the Dunning Trail (yellow), which begins to the right. Bending left, Nurian passes above Green Pond, and turns left onto the Dunning Trail at 2.3 miles. The two trails run jointly for 100 feet. Dunning then goes off to the left, while Nurian continues ahead. The Boston Mine, an interesting side trip, is 0.15 mile to the north on the Dunning Trail.

Nurian soon turns right onto Island Pond Road. It goes south on the gravel road for about 125 feet, then goes left across a pretty region, with laurels and evergreens, to meet the White Bar Trail at 2.85 miles. Nurian goes south on White Bar for about 0.1 mile, then departs down to the left to cross a small brook. It turns right and briefly follows the brook, then turns left and begins the climb up Black Rock Mountain.

Nurian ends on the Ramapo-Dunderberg Trail (red on white), 3.4 miles from the start. From here, Route 106, where some limited parking is available, is 0.4 mile to the right.

Kerson Nurian was born in Bulgaria in 1873. He was a slender man, with gray hair and a gray goatee, and was a member of ADK, AMC, GMC and the Sierra Club. During his trail-building years he was an electrical engineer, working on submarines at the Brooklyn Navy Yard. He was an eager trail marker, but never asked permission of the Park, of the Trail Conference, or of the landowners. In addition to this "Short Trail" (1929), he made the HTS (1928), the Triangle Trail (1939) and the White Cross Trail. Nurian's independence and insistence on having his own way led to several disputes with others over his trails. See p. 45 (dispute with regard to the Dunning Trail's use of a portion of the Nurian Trail), p. 51 (the "Great Ramapo Trail War," involving the HTS Trail, the Seven Hills Trail and the Trail of the Raccoon Hills), and p. 163 (dispute with regard to the Triangle Trail). Kerson Nurian died on November 19, 1948, at the age of 75.

Kerson Nurian at Camp Nawakwa

PINE MEADOW TRAIL

Length: 5.5 miles
Blazes: red square on white

Miles

0.0	Second bridge after Thruway.
0.7	Seven Hills Trail starts, right.
0.9	Reeves Meadow Visitor Center.
0.95	Reeves Brook Trail starts, right.
1.05	Reeves Brook crosses.
1.3	Turn right; Stony Brook Trail continues ahead.
1.4	Quartz Brook Trail goes right.
1.45	Gas line crosses.
2.1	HTS Trail crosses.
2.45	Footbridge across brook.
2.7	Ga-Nus-Quah Rock.
3.1	Diamond Mountain-Tower Trail, left.
3.25	Cross Pine Meadow Road West.
3.3	Path, left, to Lake Wanoksink.
3.7	Path, left, to Conklin Road.
3.75	Pumphouse ruin.
3.95	Site of Conklin's Cabin.
4.05	Conklins Crossing Trail, right.
4.45	Cross Pine Meadow Road East; Sherwood Path to right.
4.8	Many Swamp Brook crosses.
5.5	End at S-BM Trail.

The Pine Meadow Trail (PM) begins on Seven Lakes Drive in Sloatsburg, at the second bridge after the New York Thruway, 0.7 mile from Route 17. (A more convenient starting place, with parking available, is the

Reeves Meadow Visitor Center, 1.4 miles from Route 17.)

From its start at the bridge, PM goes to the right, then curves to the left and continues along the foot of the hill parallel to the road. At 0.7 mile, the Seven Hills Trail (blue on white) goes uphill, to the right. Soon afterwards PM emerges onto a field known as Reeves Meadow, where the Park has erected a visitor center (water and toilet facilities are sometimes available here). Just beyond the building, the Reeves Brook Trail (white) starts up, to the right. PM then follows Stony Brook and, at 1.05 miles, it crosses Reeves Brook.

The Pine Meadow Trail was described by Torrey and Place in the first *New York Walk Book* (1923). They advised hikers to follow Johnsontown Road, "a good dirt road through a picturesque farming country." At 1.5 miles from the Sloatsburg railroad station, the trail crossed Stony Brook on stepping stones and followed a woods road across a meadow (where the visitor center was built many years later). This meadow was part of a 125-acre farm which had been given to the Park in 1921 by wealthy George Grant Mason of Tuxedo Park (see pp. 427-28). (What is nowadays called Reeves' Meadow actually was Mason's Meadow!)

In 1922, Mason's farmhouse was occupied by Chief Park Ranger Bill Gee. During the following years, the Pine Meadow Trail, then unmarked, left Johnsontown Road in Sloatsburg and crossed a bridge (now Greenway) over Stony Brook. It went along the southerly side of Stony Brook and then skirted to the south and east of the Mason farm (which was located between Johnsontown Road and the present-day Seven Lakes Drive). It approached Stony

Brook again where the visitor center is now located.

In 1943, the trail was blazed, for the first time, by Frank Place, who used white metal discs (they were changed to red in 1945). He started it then at the cement bridge (demolished 1993) that led into the Mason farm from Johnsontown Road (*Walking News*, Nov. 1943). The trail went between the farm buildings and continued across the meadow to the area of the present-day visitor center.

In those days, Stony Brook flowed through a little pond (Allen's Pond) just south of the junction of Johnsontown Road with Washington Avenue. When the Thruway was built, that road junction was wiped out. A by-pass was made around the south side of Allen's Pond, which rejoined Johnsontown Road at the present location of the second left turn from Seven Lakes Drive onto Johnsontown Road.

In 1954, the Pine Meadow Trail was marked to enter the Park from the bypass through a trailer court (which is still there). The trail crossed Stony Brook on a little bridge. It followed the brook to the demolished Mason farm, then crossed the fields to the woods where the visitor center is now.

The route changed again in 1961, when the new Seven Lakes Drive was built. Allen's Pond was filled in, and Stony Brook was moved over to the south side of the new road where it went under the Thruway. In 1963, the trail was marked from the Sloatsburg railroad station north along the tracks to Seven Lakes Drive, and along that road to the second bridge over Stony Brook. There it turned right and went along the foot of the hill, south of and parallel to Seven Lakes Drive, as it does now.

In 1982, the trail was made to start at that second bridge, but even now the old blazes can still be seen on the poles along the railroad tracks north of station and along Seven Lakes Drive.

At 1.3 miles, PM turns right, uphill, as the un-marked Stony Brook Trail goes straight ahead. Quartz Brook is crossed at 1.4 miles. Just before that brook, an unmarked trail goes up, to the right. That was the old Quartz Brook Trail, which can still be followed for 0.9 mile to the Seven Hills Trail.

The Columbia Gas Transmission Company pipeline crosses at 1.45 miles. Here, the Pine Meadow Trail is a wide woods road, high above Pine Meadow Brook. At 2.1 miles, the Hillburn-Torne-Sebago Trail (orange) comes up from the Cascade of Slid on the left. It runs jointly with PM for a short distance and then goes up to the right. PM now levels off, following the brook and crossing it (with the Kakiat and Seven Hills Trails) on a log bridge that was first built by Adolph Hauptman, a member of the Nature Friends Club. Bending right, PM follows the brook on an eroded woods road. (If it looks like a road, it is because in the fall of 1965 the Park widened the trail to a 20-foot fire road, up to Pine Meadow Road.) At 2.7 miles, there is a pair of great boulders named Ga-Nus-Quah (Stone Giants). The Tower Trail (yellow) once started here.

A little beyond Ga-Nus-Quah, a fairly clear area can be seen on the left at the foot of the hill. In the spring, two great lilac bushes bloom there. These bushes are all that remains to mark the place where a tiny cabin stood about 1900.

The 1923 edition of the *New York Walk Book*, describ-ing the Pine Meadow Trail, says on page 102: " . . . it brings you into cleared land with rocky cliffs above you on the left. Here once stood a tiny cabin . . . ." All that can be seen there now are those great lilac bushes, with a

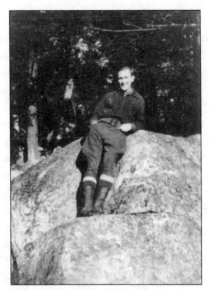

The author at Ga-Nus-Quah – 1936

piece of an old iron stove among their roots.

That land had been bought by Nicholas Rose in 1865. He also owned land up in Pine Meadow, and a farm near Sloatsburg. He was a woodcutter who carried cordwood down the Pine Meadow Trail with a four-mule team. Sometimes he lived in that little cabin beside the trail, and he undoubtedly was the one who planted those lilac bushes. Nick Rose sold the place in 1902 to Fred W. Snow. Snow was a well-to-do citizen of Hillburn, son of the founder of that town. He used the little cabin for occasional fishing trips. One day Fred Snow learned that two mountain women had been using his cabin to entertain customers. So he went up the trail and burned the cabin to the ground. In 1921, he sold the parcel to the Park.

When we pass those lilac bushes and see their blooms, we may think of those who lived there a hundred years ago. Our feelings are expressed in a poem by Jack Chard, of the Union County Hiking Club:

LILACS

Do you remember on that sunny day
We followed through the silence of the woods,
Where birds sang in the leafy green of spring,
That grassy trail where wagons once had passed;
Where grass and bushes crowded on the way;
The woods, advancing, claimed their own at last.

Suddenly lilacs met us in the wood,
Fragrant with mauve flowers of a rich delight.
Here must some long-forgotten home have stood
Where patient hands tended their simple herbs,
Some apple trees, still standing gnarled and lost,
And these sweet lilacs to adorn their life.
Some grass-grown stones recall the vanished house.
But those who lived and loved and died within,
Calling it home, their names we do not know;
Can only guess their heartbreak, joys and fears.
If men recall us at some distant day,
Long after death has closed our busy scene,
We did not live in vain if they can say:
"They left us lilacs where their life had been."

At 3.0 miles, the marked trail goes up to the left, past the foundation of a Civilian Conservation Corps building (the headquarters of the three CCC camps in the Pine Meadow area). A wide path goes straight ahead, across a level area bounded by a low stone wall (many hikers assume that the wide path is the official trail). Soon the Diamond Mountain-Tower Trail (yellow) goes off to the left.

PM now turns right, goes down to cross Christie Brook and continues along a rocky road to Pine Meadow Road West. On the right, this road crosses a dam and continues halfway around the lake. The Pine Meadow Trail now crosses the road and follows the north shore of the lake. For much of the way it follows old water and sewer pipes, usually buried but sometimes visible. This pipeline, and others around Lakes Wanoksink and Minsi, were built in 1934 to service the camps which were to be built on the lakes. The pipelines all terminate in a large (but never used) concrete septic tank on Christie Brook.

At 3.3 miles, a path leaves, left, to Lake Wanoksink. Shortly afterward a trail goes right, out to a point in the lake often used as a lunch stop. Another path goes left at 3.7 miles to Conklin Road. Until 1934, when Pine Meadow Lake was created, this was the Woodtown Road, which crossed the swampy meadow on a corduroy roadbed and went down Torne Valley to Ramapo. Just beyond is the ruin of a stone building. This is often thought to have been Conklin's Cabin, but it was actually constructed to house the pumps which were to supply water to the (never built) camps around the lakes. A path uphill behind the ruin leads to a very large water tank.

The actual site of Conklin's Cabin, 0.2 mile further on the trail, is a flat area, bounded by a steep rock on the left and the lake on the right. The cabin was next to a single large walnut tree, which stands near the middle of the area. Against the steep rock are the remains of a wall which was part of Conklin's cow barn.

The Conklin family lived there from 1779 to 1935, when the new lake was flooded. In 1933, the CCC built a camp for 200 young men across the meadow to the south. Ramsey Conklin's three sons, Steve, Nick and Theodore — then in their 30's — also worked on the new lake. When the water covered their spring and garden, the Conklins departed to Ladentown. There the town supervisor, Pincus Margulies, allowed them to live in an old schoolhouse at the corner of Camp Hill and Quaker Roads. By 1942, the cabin at Pine Meadow was in ruins (*Walking News*, Nov. 1942) despite the wire fence the Park had built around it.

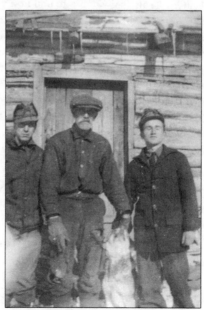

Ramsey Conklin leaving his cabin – February 15, 1935

The Pine Meadow Trail continues eastward. In sight of the end of the lake, the Conklins Crossing Trail (white) departs, down to the right, while PM goes up to the left, leaving the pipeline. At 4.45 miles, Pine Meadow Road East is crossed. Here the Sherwood Path goes right, to the Suffern-Bear Mountain Trail at Stone Memorial Shelter. Then, 0.35 mile further, Many Swamp Brook is crossed. There was once a little bridge here, called Turtle Bridge. At 5.5 miles, PM ends at the Suffern-Bear Mountain Trail (S-BM) (yellow).

To the right, the S-BM Trail leads in 0.2 mile to the start of the southbound leg of the old Pittsboro Trail (see pp. 256-58), marked there with cairns on the left. Until 1943, the Pine Meadow Trail continued eastward along with the S-BM. After 0.2 mile, PM departed steeply downhill to the right. It crossed Gyascutus Brook 0.15 mile below the S-BM crossing, and continued down another 0.3 mile to end at a woods road. That woods road is now part of the power line service road. The lower end of the old Pine Meadow Trail was abandoned after 1943, but it is still used by horse riders.

POPOLOPEN GORGE TRAIL

Length: 4.5 miles
Blazes: red dot on white

Miles

0.0	Popolopen viaduct, south end.
0.2	Old bridge site.
0.7	Go right on aqueduct.
1.4	Timp-Torne Trail joins, right.
1.45	Leave aqueduct.
2.1	Cross Queensboro Brook.
2.45	Left on Fort Montgomery Road.
2.55	Leave road, right.
2.75	Queensboro Lake on left.
3.2	1779 Trail leaves, left.
3.4	Go left on Summer Hill Road.
3.95	Anthony Wayne Trail, left.
4.5	End at Long Path.

Hikes on the Popolopen Gorge Trail (PG) often start from the Bear Mountain Inn. To reach the trailhead, take the paved path along the east side of Hessian Lake to the traffic circle near the bridge, then cross the Palisades Interstate Parkway. The blazes start on the left, in a clearing, just before reaching the Popolopen Viaduct. The trail goes down an old road to a point where there once was a bridge across the gorge.

Before the Popolopen Viaduct was opened on July 15, 1916, the road that "straggled past Highland Lake [*i.e.*, Hessian Lake] was little more than a stony track which went down to a little iron bridge over Hell Hole" (*N.Y. Post*,

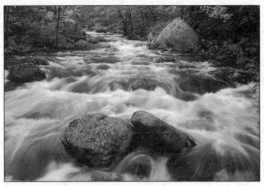
Churning waters at Popolopen Gorge

1/4/29). A dam had been built near there in 1901 to generate water power for a mill downstream. The little lake behind the dam is known as Roe Pond.

The Popolopen Gorge Trail climbs to Roe Pond and runs along it. It soon turns left and begins a steep ascent to the Bear Mountain Aqueduct, which was built in 1929-30 to bring water from Queensboro Lake to the Bear Mountain area. PG follows the aqueduct, and at 1.4 miles it joins the Timp-Torne Trail (T-T) (blue) and the two Revolutionary trails, which come up from the brook on the right.

At 1.45 miles, PG goes up left, away from the aqueduct. PG soon begins to follow Queensboro Brook, which it crosses on a footbridge at 2.1 miles. It then goes along a woods road and, after 0.35 mile, turns left on a gravel road. This is the Fort Montgomery Road, which runs from Queensboro Lake to Fort Montgomery, mostly on West Point property.

After 0.1 mile on the gravel road, PG/1779 turns right, while T-T/1777W turns left. PG/1779 soon passes Queensboro Lake (built in 1915), where a good spot can be found for a lunch stop. At 3.2 miles, the 1779 Trail leaves to the left, and 0.2 mile further PG turns left on a gravel road below the dam at Turkey Hill Lake. This road, known as Summer Hill Road, was built in 1933 by the Civilian Conservation Corps. It runs 1.4 miles from Route 6 to the north end of the lake.

Leaving the road, PG now climbs around the west end of the dam and follows the lake shore. At 3.95 miles, near the end of the lake, the Anthony Wayne Trail (white) starts to the left. PG then goes uphill, turns right on a woods road and, at 4.5 miles, ends at a junction with the Long Path (turquoise).

In 1940, Alexander Jessup marked a route with metal discs from the Bear Mountain Circle to the hikers' bridge that carried the Timp-Torne Trail across Popolopen Brook. He used the aqueduct path. The trail soon was neglected (it was wartime, and Jessup died in 1944). After the Popolopen Drive had been widened to four lanes, it was expected that the crossing of the Drive by the Timp-Torne Trail would be eliminated. As an approach to that trail, the aqueduct path was again marked by Meyer Kukle and Bob Bloom of the College Alumni Hiking Club. They used square white marks, and named it the Popolopen Gorge Trail (Trail Conference Minutes, 6/8/55). In 1960, the blazes were given a vertical red bar, and the trail was extended by Sam Wilkinson and Bill Burton to Long Mountain, passing the Queensboro and Turkey Hill Reservoirs. The bridge over Queensboro Brook was built by the Park in 1954. It carries a pipe which delivers the treated sewage from the Anthony Wayne Recreation Area into Queensboro Brook.

RACCOON BROOK HILLS TRAIL

Length: 2.95 miles
Blazes: black dot on white (black R on white at jcts.)

Miles

0.0	Leave Seven Hills Trail.
0.3	Reeves Brook Trail, left.
0.35	Start climb.
0.7	HTS Trail crosses.
1.1	Gas line crosses.
1.4	Right, on woods road.
1.55	Kakiat Trail crosses.
1.9	Viewpoint from Raccoon Brook Hill.
2.4	Viewpoint over Pine Meadow Lake from second summit.
2.45	Poached Egg Trail, right.
2.9	Caves, right.
2.95	End at Kakiat Trail.

The Raccoon Brook Hills Trail (RBH) starts east from the Seven Hills Trail (blue on white), 0.35 mile south of the junction of the Seven Hills Trail with the Reeves Brook Trail. This point is 0.1 mile north of the cliff known as Torne View. (On Bill Hoeferlin's maps after 1960, this height is labeled Reeves Mountain.) The blazes at the start of the trail, and at other junctions, have black R's on the white squares. All other blazes are just black dots on white.

Heading downhill, RBH at 0.3 mile passes the end of the Reeves Brook Trail. It then crosses a little brook and climbs up a steep fault scarp. Looking up from below, one can see a jutting rock which was called "The Pulpit" by old-time hikers. From the top of the scarp, RBH goes down a bit, then climbs again to a ridge where the Hillburn-Torne-Sebago Trail (orange) crosses on a bare rock (HTS goes south 0.25 mile to the "Russian Bear"). At 1.1 miles, a gas line crosses (Columbia Gas Transmission Company, laid in 1949). After another 0.2 mile, RBH goes fairly steeply downhill and turns right on a woods road. The woods road soon disappears into laurels, and RBH goes down to the left.

At 1.55 miles, the Kakiat Trail (white) joins from the left. The two trails run together for 125 feet, after which RBH turns left, while Kakiat continues straight ahead. RBH now climbs Raccoon Brook Hill, which has two 1,150-foot summits.

Just before the trail climbs to the first summit, it crosses an old Park boundary. Until 1963, the land from this point south to Suffern was owned by the Ramapo Land Company of the Pierson family.

The first summit, at 1.9 miles, offers a view to the south, while the northernmost summit, at 2.4 miles, affords a fine view of Pine Meadow Lake. RBH then descends. At 2.45 miles, a short rocky trail (yellow on white) leaves to the right to Pine Meadow Road West. The trail was marked by Conrad Schaefer about 1985 and is known as the Poached Egg Trail. It was officially adopted by the Trail Conference in 1989. RBH now goes up a bit, over the top of a hill, and then down again to cross Raccoon Brook. Look for caves at the foot of the hill, where Indian artifacts (now in the Bear Mountain Museum) were found. At 2.95 miles, RBH ends at the Kakiat Trail, 0.5 mile north of its first crossing of this trail.

The Raccoon Brook Hills Trail was first blazed in 1931 by Paul H. Schubert of Ridgewood (Queens), who also made the Red Disc (now Blue Disc) Trail (see p. 29). He named the trail the "Trail of the Raccoon Hills" (TRH). The original markers were half discs, red with white centers. They were later changed to red discs with vertical white bars. Schubert started his trail on Ramapo Torne, going north from there to the top of the third hill (Reeves Mountain or Torne View), where it starts today. The route from the Torne coincided with Nurian's HTS Trail and with the Seven Hills Trail which was maintained then by Jack Spivack of the New York Ramblers. When Nurian began painting out the others' blazes, a dispute arose, which was known as the "Great Ramapo Trail War" (see p. 51). Schubert gave in and started his trail from the third hill (Torne View). The extension of the Seven Hills Trail to Suffern, although reblazed, was not maintained because of opposition from the Ramapo Land Company (of the Pierson family), on whose property the trail was located.

In 1939, the TRH blazes were changed to discs which were half white/half red. In 1940, the southern 1.75 miles of the trail were closed by the landowner. Hikers then created a "northern loop" which followed the park boundary southward from the Kakiat Trail to just west of Raccoon Brook Hill, and then continued along the northern portion of the route of the original TRH for the remainder of the loop. This loop, which became known as the Raccoon Brook Hills Trail (RBH), was marked in 1942 by Frank Place with black R's on white. This situation continued until March 14, 1963, when the Park acquired 1,796 acres of Pierson land, thus permitting the reopening of the southern end of this trail (as well as other trails on the newly-acquired land).

The Woodland Trail Walkers maintained this trail from 1949 to 1991.

Ramapo-Dunderberg Trail

Length: 21.05 miles
Blazes: red dot on white

Miles

0.0	Tuxedo railroad station.
0.45	Go uphill from Grove Drive.
0.65	Triangle Trail goes left.
1.0	Viewpoint over Tuxedo.
1.25	T-MI starts, up right.
2.0	Tri-Trail Corner.
2.55	Black Ash Mountain summit.
2.95	White Bar Trail crosses.
3.25	White Cross Trail starts, right.
3.5	Triangle Trail crosses.
4.05	Victory Trail crosses.
4.2	Tom Jones Shelter, right.
4.35	Summit of Tom Jones Mountain.
4.75	Route 106 crosses.
5.15	Nurian Trail leaves, left.
6.1	Bald Rocks Shelter, right.
6.25	Dunning Trail crosses.
6.5	Goldthwaite Memorial.
6.7	Lichen Trail starts, left.
6.75	Ship Rock.
7.4	Times Square: A-SB/LP crosses.
7.5	Pothole in cliff, left.
8.15	Bottle Cap Trail crosses.
8.9	AT joins, left.
9.0	Hurst Trail ends; Fingerboard Shelter, right.
9.55	Fireplace (old FB-SK).
10.05	Arden Valley Road; go right.

10.4	Tiorati Circle.
10.75	Go left, into woods.
10.8	Start up Goshen Mountain.
11.7	Footbridge; AT joins, left.
12.5	William Brien Memorial Shelter; Menomine Trail begins, left.
12.9	Intended ski trail crosses.
13.45	Silvermine Ski Road crosses.
13.85	Summit of Black Mountain.
14.45	1779 Trail crosses.
14.65	Palisades Interstate Parkway crosses.
14.85	AT leaves, left.
15.15	Beechy Bottom East Road crosses.
15.65	S-BM Trail joins, right.
15.7	S-BM Trail leaves, left.
16.7	Timp Pass.
16.95	Summit of The Timp; T-T Trail joins.
17.15	T-T Trail leaves, right.
17.5	1777 Trail crosses.
17.9	Fireplace; Bockberg Trail, left.
17.95	Bockberg Trail leaves, right.
18.3	Summit of Bald Mountain.
18.45	Cornell Mine Trail, left.
19.35	Bockberg Trail crosses.
19.65	Intended railway grade crosses.
20.9	Route 9W crosses.
21.05	End at Jones Point.

The Ramapo-Dunderberg Trail (R-D) was the first trail in Harriman State Park to be built by the New York hiking clubs, organized in October 1920 as the Palisades Interstate Park Trail Conference. The route of the trail was suggested by Major William Welch, the General Manager of the Park.

The trail starts at the Tuxedo railroad station. Parking is permitted there on weekends; on weekdays, other parking places should be found. The trail goes south 0.1 mile along the tracks, then turns left, down the bank, to cross the Ramapo River on a steel footbridge. It passes by a town playground and turns right on East Village Road, which it follows under the Thruway. It then goes left on Grove Drive. At 0.45 mile, near the end of this paved road, R-D turns right and starts uphill on a switchback. The Kakiat Trail (white) also starts here. At 0.65 mile, the Triangle Trail begins to the left, and R-D soon starts a steep climb up Pine Hill. At 1.0 mile, there is a viewpoint to the left of the trail over the village of Tuxedo. From here, the trail descends briefly.

At 1.2 miles, R-D turns right on a woods road which comes up from below. In another 100 yards, the Tuxedo-Mt. Ivy Trail blazes (red dash on white) start to the right, up a rock face. R-D goes straight ahead, soon passing a mine down to the left and another, uphill on the right. Those mines were probably the reason for the old road, which ends near the mines. The ore must have gone to Solomon Townsend's Augusta Works at Tuxedo, about 1800.

Continuing straight ahead and downhill, R-D turns right onto a woods road that follows the south side of Black Ash Brook (the Black Ash Swamp Road). At 1.95 miles, it crosses the brook below a natural dam that backs up the water in Black Ash Swamp. In another 250 feet, R-D reaches Tri-Trail Corner, where the Victory Trail (blue V on white) and the Blue Disc Trail (blue dot on white) begin. R-D goes uphill, under a telephone line. The 1,130-foot summit of Black Ash Mountain is reached at 2.55 miles. At 2.95 miles, in the saddle between Black Ash Mountain and Parker Cabin Mountain, the White Bar Trail crosses, and 0.3 mile further the White Cross Trail leaves to the right.

R-D now climbs Parker Cabin Mountain, meeting the Triangle Trail (yellow) again at 3.5 miles. After 150 feet, Triangle leaves to the right (there is a view here of Lake Sebago), while R-D goes down the north end of the mountain to a fireplace in a notch where the Victory Trail crosses. Now the trail climbs Tom Jones Mountain (named for one of the Claudius Smith gang, who shot Parker, another horse thief, at his cabin in Parker Cabin Hollow). At 4.2 miles, the Tom Jones Shelter (built in 1927) is on the right. The 1,280-foot summit is then crossed, after which the trail goes steeply down to a brook and Route 106, which it reaches at 4.75 miles.

In 1920, when the trail was first blazed, the land south of Black Ash summit was owned by the Tuxedo Park Association. The trail was marked with their permission and was called the Tuxedo-Tom Jones Trail (from Tuxedo to Route 416 — later Route 210 and now Route 106). In those days, that road was called Seven Lakes Drive.

The trail we have described so far was blazed in November 1920 by an AMC group led by J. Ashton Allis. At that time, Allis was a bank examiner, but he later became vice-president of Grace National Bank and chairman of Fairchild Aviation Company. The trail was marked with galvanized iron squares, inscribed "T-TJ." In the beginning, T-TJ crossed the Ramapo River on East Village Road, then turned north past a group of houses. Leaving the road, it crossed Black Ash Brook and went up its north side, then crossed to its south side (where the Triangle Trail crosses now) and so to the rock dam.

On August 10, 1930, Raymond Torrey suggested to Joseph Bartha that he relocate the T-TJ Trail. At that time, the Tuxedo-Mt. Ivy Trail (T-MI) was joint with T-TJ from Tuxedo until it turned right, uphill, on an old woods road that went high above Black Ash Brook. It then left the road and turned right, up over a rock face, towards Claudius Smith Rock. Torrey's suggestion was for T-TJ to follow T-MI up the woods road and then continue down to rejoin the earlier T-TJ route near the upper crossing of Black Ash Brook. The job was soon done (*N.Y. Post*, 9/16/30). In 1932, the trail was remarked as the R-D Trail, from Tuxedo to Jones Point. The present route in Tuxedo was marked in January 1955 by the Adirondack Mountain Club after the Thruway was built. In 1997, the section of the trail just east of Grove Drive was relocated from an eroded gully to a newly constructed switchback.

Until 1935, there was a "pole" fire tower on Parker Cabin Mountain, about where the Triangle Trail crosses R-D (*N.Y. Post*, 2/20/35). During 1930, a 115-foot well was drilled near the shelter on Tom Jones Mountain and equipped with a hand pump. This pump was repaired many times after vandals broke it, and in 1967 it finally was abandoned.

After crossing Route 106, R-D gradually climbs Black Rock Mountain. Near the top, the Nurian Trail (white) departs on the left. The trail goes over the 1,280-foot summit and, at 6.1 miles, it passes near the Bald Rocks Shelter (built in 1933). 0.15 mile further, the Dunning Trail (yellow) crosses, while R-D continues north and soon goes over an open rock surface (known as the Whaleback). At 6.5 miles, a bronze plaque may be seen on a boulder to the right of the trail.

This was placed on July 13, 1964 by the Fresh Air Club in memory of George Goldthwaite (1889-1960). On December 22, 1929, he hiked the entire R-D Trail in 4 hours and 51 minutes — the record time for hiking this trail. He is also remembered for his great knowledge of Park trails and as a hike leader.

After passing through the woods beyond the memorial, R-D comes to another open rock where the Lichen Trail (blue L on white) leaves to the left. Just beyond is "Ship Rock," a boulder beside the trail that looks like a ship's prow, bottom up.

R-D now turns southeast and goes down about 40 feet, then up over Hogencamp Mountain. (When the trail was first marked in 1920, there was also a ruined fire tower here on the 1,353-foot summit; *N.Y. Post*, 4/1/21.) "Times Square," marked by a fireplace next to a great boulder, is reached at 7.4 miles. Here, R-D crosses the Arden-Surebridge Trail (red triangle on white) and the Long Path (turquoise).

Continuing north, 0.1 mile from Times Square R-D climbs a rocky ledge. On this ledge, to the left of the trail, a large pothole was discovered by Frank Place on March 9, 1924 (*N.Y. Post*, 4/22/30). At 8.15 miles, as R-D goes down through a hemlock grove, the Bottle Cap Trail crosses. After climbing several more ledges, R-D swings east and joins the Appalachian Trail (AT) (white) on Fingerboard Mountain. The joint trails go north, passing the Fingerboard Shelter (built 1928; *N.Y. Herald Tribune*, 10/7/28). Just beyond the shelter, at 9.0 miles, the Hurst Trail (blue) leaves to the right.

At 9.55 miles, R-D/AT passes a stone fireplace. The old Fingerboard-Storm King Trail (FB-SK) (built in

1922) used to start here. In 1964, its route was taken over by the new Long Path. Descending gradually now, R-D/AT reaches Arden Valley Road at 10.05 miles. Across the road, a path leads to the site of the Fingerboard Fire Tower (erected 1922; removed in 1987). The AT crosses the road and re-enters the woods to the left, while R-D turns right and follows the road down to the Tiorati traffic circle.

The trail from Route 106 up Black Rock Mountain and over Hogencamp Mountain was first blazed on December 11, 1920 by J. Ashton Allis and William W. Bell, both of the AMC. Then on December 18th they marked the trail from Surebridge Mine Road (Times Square) to Arden Valley Road. Also, in December 1920 a team from the Tramp and Trail Club (Frank Place) blazed the trail from Tiorati Circle to Beechy Bottom.

In 1920, Arden Valley Road going west from Tiorati Circle was a dirt road 12 feet wide (*N.Y. Post*, 5/18/23). Going east from the circle, Tiorati Brook Road was "being improved."

From Tiorati Circle, R-D follows Tiorati Brook Road around the north end of the lake for 0.35 mile, then turns left into the woods. At 10.8 miles, shortly after leaving the road, the trail starts up Goshen Mountain, going northeast along the 1,320-foot ridge, then down to a footbridge. Here the AT comes in from the left and the unmarked Bockey Swamp Trail comes up from below, crosses R-D/AT, and continues south. After some ups and downs, R-D/AT reaches the William Brien Memorial Shelter at 12.5 miles. Here the Menomine Trail (yellow) begins. It goes down 1.35 miles to the Silvermine Ski Area on Seven Lakes Drive.

On current trail maps, the unmarked Dean Trail starts at this shelter, going downhill 0.85 mile to the Red Cross Trail. This section of the Dean Trail was once (1922) part of the Boy Scouts' White Bar Trail system. The Dean Trail is an old trail that went down to Stillwater Brook and then southeast to Bulsontown. The broad road that comes up to the shelter from Seven Lakes Drive was built in 1935 by the Civilian Conservation Corps.

The shelter here, built in 1933, was known as the Letterrock Shelter. William Brien, a naturalist, was the first president of the New York Ramblers (1923). He died on October 12, 1954. In his will, he left funds to build a new shelter in the Park. Such a shelter was built at Island Pond in 1957, but because of later vandalism it was demolished in 1973, and the Letterrock Shelter was renamed in his memory.

Originally, this mountain was called "Lettered Rock Mountain." In the early Park days, a Weyant family lived in Beechy Bottom near Queensboro (their graves are still there, in the road maze at Long Mountain Circle). They told a tale (*N.Y. Post*, 6/12/24) about a Frenchman who made periodic trips from Caldwell's Landing (Jones Point) into the mountains with his slave, returning with sacks of silver coins. In his cups, he boasted of the "lettered rock" and of a silver hoard that lay due east of that rock. No one could find that lettered rock — until 1934. In that year, a group of four treasure hunters was arrested after they had spent months blasting various places on Letterrock Mountain (*N.Y. Times*, 11/30/34). They had obtained a 1690 map from the Morgan Library, old, yellowed and cracked, that gave directions to the mine where Spaniards had hidden a silver treasure. They pointed to marks on a great boulder, but William Carr of the Trailside Museum said the marks had been caused by weathering.

R-D/AT climbs over rocks behind the shelter and continues northeast. About ten minutes from the shelter, a faint trail crosses. Followed to the right, this eventually becomes the wide ski trail that goes down to Silvermine Lake. To the left (indistinct) it becomes a woods road that slabs down off the mountain to join the CCC trail out to the Seven Lakes Drive. R-D/AT then descends to a valley where, at 13.45 miles, it crosses a wide gravel road — the Silvermine Ski Road. Before it was "paved" in 1934 by the Temporary Emergency Relief Administration, it was known as the Black Mountain Trail (red blazes). R-D/AT now climbs steeply up Black Mountain, passing over ledges which afford beautiful views of Silvermine Lake. The trail levels off along the top at 13.85 miles, with grand views toward the south and east. In the shrubbery to the left as the trail starts down, one can find a prospector's hole and, a little further along, a much deeper, water-filled hole. This hole came to be called the "Spanish Silver Mine," although there is not a trace of silver there. It was

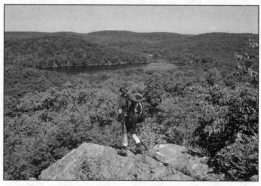

View of Silvermine Lake from Black Mountain

sufficiently romantic, however, to give its name to a nearby ski slope that was opened in 1936, and later to the lake beside the ski slope.

Now the trail starts steeply down the east end of Black Mountain. After going up and over a low ridge, the 1779 Trail crosses and, soon afterwards, R-D/AT crosses the Owl Lake Road (rather vague just here) and then the Palisades Interstate Parkway. About 0.2 mile after going up steps on the east side of the Parkway, the AT leaves sharply to the left, while R-D goes down to Beechy Bottom Brook. Against the high bank, just west of the brook, Major Welch built the first trail shelter — a half-hexagon of corrugated iron (*N.Y. Post*, 11/25/21). It was removed in 1936, after extensive damage by the CCC boys.

Beyond the brook, R-D turns left and briefly follows the Anthony Wayne South Ski Trail, now blazed as a bike trail, with blue-on-white plastic markers. Then, at 15.05 miles, R-D turns off to the right and soon crosses the Beechy Bottom East Road (made into a fire road by CCC), also marked as a bike trail. On the way up West Mountain, R-D passes an old iron mine, and then meets the Suffern-Bear Mountain Trail (S-BM) (yellow) at the top of the Cats Elbow. There are good views here. The two trails are joint for about 300 feet. On a ledge, at 15.7 miles, S-BM leaves to the left. R-D climbs around another spur, then drops down to Timp Pass where it meets the Red Cross Trail. Here the unmarked Timp Pass Road goes left, down to Doodletown. R-D now goes up the picturesque steep rock face of The Timp, rising 280 feet above the pass.

The R-D on the south crown of West Mountain was marked in 1920 by A.B. Malcolmson; the route up the Timp face, known then as the Six Chins Trail, had been located and named by Frank Place in 1917. Both men were from the Tramp and Trail Club. From The Timp to Jones Point, the trail was blazed in January and February 1921 by E. Cecil Earle and A.B. Malcolmson of the Tramp and Trail Club and J. Ashton Allis of AMC.

The R-D's route up The Timp has become badly eroded, and a relocation is scheduled to be opened in the fall of 1999.

On the Timp summit, just to the left of the trail, a stirring panorama spreads to the north, west and south. R-D now joins the Timp-Torne Trail (T-T) (blue), and both trails continue east. At 17.15 miles, Timp-Torne leaves to the right, briefly following the route of the older Red Timp Trail.

0.35 mile further, R-D crosses the 1777 Trail. In the past, this old road was called the Lumberjack Trail and Steep Street. It is the route taken by the British troops in 1777 from Stony Point to attack Forts Clinton and Montgomery. Going now northeast, R-D climbs through laurels, then descends to a brook where there is a fireplace. The road which comes from the hill ahead, and departs down left, is the Bockberg Trail. R-D follows it briefly uphill, leaves it, then briefly rejoins it. At 17.95 miles, the Bockberg Trail departs to the right for the second time, while R-D continues its steep climb to the 1,115-foot summit of Bald Mountain (the Bockberg), with great views. The Cornell Mine is passed 250 feet beyond the summit, and the end of the Cornell Mine Trail (blue) is reached at 18.45 miles.

Continuing now toward Dunderberg proper, R-D at 19.35 miles meets the Bockberg Trail again, and then crosses an intended grade of the old Dunderberg Spiral Railway, started in 1890 (see pp. 341-46). R-D now climbs gently over the 930-foot summit and descends the eastern face. On the way down, it crosses the completed railway grade twice and passes by several beautiful viewpoints. At 20.9 miles, Route 9W crosses, and the trail drops steeply down, past the edge of a sand pit, to end at Jones Point, 21.05 miles from Tuxedo.

The old road at Jones Point that goes around Dunderberg at the river level was built in 1907, 12 feet wide. The new road was built 30 feet wide, higher up, in 1930 (*N.Y. Times*, 6/29/30). Until 1930, the road was designated N.Y. Route 3. An even older road, the Dunderberg and Clove Turnpike, had been built in 1809.

Jones Point and part of the mountain, including much of the spiral railway, were purchased by the Park in 1928 from Mary E. Jones and Charles and Anna Jones. They were a wealthy Westchester/Long Island family. Their ancestor, Joshua T. Jones, bought 100 acres in 1836 at what was then known as Caldwell's Landing.

On Thursday night, May 11, 1967, a single-engine plane crashed on Dunderberg Mountain. The pilot, Arnold Shaefer of New York City, was killed. Three hikers found the wreck on the following Saturday morning (*Journal News* (Nyack, N.Y.), May 15, 1967). Part of the wreckage may still be seen a little way north of the R-D, about 0.5 mile from Route 9W, just west of where the R-D crosses a loop of the spiral railway.

RED ARROW TRAIL

Length: 1.45 miles
Blazes: red arrow

Miles

0.0	Start up from T-MI.
0.15	Old Limekiln Mountain Trail, right.
0.35	S-BM joins, left.
0.5	Cross Woodtown Road.
0.8	Summit of Ladentown Mountain.
1.1	Third Reservoir.
1.25	Breakneck Mountain Trail, left; S-BM departs, right.
1.45	End at camp road.

This short trail presently connects the Tuxedo-Mt. Ivy Trail (T-MI), which comes up from Ladentown, with the Suffern-Bear Mountain Trail (S-BM), which descends Circle Mountain.

Going up T-MI from Ladentown, Red Arrow starts steeply up to the right at 0.95 mile. At 0.15 mile from the T-MI, Red Arrow goes uphill, to the northwest, beside a stone wall. Off to the right is another stone wall, which goes uphill to the north. The old Limekiln Mountain Trail begins on the east side of that stone wall.

Further along the Red Arrow Trail, at 0.35 mile, the S-BM joins from the left. The Red Arrow Trail now officially ends here.

Old Red Arrow blazes can still be seen occasionally, joint with S-BM, going over Ladentown Mountain, down past the Third Reservoir, and up to Breakneck Mountain. Here the S-BM departs to the right, up over a big rock, and the Breakneck Mountain Trail (white) starts to the left. Red Arrow, now unmarked at the request of the camp below, continues straight ahead, and soon goes steeply down to the Camp Lanowa Road, where it ends, 1.45 miles from the T-MI.

In older editions of the *New York Walk Book*, the Red Arrow Trail was described as a "fisherman's short-cut from Ladentown to Breakneck Pond." It is not known how the trail was first marked. About 1931, the Interstate Hiking Club cleared and re-marked it (*Paterson Morning Call*, 9/20/35). It was restored again by Frank Place in 1943, then maintained by Joseph Bartha until the NYU Club took it over in 1948.

RED CROSS TRAIL

Length: 7.9 miles
Blazes: red cross on white

Miles

0.0	Start from A-SB on Pine Swamp Mountain.
0.45	Cross Seven Lakes Drive.
1.15	Telephone line crosses.
1.35	Hasenclever Mountain Trail, left.
1.65	Turn left on woods road from Lake Askoti.
1.9	Hasenclever Road joins, right.
2.45	Cross Tiorati Brook Road.
2.55	Cross Tiorati Brook.
3.1	Bockey Swamp Trail crosses.
3.2	Beech Trail starts, right.
4.45	Dean Trail, left.
4.75	Stillwater Trail, right.
5.65	Cross Palisades Interstate Parkway.
5.85	1779 Trail joins, left.
5.95	S-BM joins, left.
6.02	S-BM leaves, right.
6.05	Red Cross turns left.
6.55	Cross Beechy Bottom Road.
7.0	Turn left onto woods road.
7.15	Turn left onto Horn's Route.
7.4	Turn left onto North "Ski Trail."
7.45	Turn right onto stone road.
7.9	End at Timp Pass.

The Red Cross Trail was first blazed in April 1944, but it has been relocated several times since then. It now starts from the Arden-Surebridge Trail (A-SB) on

Pine Swamp Mountain, 0.25 mile from the parking area at Lake Skannatati. After ascending briefly, parallel to the A-SB, it descends the mountain and crosses Seven Lakes Drive. Red Cross then passes the north end of Lake Askoti and climbs up the ridge on the far side of the lake. About 0.2 mile after Red Cross crosses a telephone line, the Hasenclever Mountain Trail begins to the left. Red Cross crosses a swampy area on a wooden bridge and, at 1.65 miles, turns left onto a woods road which comes from Lake Askoti. It follows this woods road for 0.25 mile and then turns left onto the Hasenclever Fire Road. Just beyond the junction, the old water-filled Hasenclever Mine is visible on the right.

In 1765, Peter Hasenclever, a German mining engineer working for a London company, discovered this mine on the old woods road. In the years before the Interstate Park was created, this road, then known as Cedar Ponds Road, was maintained by the Town of Stony Point. An occasional cement town marker may be seen in the grass by the roadside. The history of "Baron" Hasenclever and his mine is related in J.M. Ransom's *Vanishing Ironworks of the Ramapos* (pp. 130-35).

After crossing Tiorati Brook Road at 2.45 miles, the trail goes across an unused ballfield, enters the woods and goes down to Tiorati Brook. A little way up the brook, hidden in weeds, is an earth mound. This is all that remains of the Orange Furnace, planned by Hasenclever but built by James Brewster about 1800. The trail crosses the brook and proceeds with Goshen Mountain on the left. Going gently downhill, it crosses a little brook coming from the left. Just past the brook, an unmarked woods road starts to the left. That old road crosses the brook again and goes north for about 0.9 mile, with Goshen Mountain on the left and swamps on the right.

Red Cross now rounds the south end of Letterrock Mountain. At 3.1 miles, the Bockey Swamp Trail (unmarked) crosses. The junction is marked by a cairn. The Beech Trail (blue) starts to the right in another 0.1 mile. Red Cross then goes down a long valley, with Letterrock Mountain on the left and Flaggy Meadow Mountain on the right, and crosses several streams. At 4.45 miles, the Dean Trail (white) comes in to the left. In another 0.1 mile, the cellar hole of the Burnt House is visible to the left of the trail. A local story relates that this was the home of a boss woodcutter named Jonas Lewis.

Before it was marked with red crosses, the trail down from Tiorati Brook had been called the Burnt House Trail. Here it briefly coincided with the Dean Trail, then crossed to the right side of Stillwater Brook and followed that brook around the end of Flaggy Meadow Mountain, ending on Tiorati Brook Road. (The lower end of the trail, from the crossing of the brook to Tiorati Brook Road, is now known as the Stillwater Trail.) About 1920, the Boy Scouts made it part of their White Bar Trail system. In 1965, the Park widened the Red Cross Trail to 20 feet, from the Hasenclever Mine to the Burnt House.

At 4.75 miles, the Stillwater Trail (unmarked) leaves, to the right, to cross the brook on a sturdy footbridge. Red Cross continues east and passes a swamp to the right. At 4.95 miles, it crosses a wet region where Owl Swamp Brook comes down from the left. On the west side of that brook are traces of an (intended) old road, started in 1934 but abandoned. At 5.6 miles, the trail reaches the Palisades Interstate Parkway. It turns left along the southbound lanes for 150 feet, then crosses the road opposite the end of the guardrail and enters the woods on the median strip. Red Cross then crosses the northbound lanes and turns left. Again, it runs along the guardrail for 150 feet, then turns right and enters the woods. East of the Parkway, it passes through a level region, with the 1779 Trail joining from the left at 5.85 miles. (This point is the end of the old Black Mountain Trail.) Soon the Suffern-Bear Mountain Trail (yellow) comes in from the left and departs again after 400 feet. About 150 feet further along, Red Cross suddenly turns left, while the 1779 Trail goes on down the wide old Dean Trail.

For the next mile, Red Cross follows a route that was first marked about 1940 by J. Ashton Allis, who was then treasurer of the Trail Conference. On the way, Red Cross crosses Beechy Bottom Road (built in 1740 from Stony Point to Central Valley). Red Cross then descends steadily and, at 7.0 miles, turns left onto an old woods road, once known as the Bulsontown-Timp Road. In another 50 feet, a trail marked with "A-B" blazes (by the Addisone Boyce Girl Scout camp) joins from the right. To the right, the A-B blazes go across a stone wall and continue down to Mott Farm Road. Red Cross once followed that route, but it now goes north on the old road for 0.15 mile, crosses a stream, and then turns left at a T-junction onto another old road (Horn's

Route). A little way up that road, a faint trail goes off to the left near the ruin of an old cabin. After another 0.2 mile, Red Cross departs to the right from Horn's Route, crosses a little brook and then an old woods road, and turns left onto the North "Ski Trail" at 7.4 miles. In another 275 feet, it turns sharply right onto another "stone road" which, for much of its distance, is a real "ankle-breaker"! This "stone road" climbs (often steeply) to Timp Pass, which it reaches at 7.9 miles. Here the Red Cross Trail ends at a junction with the Ramapo-Dunderberg Trail and the unmarked Timp Pass Road.

When it was first blazed in 1944, Red Cross started from the Dunning Trail (now Long Path) near a shaft of the Hogencamp Mine, and followed an older Boy Scout trail to Lake Skannatati (the first dam of which was built in 1938). The trail went around the south end of Lake Askoti and climbed the hill to the east on an old woods road. That road, which more or less followed the county line, joined the present route near Hasenclever Mine. From there the route was the same as now, except at the eastern end. There, instead of turning up toward Timp Pass, it went on down to Bulsontown Road (now known as Mott Farm Road). In 1951, when the Rockland County Girl Scouts began to build Camp Addisone Boyce, they asked that the Red Cross Trail be relocated. This was done in 1952, sending the trail to the road across the dam of the new lake. Finally, in 1964, Red Cross was sent uphill to end at Timp Pass.

In 1947, the western end of the trail was relocated. It was made to start from Seven Lakes Drive, at the entrance to Camp Thendara. That made the trail one mile shorter. The original western end, from near the Hogencamp Mine shaft to

Lake Skannatati, was demarked but still maintained (Trail Conference Minutes, 2/6/57), and it became the Skannatati Trail in 1961. (In 1981, the Skannatati Trail became part of the Long Path.)

In 1978, the beginning of Red Cross was again relocated, this time to the route it follows at present. That was done to avoid parking congestion and vandalism at Camp Thendara.

RED TIMP TRAIL

Length: 0.5 mile (to old T-T Trail)
Blazes: two red T's and red cross on white, in a red circle, or silver hiker symbol on red background

This trail, which is not an official Conference trail, was blazed by the Girl Scouts of Camp Addisone Boyce on Mott Farm Road. It is a very old trail, which was known on the Park's 1927 topo map as the Timp Trail. For many years it was known to hikers as the Timp Bypass, since, when used together with the old Timp-Torne Trail (T-T), it permitted hikers to bypass the very steep descent of The Timp on the Ramapo-Dunderberg (R-D) Trail. Now that a new trail route, which allows for a gentle descent of The Timp to the north of the former route, has been completed, it is no longer necessary to use the Red Timp Trail for this purpose.

The Red Timp Trail starts from the R-D Trail 0.2 mile east of the Timp summit. For 175 feet, it runs jointly with T-T (blue). T-T then turns left, while Red Timp zig-zags down nearly 400 feet in 0.5 mile. There it meets the old T-T in a region that was lumbered in 1986.

Here, Red Timp turns right (west) and runs jointly with the old T-T (with its blue-on-white blazes still visible) for 0.15 mile, with a swampy area on the left. It then goes left, away from the old T-T, and around a great cliff called the Boulderberg. The trail soon enters

Girl Scout property and follows an old road, along a stream, down into their camp on Mott Farm Road.

The route of the old T-T Trail, a woods road still marked with blue-on-white blazes, may be followed to the northwest all the way up to its intersection with the R-D Trail just east of Timp Pass. Although this route is no longer needed as a bypass around The Timp, it makes it possible to hike the Red Timp Trail without retracing one's steps and without entering the private Girl Scout property. To the east of the junction with the Red Timp Trail, the old T-T (which was on private property) has largely been obliterated due to logging operations.

REEVES BROOK TRAIL

Length: 1.65 miles
Blazes: white

Miles

0.0	Reeves Meadow.
0.2	Reeves Brook, left.
0.5	Woods road leaves, right.
1.35	Seven Hills Trail crosses.
1.65	End at Raccoon Brook Hills Trail.

The Reeves Brook Trail starts near Seven Lakes Drive, at the far edge of Reeves Meadow. (To reach the beginning of the trail from the visitor center parking lot, turn left on the Pine Meadow Trail and follow it for 300 feet to the start of the Reeves Brook Trail, which goes off to the right.) Going uphill on a woods road, the trail approaches Reeves Brook at 0.2 mile. Then at 0.5 mile the woods road (once known as the Fishline Trail) departs to the right. The Reeves Brook Trail goes straight ahead, fairly steeply up, following the brook which flows down along a geologic fault. At 1.35 miles, the Seven Hills Trail (blue on white) crosses, and at 1.65 miles the Reeves Brook Trail ends at the Raccoon Brook Hills Trail (black dot on white). 0.1 mile north, on top of a cliff, is the rock known as "The Pulpit."

The Reeves Brook Trail was first mentioned in the Trail Conference minutes of April 4, 1956, which stated that this "unofficial trail" had "not been accepted by the Park." When the Park purchased 1,796 acres of Pierson land in 1963, the Reeves Brook Trail was made a Conference trail, and Bob Bloom of the College Alumni Hiking Club, who probably first blazed it, became its maintainer. Bloom, who served for many years on the Board of the Trail Conference, maintained the trail until his death on April 4, 1986.

SEVEN HILLS TRAIL

Length: 6.65 miles
Blazes: blue on white

Miles

0.0	Entrance to Sebago parking area.
0.35	Buck Trail goes left.
0.6	Turn left, up Woodtown Road (West).
0.7	Turn right, off road.
0.9	T-MI crosses.
1.1	Fire road joins, left.
1.4	Tower Trail, left.
1.5	HTS joins, right.
1.75	Diamond Mountain-Tower Trail, left.
1.77	Diamond Mountain summit.
1.8	HTS leaves, right.
2.5	Cross Pine Meadow Brook.
3.0	HTS crosses.
3.3	Gas line crosses; Quartz Brook Trail, right.
3.7	Reeves Brook Trail crosses.
4.05	RBH Trail starts, left.
4.15	Torne View.
4.5	HTS joins, left.
4.7	HTS leaves, left; 7H turns down, right.
5.25	Foot of hill; go right.
6.3	Fishline Trail crosses.
6.65	End at Pine Meadow Trail.

The Seven Hills Trail (7H) starts opposite the entrance to the Lake Sebago hikers' parking area on Seven Lakes Drive, four miles from Route 17. For 0.3 mile, the trail goes fairly steeply up Conklin Mountain on an old woods road, once known as the Monitor Trail. (In November 1988, the lower end was slightly relocated.) Near the top of the climb, a trail, marked by a cairn, bends left toward the hilltop. This is the Buck Trail, which is 1.6 miles long, and ends at Pine Meadow Road.

The Seven Hills Trail goes down the slope of Conklin Mountain and, at 0.6 mile, turns left, up Woodtown Road (West). Here the trail crosses Diamond Creek, and after going up 0.1 mile, it leaves the road and turns sharp right. On the left at this point, a white-blazed trail goes about 300 feet to a ledge on which there is a large quartz boulder known as Monitor Rock.

When the Seven Hills Trail was first blazed, it started from Monitor Rock. The rock was so named by the Fresh Air Club when they found tucked under it a copy of the *Christian Science Monitor* newspaper. The road up to the rock from the parking area at Old Sebago Beach was named the Monitor Trail. That trail was forgotten until hiker parking at Sebago Dam was ended in 1977. At that time, 7H was rerouted down to the present parking area.

Woodtown Road (West) is a very old road that started at the Burnt Sawmill Bridge (where Sebago Dam is now).

It crossed the saddle between Conklin and Diamond Mountains, then went across the south end of a swamp on Christie Brook (now Lake Wanoksink) to join the main Woodtown Road which ran from Willow Grove to Ramapo.

Diamond Mountain, too, has changed its name. The 1923 edition of the *New York Walk Book* showed it as Halfway Mountain. Then in 1927 the Park's large topographic map named the higher eastern end Diamond Mountain, while the western end remained Halfway Mountain.

Seven Hills Trail now goes along the ridge of Diamond Mountain. At 0.8 mile, it passes a great boulder, called the "Cracked Diamond," and at 0.9 mile, the Tuxedo-Mt. Ivy Trail (red dash on white) crosses. At 1.1 miles, 7H briefly joins a fire road (which goes from Pine Meadow Road up to the site of the fire tower). A little further, at 1.4 miles, the Diamond Mountain-Tower Trail (yellow) leaves to the left. There was once an 80-foot steel fire tower, 75 yards east of this junction, erected in 1935 from the steel of the tower that stood on Bear Mountain. It was removed in 1955, erected again in 1966, and removed again in 1986.

At 1.5 miles, the Hillburn-Torne-Sebago Trail (HTS) (orange) joins from the right. The Diamond Mountain-Tower Trail (yellow) ends on the left at 1.75 miles, just before 7H reaches the 1,242-foot summit of the mountain. At 1.8 miles, HTS departs to the right, while 7H goes steeply down to Pine Meadow Brook, where it turns left briefly on the Kakiat Trail (white). Both trails (along with the red-blazed Pine Meadow Trail) cross the brook on an often-washed-away log bridge. Kakiat then departs to the left, following Raccoon Brook, while the Pine Meadow Trail goes right, down along Pine Meadow Brook. 7H follows the Pine Meadow Trail for about 450 feet beyond the bridge, and then turns left at a fireplace and begins to climb Chipmunk Mountain.

At 3.0 miles, HTS again joins from the right, and leaves left 100 feet further on. 7H turns right onto the route of a buried gas pipeline at 3.3 miles, and in another 100 feet 7H turns left and soon crosses Quartz Brook. The Quartz Brook Trail, abandoned in 1969, went down the left side of the brook to the Pine Meadow

Trail. Until 1963, this trail was on private property, as was the Seven Hills Trail south of the summit of Chipmunk Mountain.

At 3.65 miles, 7H drops very steeply down from a fault scarp (good view) to cross the Reeves Brook Trail (white). Climbing again, 7H passes the start of the Raccoon Brook Hills Trail (black R on white) to the left at 4.05 miles. Shortly afterwards, 7H reaches a viewpoint from the south end of this hill, known as Torne View (1,170 feet). 7H then drops steeply down into a gully, and climbs back up to meet HTS once again at 4.5 miles. In another 0.2 mile, at a dip in the ridge, 7H bears right, while HTS turns left and continues ahead to Ramapo Torne.

This is a good place to relate the early history of the Seven Hills Trail. It was first blazed by J. Ashton Allis about 1922. At that time, he was President of the Fresh Air Club, which had been organized in 1876 by "Father Bill" Curtis (there is a monument on the way up Slide Mountain to Curtis and his companion Allen Ormsbee, both of whom died in June 1900 in a snowstorm on Mt. Washington). Allis was a compulsive trail blazer. His marks were tiny nicks, called "bird's eye blazes," and his cairns were soon hidden by weeds. His trail started in the village of Ramapo, went up the Torne, and continued over Torne View and Chipmunk, Halfway, Diamond and Conklin Mountains, ending at Monitor Rock.

After he marked the trail, Allis broached the idea to Major Welch who, in 1923, suggested the need for such a trail, landowners permitting. (*N.Y. Post*, 11/29/23). In 1926, Allis' faint trail was discovered by Jack Spivack of the New York Ramblers. On December 18, 1927, with two friends, Spivack blazed Allis' trail white from the Torne to

Pine Meadow Brook. He later continued the blazes to Monitor Rock (*Mountain Magazine*, Jan. 1928). Spivack intended to start the trail up Nordkop Mountain at Suffern, then over the hill above Hillburn to the Torne. It was Spivack who named it "Trail of the Seven Hills." The seven hills he had in mind were: (1) Nordkop Mountain (above Suffern); (2) Hillburn Mountain (above Hillburn); (3) Ramapo Torne; (4) Torne View; (5) Chipmunk Mountain; (6) Diamond Mountain; and (7) Conklin Mountain.

During 1928, Kerson Nurian blazed the HTS Trail from Hillburn partly on Allis' older route, and used Spivack's trail for 0.2 mile north of the Torne. Eight years later, in the fall of 1936, Spivack at last extended his Seven Hills Trail (now blazed blue) to Suffern, using part of Nurian's HTS and part of the S-BM. In that year, there began the "Great Ramapo Trail War," as a result of which parts of the Seven Hills Trail were painted out by Nurian (see p. 51). When the "war" was over, Spivack repainted his blue blazes to Suffern. But the Seven Hills Trail, as well as other trails in the area south of the Park boundary (just south of Pine Meadow Brook) were closed in 1940 by order of the Ramapo Land Company (Pierson Estate).

From the saddle in the Torne ridge, 7H turns down right on a woods road. At the bottom (5.25 miles), the trail turns right (the road going left was once the route of 7H into Sloatsburg). The trail passes a beaver swamp, crosses Beaver Brook, and goes down around the north side of Middle Hill, now following the old Mason Trail. At 6.3 miles, the Fishline Trail crosses, and at 6.65 miles the Seven Hills Trail ends at the Pine Meadow Trail.

James R. Pierson, president of the Ramapo Land Company, died on May 3, 1959, at the age of 85. In 1963, after several years of negotiation, the Park acquired 1,796 acres of Pierson land by condemnation. This included the land south to the Ramapo Torne, and enabled all trails in this area to be reopened. The Seven Hills Trail was extended to Suffern, using Spivack's old route. But the extended trail still passed over some private land, so by 1965 it had been rerouted onto the woods road at the foot of the Torne. That road went to the Thruway fence (the "Going East" Trail), and then continued north along the fence to Greenway, the first street in Sloatsburg east of the Thruway. Local residents protested (since there was no room to park near the trailhead), and in November 1976 the Seven Hills Trail was given its present route from Ramapo Torne to the Pine Meadow Trail, where it ends, 0.2 mile south of the visitor center on Seven Lakes Drive.

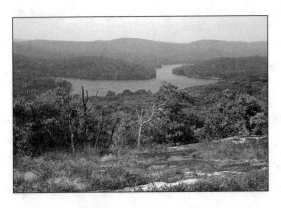

Lake Sebago from Diamond Mountain

SUFFERN-BEAR MOUNTAIN TRAIL

Length: 23.45 miles
Blazes: yellow

Miles

0.0	Suffern; Route 59.
0.2	Viewpoint.
0.35	Viewpoint to right; woods road joins.
0.6	Gas line crosses.
0.8	Summit of Nordkop Mountain.
1.0	Seven Hills Trail went left (1944-63).
1.3	Seven Hills Trail went left (1936-44).
1.45	Climb Kitchen Stairs.
1.9	Gas line crosses.
2.15	Cross outlet of Cat Swamp.
2.75	Power line crosses.
3.15	Cross Os-Sec Brook in Valley of Dry Bones.
3.7	Sky Sail Farm.
4.2	Gas line crosses.
4.4	MacIlvain's Rocks; Grandma and Grandpa Rocks.
4.5	Kakiat Trail crosses.
4.65	Summit of Cobus Mountain.
5.6	Conklins Crossing Trail, left.
5.75	The Egg.
5.95	Stone Memorial Shelter; cross Sherwood Path.
6.5	Hawk Cliff.
6.8	Pittsboro Trail joins from right.
7.0	Pine Meadow Trail, left.
7.2	Old Pine Meadow Trail goes right.
7.45	Gyascutus Brook crosses.
7.7	Summit of Panther Mountain.
8.3	Many Swamp Trail crosses.

8.65	T-MI Trail (Two Bridges Road) crosses.
9.4	Red Arrow Trail, right.
9.5	File Factory Brook crosses.
9.55	Woodtown Road crosses.
10.15	Third Reservoir, right.
10.3	Breakneck Mountain Trail, left.
11.15	Big Hill Shelter; Long Path joins.
11.35	Long Path leaves, right.
11.5	Old Turnpike crosses.
12.1	Fire tower.
12.8	Ruins of ORAK.
13.2	Gate Hill Road crosses.
13.75	Irish Potato.
15.55	Turn right on Lake Welch Drive.
15.75	Palisades Interstate Parkway crosses.
15.95	Scutt Memorial tablet.
16.45	Pingyp summit.
17.0	Brook crosses; fireplace.
17.25	Pines summit.
17.6	Turn left onto Red Cross/1779 Trail.
17.65	Leave Red Cross/1779 Trail.
18.2	Beechy Bottom Road crosses.
18.3	Horn Hill summit.
18.6	North-South Connector crosses.
18.75	North "Ski Trail" crosses.
19.1	Cats Elbow; R-D Trail joins.
19.15	R-D Trail leaves, right.
19.55	Fire Escape, right.
19.8	Timp-Torne Trail joins, left.
20.1	Timp-Torne leaves, right.
20.7	Knob of West Mountain.
21.1	Doodlekill crosses.
21.5	Turn left onto Bridle Path.
21.65	Turn right, leaving Bridle Path.

21.85 Rejoin Bridle Path at Doodletown Road.

22.35 Turn left, leaving Bridle Path.

22.5   Seven Lakes Drive crosses.

22.95 AT joins.

23.45 End, near Bear Mountain Inn.

The Suffern trailhead of the Suffern-Bear Mountain Trail (S-BM) is on Route 59, about 500 feet north of the Thruway crossing. The trail leaves the sidewalk and goes steeply up a ravine, over rocks, to a good viewpoint. It continues to climb steeply until it reaches another viewpoint to the right. S-BM then joins a woods road and, at 0.6 mile, crosses a gas pipeline. After reaching the summit of Nordkop Mountain, the trail passes under a power line and descends into a hollow. Near this location, from 1944 to 1963, the Seven Hills Trail joined S-BM. (The route of this old trail is no longer obvious.) From this hollow, S-BM climbs a broken fault face which Frank Place in 1925 named the Kitchen Stairs. Beyond the Stairs, S-BM goes up and continues across a fairly level area. At 1.9 miles, it crosses another gas line, with an especially wide right of way. To the west, this gas line comes down in Hillburn, near where Route 59 crosses the Ramapo River. The trail then dips down across the outlet of a cattail swamp, goes up again over irregular ridges, and passes beneath a power line. At 3.15 miles, a deep notch, full of boulders, is crossed. Frank Place called this area the "Valley of Dry Bones" (a reference to the Bible — Ezekiel, chapter 37) because he felt that some rocks resembled animals. The little stream through this notch was named Os-Sec Brook.

After climbing the next hill, S-BM runs along the eastern edge of the Ramapo Rampart, passing the stone walls of the long abandoned Sky Sail Farm. In another 0.5 mile, the Columbia Gas Company pipeline crosses, and the trail passes through boulders known as MacIlvain's Rocks. At 4.5 miles, just beyond two great boulders that have been named "Grandma and Grandpa Rocks," S-BM crosses the Kakiat Trail (white). To the right on this trail, it is 1.5 miles to Route 202. S-BM now climbs over Cobus Mountain (1,130 feet), named after Jacobus Smith, said to have been the brother of Claudius Smith, the bandit (see p. 60). After climbing the next hill, with views down into the glacial cirque behind Horse Stable Mountain, the trail descends to the Conklins Crossing Trail (white), which ends here.

The S-BM Trail was proposed in 1924 by Major Welch, General Manager of the Palisades Interstate Park, as a project for the Trail Conference. Under the general direction of Frank Place, the trail builders divided the task into sections. Place himself, with Torrey's help, took the southern portion from Suffern to Conklin's Crossing. He reported: "I have already started scouting over the ridges at the lower end of the Ramapo Rampart . . . " (*N.Y. Post*, 10/28/24). It was Frank Place who, in 1925, named the Kitchen Stairs, the Valley of Dry Bones, and the Grandma and Grandpa Rocks.

The pipeline over Nordkop Mountain was built in 1952 by the Algonquin Company. Before crossing the mountain, this pipeline goes south from Ladentown along the foot of the hills, parallel to Route 202. The Columbia Gas Transmission Company pipeline, crossed by S-BM near the Kakiat Trail, was built in 1949.

The trail makers named MacIlvain's Rocks after William J. MacIlvain of the Fresh Air Club. They said he had chosen the most difficult route possible through those rocks (*N.Y. Post*, 5/1/27).

Until 1963, the Park boundary was 0.5 mile north of the Kakiat Trail. The first 5.0 miles were on land belonging to the Ramapo Land Company (of the Pierson family). At times they closed their land to hikers who, when allowed to hike on the property, were required to pay a fee for a permit to hike the S-BM, Kakiat, HTS and Seven Hills Trails.

Continuing north from the Conklins Crossing Trail, S-BM passes a great boulder named "The Egg." It then descends to cross Many Swamp Brook and climbs up a ledge to the E.D. Stone Memorial Shelter (built 1935), which it reaches at 5.95 miles. Just beyond the shelter, the unmarked Sherwood Path, a wide woods road, crosses. S-BM now climbs gently for 0.3 mile. It then crosses back to the edge of the ridge and passes along a height called Hawk Cliff. The land on the hillside below this cliff was once terraced for the gardens of Albert and Grace Pitt, a mountain couple who lived in a shack nearby.

Going down now, S-BM at 6.8 miles joins the Pittsboro Trail (unmarked) which comes up from the right. At the junction is the Witness Oak, a great white oak with a hollow trunk. In generations past, this tree marked the boundary of long-forgotten mountain farms. In another 0.1 mile, S-BM bends to the right, while the Pittsboro Trail (now invisible) continues straight ahead. At 7.0 miles, the Pine Meadow Trail comes in from the left (it ends here). S-BM now crosses Pittsboro Hollow Brook and continues along an old woods road.

In another 0.2 mile, S-BM turns left from the old road and descends into the gully of Gyascutus Brook. (The woods road, which was formerly the continuation of the Pine Meadow Trail, crosses the brook further down and continues to the service road of Orange and Rockland Utilities. It is now used by horse riders.) Just before reaching the brook at 7.45 miles, S-BM crosses another woods road which comes up along the brook from below the S-BM. This road becomes indistinct after going up another quarter mile.

S-BM now goes steeply up to the 1,124-foot summit of Panther Mountain, passing several viewpoints on the way. The best view is from the summit, which affords a beautiful panoramic vista. The Hudson River and its surrounding villages are visible to the left, and on a clear day the skyscrapers of New York City may be seen to the right. The trail swings around the end of the mountain and descends across a hollow where it crosses the Many Swamp Trail (unmarked, indistinct). It passes through a region of large boulders, then crosses one of the brooks that drain Squirrel Swamp and, at 8.65 miles, arrives at a fireplace on Two Bridges Road. This woods road, which nowadays is the route of the Tuxedo-Mt. Ivy Trail (T-MI) (red dash on white), connects Woodtown Road with Ladentown, in the valley below.

S-BM now climbs gradually to the 1,222-foot summit of Circle Mountain, and on the way down meets the Red Arrow Trail. The Red Arrow Trail starts at the T-MI, 0.35 mile downhill, and presently ends here at S-BM. Now S-BM descends gently, crosses File Factory Brook, and at 9.55 miles crosses Woodtown Road. 0.9

mile to the right is the Second Reservoir. S-BM then goes over 1,252-foot Ladentown Mountain and steeply down an eroded path through laurels to the Third Reservoir (built in 1951). Swimming in these reservoirs is strictly forbidden.

After a short climb, Breakneck Mountain is reached at 10.3 miles. Here the Breakneck Mountain Trail (white) starts to the left, and the old Red Arrow Trail used to go straight ahead, down to Camp Lanowa. S-BM turns right, goes up over a rock and continues north 0.85 mile to Big Hill Shelter (built October 1927), where the Long Path joins briefly. The trail drops over ledges, crosses a woods road (which goes down to the Second Reservoir), and reaches the wide Old Turnpike. This road carries a coaxial cable (buried there in 1969). Across the road, S-BM climbs gradually to the 1,276-foot summit of Jackie Jones Mountain, which it reaches at 12.1 miles. The fire tower there is no longer in use. The

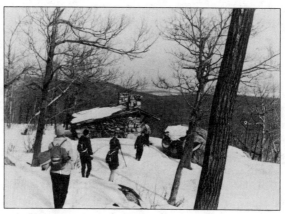

Big Hill Shelter – 1963

trail then goes down a gravel road for 0.2 mile and, opposite the AT&T microwave relay towers, turns right and soon crosses a bare rock outcrop with a view to the east. S-BM then descends steeply to a woods road. After several turns, it goes by the ruins of ORAK, the old Buchanan mansion, reaching Gate Hill Road (Route 106) at 13.2 miles.

The trail from Conklins Crossing to Gate Hill Road was scouted in 1924 by Archibald T. Shorey. He was a member of ADK, and a Brooklyn Boy Scout leader. He later, in 1931, joined the New York State Conservation Department. In that capacity, he scouted and blazed trails in the Catskills: Devil's Path, Giant Ledge/Panther, Escarpment, Mary's Glen, etc. He also built Adirondack trails.

The Stone Memorial Shelter was dedicated on April 28, 1935 in memory of Edgar D. Stone, who died on June 29, 1932. Stone was a mining engineer who, with his wife Jessie, founded the Tramp and Trail Club of New York in 1914. Jessie Stone died in 1936.

Gyascutus Brook was named by Frank Place (*N.Y. Post*, 2/12/26). The "gyascutus" described in Tacitus' *Germania* was a sort of deer or chamois with legs longer on one side than on the other. Torrey had earlier called attention to the similar Dingmaul (*N.Y. Post*, 12/31/23).

During the fall of 1925, Shorey gave up his work on S-BM. Frank Place and Leon Walker, of South Orange, New Jersey, took over. Various routes were considered: south along Breakneck Mountain to T-MI, joint with T-MI to Woodtown Road, then over Squirrel Swamp Mountain to Hawk Cliff, etc. (*N.Y. Post*, 11/19/25), but by January 1926 the route the trail presently follows had been worked out. The shelter on

Big Hill was scouted by R.H. Torrey and Park officials Raymond Adolph and John Tamsen in March 1927 (*N.Y. Post*, 3/18/27). A steel fire tower was erected in 1928 on Jackie Jones Mountain to replace an older one made of wood. The AT&T microwave tower was built early in 1947.

The original route of S-BM came down from the Jackie Jones Mountain fire tower almost due north, reaching Gate Hill Road about where the dam was later built. In 1954, it was rerouted to go down the road from the new relay tower. In 1993, it was rerouted through ORAK.

ORAK was a mansion on the east side of Jackie Jones Mountain that belonged to George Briggs Buchanan, a vice-president of the Corn Products Refining Co., which made KARO syrup. Buchanan bought the land and built his house in 1923. He named his estate for KARO, which he spelled backwards. The dining room of the house resembled a ship's cabin, with portholes for windows, and a floor that rocked gently to simulate a ship's motion. Buchanan died on April 13, 1939, and his heirs sold the property to the Park in 1947. The home, gardens and outbuildings were rented to Park employees until 1973, when the main house and hothouse were demolished. The foundations are still impressive.

S-BM turns right on Gate Hill Road to cross a brook. It immediately turns left and follows a woods road for about 0.15 mile, then turns right and goes up Irish Mountain. (The woods road continues to the tent camp area northeast of Lake Welch.) At the summit of Irish Mountain (1,174 feet), the trail passes a huge boulder, named the Irish Potato by Bill Hoeferlin. Here, S-BM turns right and descends gently from the summit. On the way down, Upper Pound Swamp, which usually looks like a lake rather than a swamp, can be seen below, to the right of the trail.

At 15.55 miles, S-BM reaches Lake Welch Drive. It follows this road east for about 0.15 mile and then bears left and crosses the southbound lanes of the Palisades Interstate Parkway and a brook on an overpass. It turns left, crosses the northbound lanes of the Parkway, and then turns left again and, for a short distance, goes north along the Parkway. Watch carefully for the yellow blazes — about 50 yards from the overpass, the trail suddenly turns right and goes up over rocks.

Here, the climb of the Pingyp begins. The way up is over steep ledges. After about 0.15 mile (and a climb of 300 feet!), if you can manage to look up (rather than at your feet), you may notice on a rock face, just above the trail, a memorial plaque to Harold B. Scutt, who first scouted this trail in May 1925. The grade moderates soon after the plaque is passed. After continuing upward for another 0.5 mile, the 1,023-foot summit of Pingyp is reached, with a grand view down the Hudson River.

Now the trail drops down the north side of the mountain to a woods road in the valley between Pingyp and The Pines. It turns right briefly on this road (the Pines Trail), parallel to a little brook. To the east, this road goes to Bulsontown; to the west, it goes to Stillwater Brook at the Palisades Interstate Parkway. After about 300 feet, S-BM turns left, crosses the brook, passes a fireplace, and climbs 250 feet to the summit of The Pines. As it begins to go down the north side, S-BM passes a ledge which affords a nice view of West Mountain and The Timp.

At 17.6 miles, S-BM turns left on the Red Cross/1779 Trail. After 400 feet, it turns right again, and soon crosses two streams and goes steeply up a rocky ledge. About 0.5 mile from the Red Cross Trail, it crosses a small brook and then crosses old Beechy Bottom Road, now marked with blue-on-white plastic blazes as a bike path. From here, a 120-foot climb leads to the summit of Horn Hill (930 feet). S-BM then descends gradually. It crosses the North-South Connector (also marked as part of the bike path) and then crosses a "stone road," known as the North "Ski Trail." S-BM now goes up the southern spur of West Mountain. After a climb over steep ledges, at 19.1 miles S-BM joins the Ramapo-Dunderberg Trail (R-D) (red) at the top of a curve called the Cats Elbow.

This section of S-BM, from Gate Hill Road to Cats Elbow, was scouted in the spring of 1925 by Harold B. Scutt of Douglaston, L.I., who also had a summer home in Tomkins Cove (*N.Y. Post*, 5/25/25). He died on April 2, 1930 in an airplane accident at Attica, N.Y. Scutt was a member of AMC and GMC. He and Torrey had been the first to go over the route proposed for the Northville-Lake Placid Trail which ADK was building. In Harriman Park he also worked on the Timp-Torne Trail (*N.Y. Post*, 8/11/22). At 11:00 a.m. on Sunday, October 19, 1930, the tablet on Pingyp was dedicated in his memory by his friends. Thirty people were present.

Gate Hill Road was built in 1824 as the "new turn-pike" from Monroe to Haverstraw. It replaced the Old Turnpike, which was the route of the Long Path from 1981 to 1992. The new turn-pike was a toll road, with a toll gate just east of the bridge over Minisceongo Creek — hence the name "Gate Hill Road."

When first built in 1925, S-BM crossed Gate Hill Road near the location of the present-day dam. The Hasenclever Fire Road also crossed at this point. That road has been cut off by the Lake Welch Drive and drowned by Lake Welch.

Scutt followed a suggestion by Herb Hauptman of ADK (*N.Y. Post*, 12/24/24) to cross the brook on stepping stones. (In 1949, the brook crossing was moved 0.2 mile east of the dam.) S-BM then proceeded across the fields east of Hasenclever Road (where the tent camping area was built in 1953), entered the woods at the foot of Grape Swamp Mountain and followed a woods road around the north side of Grape Swamp to a fireplace at a junction with an unmarked trail above the south side of Tiorati Brook. S-BM turned right on this trail and, in another 0.3 mile from the fireplace, it crossed Tiorati Brook on a wooden footbridge and reached Tiorati Brook Road a short distance west from where the trail presently arrives at the road. The abutments of that bridge are still there. The trail then went to the right on Tiorati Brook Road. In 0.2 mile, the road crossed Tiorati Brook, and 0.25 mile further, S-BM turned left off the road, crossed Stillwater Brook on stepping stones, and started up Pingyp. In 1953, when the Lake Welch tent campsites were built, the trail was rerouted over Irish Mountain. After reaching the Irish Potato near the summit, it went down to the northwest. It passed the campsites and went around the east side of Grape Swamp to a junction with the older route of the trail. Most of this portion of the trail has been obliterated by Lake Welch Drive.

In 1969, when Lake Welch Drive was being built, S-BM was rerouted to the northeast. It went over Pound Swamp Mountain and down along Grape Swamp Brook until it reached the paved road. About 1972, it was relocated to the hillside above the brook.

At present there is a level area just south of the brook, near the junction of Lake Welch Drive with Tiorati Brook Road. On old maps this was labeled the "Jimmy Stalter Place," a reference to the Stalters, a family of woodcutters. The Boy Scouts adopted this area in 1922 for their Camp Pathfinder, part of their White Bar Trail system.

Pingyp is a name which was put on the first park map in 1920 by Major Welch. It is a very old name, which he had heard from local residents. There had been a wooden fire observatory on the summit, but by 1925 it had fallen down. After descending from Pingyp, S-BM climbs The Pines where, according to the fifth edition of the *New York Walk Book* (p. 90), "there is not a single pine tree to be found." When the trail was made, this was private land, but even then there were only a couple of pines on it (*Paterson Morning Call*, 6/3/32). In 1945, the owner cut down all the trees and sold the land to the Park. Then, on April 25, 1948 (Arbor Day), led by Trails Chairman Joseph Bartha, sixty

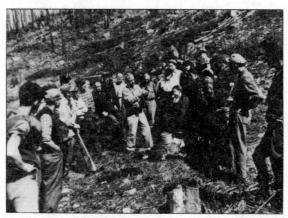

Tree planting on The Pines – 1948

Trail Conference members planted eight-inch trees on The Pines. This was repeated in 1949 and 1950.

After The Pines, S-BM briefly joins the Red Cross/ 1779 Trail. This woods road, once known as the Dean Trail, is now thought to have been the route followed in 1779 by General Anthony Wayne and his men on their way to attack the British at Stony Point. A half mile further, S-BM crosses Beechy Bottom Road. This was the first road built across the Highlands in 1740 from Stony Point to the Queensboro Road. After going over Horn Hill, S-BM crosses a "stone road" known as the North "Ski Trail." This once was a trail marked with aluminum H's by Jim Horn, Vice President of the Fresh Air Club (*N.Y. Post*, 9/9/21). In 1934 it was "paved" by the CCC as a fire road, and it was subsequently marked as a ski trail. The Cats Elbow, where S-BM meets the R-D Trail, was named by Frank Place (*N.Y. Post*, 6/8/28).

The section of S-BM from Cats Elbow to Bear Mountain Inn was first scouted by Raymond Torrey in 1926. From the Cats Elbow ledge, S-BM and R-D run together for a short distance. R-D then goes off to the east, while S-BM turns north to cross the hollow between two summits of West Mountain. It formerly went up a steep route, named the Fire Escape by Torrey, but has been rerouted to climb on a more moderate grade. On the crest of West Mountain, the Timp-Torne Trail (T-T) (blue) joins for 0.3 mile. T-T then departs right to the West Mountain Shelter, while S-BM goes northwest to a knob. A rocky descent, soon followed by a steep ascent, leads to another knob, a high point of West Mountain. From here, S-BM goes steeply down and continues to descend along an old woods road, following the gully of the Doodlekill. After crossing the brook, S-BM turns left onto the Doodletown Bridle Path at 21.5 miles. Both run together for 0.15 mile. S-BM then turns right, goes over a low ridge, crosses two branches of a brook and goes up a bank to rejoin the Bridle Path at the old Doodletown Road. The 1777W Trail crosses here. After 150 feet, S-BM and the Bridle Path turn left and leave Doodletown Road. S-BM follows the Bridle Path northeast for 0.5 mile until, at a bend in the path, the yellow blazes turn left uphill to Seven Lakes Drive.

From the Drive, S-BM ascends the shoulder of Bear Mountain, following a telephone line. Soon the Appalachian Trail (white) joins from the left, and the joint trail descends toward the Bear Mountain playground. The joint trail follows a paved path which crosses under the ski jump and goes down toward the Bear Mountain Inn, where S-BM ends at 23.45 miles.

S-BM originally climbed West Mountain on a very steep route up a cliff, known as the Fire Escape. In 1985, Chief Ranger Tim Sullivan requested that the trail be rerouted because the Fire Escape's precipitous descent made it dangerous in winter conditions. The new route, which is much less steep, adds about 0.5 mile to the trail.

Coming down northeast from West Mountain, or southwest from Seven Lakes Drive, S-BM encounters the Doodletown Bridle Path (now a ski trail). In 1926, when Torrey described his section of S-BM from Bear Mountain to the Fire Escape (*N.Y. Post*, 12/17/26), the Bridle Path had not yet been built. His trail crossed Doodletown valley just about where it does now. From Doodletown Road, near the last house, Torrey cut a new trail which roughly paralleled the Seven Lakes Drive for half a mile, then went uphill to cross the Drive (*New York Walk Book*, 1936 ed., p. 192).

In 1934-35, a path was built around Doodletown by men of the Temporary Emergency Relief Administration. Known as the Doodletown Bridle Path, it was used as a bridle path for some years, but also became popular as a cross-country ski trail. This new path used part of the route of Torrey's S-BM Trail from where it came down from the Drive to the junction with Doodletown Road. For years, S-BM followed its original line, but in 1949, at the suggestion of Park Police Chief Hlavaty, the northern loop of the Bridle Path was included in the S-BM. This made the trail 1.1 miles longer. About 1965, the northern loop was again left out.

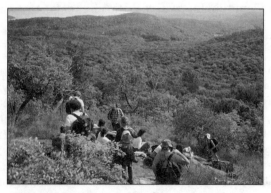

Hikers at the top of the Cats Elbow

TIMP-TORNE TRAIL

Length: 11.15 miles
Blazes: blue

Miles

0.0	North end of Popolopen Viaduct.
0.35	Left on Mine Road.
0.7	Go left on West Point Aqueduct.
1.35	Turn up right.
1.95	Summit of Popolopen Torne.
2.25	Cross Mine Road.
2.35	Right on Aqueduct path.
2.45	Left, down across brook.
2.5	Join Popolopen Gorge Trail.
3.2	Cross Queensboro Brook.
3.55	Left on Fort Montgomery Road.
3.7	T-T/1777W goes up, left, from road.
3.9	Rejoin road; pass water plant.
4.1	Palisades Parkway overpass.
4.3	Anthony Wayne Trail, right.
4.55	Fawn Trail crosses.
5.3	AT joins, left.
5.4	First view to west.
6.05	AT leaves, right.
6.2	S-BM joins, right.
6.5	S-BM leaves, left.
6.6	West Mountain Shelter.
6.95	Cross brook; fireplace to left.
7.2	Turn left onto Timp Pass Road.
7.25	Turn right, leaving Timp Pass Road, and ascend.
7.7	Viewpoint over Bear Mountain Bridge.

7.8	Summit of The Timp.
8.0	Go right on Red Timp Trail.
8.45	1777 Trail crosses.
8.85	Cairns, right, to Escalator.
9.95	Jones Trail crosses.
10.10	Upper tunnel.
10.15	Down, right, to lower grade.
10.4	End of grade; go right.
10.65	View to river.
10.95	Pass lower tunnel.
11.15	Route 9W; left to parking.

The Timp-Torne Trail (T-T) starts on the west side of Route 9W at the north end of the Popolopen Viaduct, 0.8 mile north of the Bear Mountain Inn. At first, it runs jointly with the 1777W and 1779 Trails. T-T/1777W/1779 soon turns left onto a paved residential street, then goes down and continues along an old woods road. At 0.35 mile, the joint trails reach Mine Road (old Forest of Dean Road), which they follow northwest for 0.35 mile. They then turn down left on a path which is the route of the West Point Aqueduct.

At 1.35 miles, T-T turns right and leaves the aqueduct. (1777W and 1779 continue straight ahead along the aqueduct.) T-T climbs steeply, crosses Mine Road at its intersection with Fort Montgomery Road, and climbs 500 feet to the summit of Popolopen Torne (941 feet), which it reaches at 1.95 miles. There is a good view toward the Bear Mountain Bridge and Anthony's Nose, to the southeast, and toward Crown Ridge, to the north.

The trail now goes down the steeper face of the Torne and crosses in quick succession the Mine Road, the bed of the old Forest of Dean Iron Ore Railroad and the Fort Montgomery Road. At 2.35 miles, it turns right onto the West Point Aqueduct, rejoining the 1777W and 1779 Trails. In another 0.1 mile, all three trails go down to the left to cross Popolopen Brook on a footbridge. Passing a fireplace, the trails go up and turn right onto the Bear Mountain Aqueduct, which is also the route of the Popolopen Gorge Trail (PG) (red dot on white). The four trails follow the aqueduct path along the brook for about 100 yards. They then turn left, leaving the aqueduct route, and continue along a rougher trail. At 3.2 miles, the trails turn right and cross Queensboro Brook. The pipe that the footbridge uses here was built to carry treated waste water from the Anthony Wayne Recreation Area to Queensboro Brook.

T-T/1777W/1779/PG now follows a woods road and, in another 0.35 mile, turns left onto Fort Montgomery Road (a short distance to the right, this road enters West Point land and is closed to hikers). At 3.7 miles, PG/1779 turns right, while T-T/1777W goes left, avoiding a pistol range. T-T/1777W soon rejoins the road and passes the water treatment plant (built in 1929) at Queensboro Dam. After crossing the Palisades Interstate Parkway on an overpass, 1777W departs to the left, while T-T goes up a bank to start the climb up West Mountain. 0.2 mile from the Parkway, the Anthony Wayne Trail (white) starts to the right. After climbing a small knob, with a good view, T-T crosses the Fawn Trail (red F on pink). T-T now climbs more steeply, with more views along the way, to a junction with the Appalachian Trail (AT) at 5.3 miles.

The Timp-Torne Trail was the second trail built by the new Palisades Interstate Park Trail Conference, in the winter of 1921. It was considered to be a branch of the R-D Trail, which had been built in 1920 (*N.Y. Post*, 12/9/21). Most of the scouting for the new skyline trail was done by William W. Bell of the AMC. At the beginning, the markers were 3x3-inch galvanized iron squares, with a red square and a "TT."

The trail started at Timp Pass and went up West Mountain. A western leg came up from Beechy Bottom; this later became the route of the AT. The trail descended to Doodletown Road (following the route of the present-day AT). It climbed Bear Mountain on the route adopted by the AT in 1922, then descended the north face, on the route presently used by the Major Welch Trail, down to Perkins Drive. There was no Perkins Drive there then, and the trail continued down to Popolopen Brook. It crossed the brook on a footbridge that was built by Major Welch in April 1922. T-T then climbed to the Torne, where it ended.

In March 1948, the New York Hiking Club marked the trail down the east side of the Torne, with permission of the landowner, Mr. King James Weyant, Jr. (the Weyant family cemetery is on the edge of the Long Mountain traffic circle). Their trail crossed the northernmost bend of Mine Road and went 0.3 mile down to the dam on the brook at Roe Pond. From the dam, hikers scrambled up to the abutment of the old Hell Hole Bridge. From that point, a narrow road went 0.15 mile to a junction — up left to Old Mine Road, or straight ahead to Route 9W (the Timp-Torne Trail follows the latter route today).

From the dam at Roe Pond, a 20-inch iron pipe went downstream along the north side of the brook. It carried water to a gristmill that was just a bit upstream of the present viaduct. That old mill and the Hell Hole Bridge were demolished in the 1950s. One

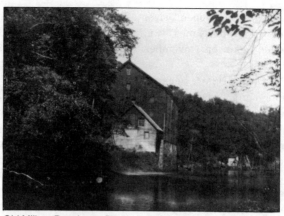
Old Mill on Popolopen Brook – 1925

of the millstones was salvaged from the brook a few years ago. It was erected at the edge of Garrison Pond (near the dam) in Fort Montgomery, with a plaque that reads: "Built in 1799 by Eugene Lucet, who lived in a mansion at the site of Fort Clinton."

One person interviewed by the author remembers that, in 1918, when she was 10 years old, her parents took her to stay in the mill for a week. A German couple named Krieger were the proprietors until 1920 (there is a short Krieger Road in Fort Montgomery). She says that the place had previously been used as an electric generating station. That hydroelectric plant, and another electric generating station in Highland Falls, had been operated by George W. Flood. He was bought out in 1917 by Roscoe Smith, president of the recently organized Orange and Rockland Electric Co.

In 1925, only four years after T-T had been blazed, the Park started construction of Popolopen Drive. It opened in 1927, and was widened to three lanes in 1934. In 1947, the construction of the Palisades Interstate Parkway was begun. Popolopen Drive, widened to four lanes, was opened again on November 30, 1953.

Gradually, it became clear that crossing that high-speed road was dangerous for hikers, especially after August 28, 1958, when the Parkway was opened all the way to the George Washington Bridge. So the Trail Conference rerouted T-T to avoid that crossing. From West Mountain, where T-T/AT had gone down to Doodletown Road, there was an old white-blazed Queensboro-West Mountain Trail (Q-W) that went down the ridge line. This had been scouted and cairned in 1934 by Frank Place and the Tramp and Trail Club as a short cut to the T-T/AT (*N.Y. Post*, 3/18/35). In June 1960, T-T was routed down the old Q-W Trail to the Fort Montgomery Road at the water treatment plant. It followed that road, past the Queensboro Furnace, to the old route coming up from the footbridge across the brook. This arrangement lasted until 1971, when West Point closed the Fort Montgomery Road. T-T was then made to join the Popolopen Gorge Trail (vertical red bar on white), which had been marked in 1960 to Long Mountain by Sam Wilkinson and Bill Burton. Once again, T-T crossed the creek on the often washed-out footbridge.

Shortly after the junction with the AT, the trail arrives at a viewpoint over Bear Mountain and the Hudson River. T-T/AT then crosses to the west side of West Mountain, where there is an excellent view of Beechy Bottom and the Anthony Wayne Recreation Area. For the next 0.65 mile, the joint trails run along the ridge, with a number of additional viewpoints. T-T then turns left as the AT continues straight ahead and begins its descent (that was the original "western leg" of T-T). At 6.2 miles, the Suffern-Bear Mountain Trail (S-BM) (yellow) comes in from the right and runs jointly with T-T for 0.3 mile. S-BM then departs to the left. At 6.6 miles, the trail passes the West Mountain Shelter. This shelter was built in 1928, with burros being used to carry up the lumber and cement. A gradual descent (there are some steep sections), with good views to the south, brings the trail to a fireplace at a brook. T-T then continues down an eroded road.

At 7.2 miles, T-T turns left and goes down to Timp Pass Road. It turns left again and follows the road for 300 feet. (To the right, Timp Pass Road leads in 350 feet to Timp Pass, and a junction with the Ramapo-Dunderberg and Red Cross Trails.) T-T then turns right and begins its climb to the summit of The Timp. At 7.7 miles, it reaches a beautiful viewpoint over the Bear Mountain Bridge, and then, in another 500 feet,

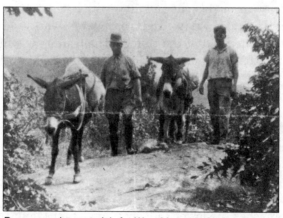

Burros carrying materials for West Mountain Shelter – Oct. 1928

it comes out at the 1,080-foot summit of The Timp, with a view over Haverstraw Bay to the south.

T-T now joins the Ramapo-Dunderberg Trail (R-D) (red), and both trails continue east, descending gently. At 8.0 miles, T-T/R-D reaches the Red Timp Trail. This was blazed by Girl Scouts from Camp Addisone Boyce, following the route of an old trail once called the Timp Bypass. Here, T-T leaves R-D, follows the Red Timp Trail for 175 feet, and then turns east. It soon passes a good viewpoint from the top of a large rock. The 1777 Trail crosses at 8.45 miles. At 8.85 miles, several cairns on the right show the way down to the Escalator, a steeply slanting crack in the face of the cliff. Now zig-zagging downward, with a number of good views along the way, T-T crosses the Jones Trail and a little brook at 9.95 miles. Ahead and a bit to the left is one end of the unfinished upper Dunderberg Spiral Railway tunnel. The trail follows the descending grade of the railway through a cut and fill —with a beautiful view over Haverstraw Bay—and then follows a work road up to the other end of the tunnel. The trail crew which blazed the trail here also cleared the debris from this quite impressive tunnel. Unfortunately, it is likely to be water-filled in wet weather.

A few yards further along, the trail goes down tumbled rocks to the next lower descending railway grade, which it follows for 0.25 mile. At 10.4 miles, the grade ends, and T-T goes down to the right. Again zig-zagging downward, at times steeply, and passing a beautiful viewpoint that invites family picnics, the trail approaches the lower railway tunnel. Steps built into the hillside lead down past the tunnel, and, at 11.15 miles from the beginning, T-T ends at Route 9W, just south of Jones Point.

When it first was blazed, the Timp-Torne Trail, a high-line branch of the R-D Trail, started from the R-D at Timp Pass. In 1947, it was extended from Timp Pass to Tomkins Cove (Trail Conference Minutes, 4/2/47). It went down from Timp Pass on the 2.6-mile-long, white-blazed Timp Trail which went around the east side of a 680-foot knob known as the Little Timp, or Boulderberg. At Mott Farm Road the trail turned east and was blazed all the way to the railroad station at Tomkins Cove.

The land where the T-T and Red Cross Trails met Mott Farm Road was acquired in 1951 by the Rockland County Girl Scout Council, who built a camp and a lake there. They asked that the trails be rerouted. In 1952, T-T was rerouted from the foot of the Boulderberg, paralleling the Park boundary until it intercepted the Jones Trail. It followed that trail out to Route 9W, 0.5 mile south of the Anchor Monument. In 1967, slight relocations were made to move the trail away from homes in the Tomkins Lake Colony. Then, in 1986, disaster struck! Lumberjacks were clear-cutting the south side of Dunderberg Mountain. Even the trees with the T-T blazes were cut, from the Red Timp Trail to the 1777 Trail. It turned out that the trail had been blazed outside the Park boundary and was actually on private property!

With the help of the Park authorities, a new route for the Timp-Torne was devised: the one described above. The new section, from Jones Point to a junction with the R-D Trail just east of The Timp, was built in the fall of 1987 by an AMC crew led by Bob Marshall and Tom McCarthy. The new section of the Timp-Torne Trail was designed to include many viewpoints, a section of the old railway bed, and both tunnels of the spiral railway.

Then, in 1998, the route of the Timp-Torne in the area of The Timp was changed again. The 1987 relocation had rerouted the T-T onto the R-D Trail for the descent of The Timp. But this very steep trail had become badly eroded, so it was decided to construct new routes down The Timp for both the T-T and R-D Trails. A new route for the T-T was located north of Timp Pass, and the trail was constructed by the West Hudson Trail Crew, under the direction of Bob Marshall, and opened in the summer of 1998. A relocation of the R-D descent of The Timp is planned for the summer of 1999.

Triangle Trail

Length: 5.25 miles
Blazes: yellow triangles

Miles

0.0	Start at R-D Trail.
0.5	Telephone line.
0.95	Cross Black Ash Brook.
1.25	Cross Deep Hollow Brook.
1.7	Old Park boundary.
2.5	Cross brook, bear right and ascend.
2.6	White Bar Trail joins.
2.75	Turn left and leave White Bar Trail.
3.3	Parker Cabin Mountain; R-D Trail crosses.
4.0	Telephone line.
4.1	Victory Trail crosses.
4.2	Cross brook; swamp to right.
4.5	Cross into Rockland County.
4.8	Trail, left to ADK camp.
5.05	Trail, left, to ADK camp.
5.2	Old Rectangle Trail, right.
5.25	End at White Bar Trail.

The Triangle Trail starts at the Ramapo-Dunderberg Trail (R-D),0.2 mile from Grove Drive in Tuxedo. After 0.5 mile, it briefly runs along a telephone line, and then turns right onto a woods road. After again passing under the telephone line, it turns left onto the woods road that runs along Black Ash Brook. This road was once the route of the R-D Trail. It then crosses the brook and soon turns right onto another woods road. Triangle continues gently uphill and, at 1.25 miles, crosses Deep Hollow Brook. As the trail goes north, Black Ash Mountain is on the right. At 1.7 miles, the trail crosses the old boundary line on Fox Mountain between Harriman Park and the Tuxedo Park Association. After crossing a fairly level region, the trail crosses a stream at 2.5 miles and goes up to join the White Bar Trail, which comes in from the left. Soon Triangle leaves White Bar and climbs up Parker Cabin Mountain. It joins the R-D Trail briefly on the summit. Until 1935, there was a wooden fire tower here.

Triangle then leaves the R-D Trail and goes to the eastern edge of the summit for a view of Lake Sebago — a favorite lunch stop. The trail now goes steeply down for a short distance, and then continues to descend more gradually. At 4.1 miles, Triangle crosses the Victory Trail (blue V on white) near Lake Skenonto. Soon afterwards, it crosses a brook that drains a swamp on the right. At this point, a woods road goes right; in 0.6 mile it reaches the White Bar Trail. After skirting the south end of Lake Skenonto, Triangle goes over several small ridges and comes down near an arm of Lake Sebago. It joins the Sloatsburg Trail that goes along the western edge of the lake. Near this point, an unmarked trail goes left along the lake edge to ADK Camp Nawakwa. A little further along, by a huge boulder, another unmarked trail goes to Camp Nawakwa. At 5.2 miles, someone has recently re-marked the old Rectangle Trail (white blazes and cairns) which goes northwest to the Victory Trail. In another 250 feet, the Triangle Trail ends at the White Bar Trail. The Dutch Doctor Shelter is 0.15 mile farther down the White Bar Trail, about 100 feet up to the left.

The Triangle Trail was first marked in 1939 as the Yellow Bar Trail. It was blazed by Kerson Nurian, with yellow bands around the trees, starting from the the woods road along Black Ash Brook, the former route of the R-D Trail. Nurian used already existing roads and trails, ending on Parker Cabin Mountain. In October 1939 he offered his trail to the Trail Conference. They accepted, and assigned Harry Zilverman as its maintainer.

Early in 1942, the Conference marked a Yellow Triangle Trail from Parker Cabin Mountain to the arm of Lake Sebago, and continuing to ADK Camp Nawakwa. At the lake edge it crossed an older trail that ran past the Old Dutch Doctor's place to Johnsontown at the northwest end of Lake Sebago (the Sloatsburg Trail). Nurian was a Bulgarian electrical engineer who worked on submarines at the Brooklyn Navy Yard (see p. 89). In 1943, he returned to Bulgaria, and the Conference then decided to mark the whole trail, from Black Ash Brook to Lake Sebago, with yellow metal triangles (Trail Conference Minutes, 4/4/44). By 1946, it was marked to the Dutch Doctor Shelter. The Conference (probably Joe Bartha) also eliminated an 0.75-mile loop which followed the old Park boundary on Fox Mountain.

Then, in 1947, Nurian returned! Joseph Bartha's Trail Committee minutes for September 24, 1947 reported that all 80 metal markers had been removed from the Triangle Trail from Black Ash Brook to Parker Cabin Mountain (that had been the route of Nurian's Yellow Bar Trail). By the spring of 1948, it was clear who had done it, because the yellow bars had been repainted around the trees. After heated discussions with Bartha and the Conference, Nurian agreed to leave the trail alone, provided that painted triangles were used instead of metal ones. And so it was. Nurian died on November 19, 1948, at the age of 75.

In 1951, 1,200 acres of land were sold by the Tuxedo Park Association to the Interstate Park. Half of the required funds were supplied by New York State, and half by Commissioners W. Averell Harriman and George W. Perkins. Now the R-D, Kakiat, Blue Disc and Triangle Trails were no longer on private property. In 1954, the new Thruway cut off the original R-D route from Tuxedo up Black Ash Brook. Although R-D had not used that route since 1930, the Triangle Trail did start there until 1955. In the spring of 1955, Triangle was relocated onto its present route.

Tuxedo-Mt. Ivy Trail

Length: 8.2 miles
Blazes: red dash on white

Miles

0.0	R-D Trail, 1.25 miles from Tuxedo station.
0.35	Claudius Smith Rock.
0.7	Horseshoe curve at swamp.
1.55	Join White Bar Trail.
1.65	Turn left, uphill.
2.05	Camp road crosses.
2.4	Sebago Dam.
2.65	HTS Trail crosses.
2.8	Diamond Creek crosses.
3.35	Seven Hills Trail crosses.
3.55	Woodtown Road (West) crosses.
4.3	Pine Meadow Road West crosses.
5.1	Pine Meadow Road East crosses.
5.15	Breakneck Mountain Trail, left.
6.0	Woodtown Road; go right.
6.05	Turn left, leaving road.
6.65	Fireplace; S-BM Trail crosses.
7.25	Red Arrow Trail starts, left.
7.8	Power line; go left, then right.
8.1	Turn left onto dirt road.
8.2	End at road to power substation.

The Tuxedo-Mt. Ivy Trail (T-MI) starts from the Ramapo-Dunderberg Trail (R-D). It begins 0.8 mile from Grove Drive, and 1.25 miles from the Tuxedo railroad station. Both T-MI and R-D have red blazes on white backgrounds (although T-MI is blazed with a red *dash*, while R-D is blazed with a red *dot*). After 0.35 mile, the trail reaches the base of Claudius Smith Rock. It then curves to the left and climbs up towards the top of the rock. On the way up, the Blue Disc Trail (blue dot on white) crosses. At the top, a path to the left leads to a viewpoint. In another 125 feet, the White Cross Trail starts to the left.

Claudius Smith was of English stock, born in Brookhaven, Long Island. He was descended from Richard Smith, the founder of Smithtown. His father bought 200 acres in Orange County at Smith's Clove, later named Monroe. Claudius, a man of large stature, married and had three sons: William, Richard and James. The sons, and perhaps a dozen others, formed a gang of thieves who operated in the southern part of Orange County around Suffern and Haverstraw. They robbed local farms, and during the Revolution they hijacked the arsenal trains of the Continental Army. They hid out in places like this cave on Horse Pond Mountain near Tuxedo, and Horsestable Mountain near Ladentown.

Claudius was captured and jailed at Kingston on July 17, 1777, but he escaped. With a reward posted for the arrest of him and his three sons, Claudius fled to the British in New York City. Later he settled near Smithtown. He was recognized there by Major John Brush of the Continental Army. On a December night in 1778, Brush and five comrades crossed Long Island Sound and found Claudius asleep in bed. They took him prisoner and transported him to the jail in Goshen. There he was hanged on Friday, January 22, 1779.

Sons Richard and James were later captured and hanged. Son William died in the Goshen jail of wounds inflicted by Continental soldiers who chased the gang on Schunemunk Mountain. The

rest of the gang fled to   the *New York Sun* of October
Canada. (This story is from   26, 1927.)

Going gently downhill now, T-MI at 0.7 mile makes a horseshoe turn around the right end of a swamp. From the south end of that swamp, a faint old road goes up a slope. In 0.4 mile, this road forks. To the right, it goes to the Blue Disc Trail at the point where the gas pipeline crosses. To the left, it goes more steeply down, with many turns, to the old Johnsontown Road.

T-MI now goes over a low ridge and down to a woods road, the route of the White Bar Trail. (0.1 mile to the left is the Dutch Doctor Shelter, built in 1935.) T-MI turns right on this road, which was once known as the Sloatsburg Trail.

In another 0.1 mile, T-MI leaves the White Bar Trail to the left and goes uphill over another ridge. T-MI then goes down to Lake Sebago. It crosses the paved camp road that serves the American Canoe Association and the Adirondack Mountain Club (Nawakwa) camps, and then runs along the southwest shore of the lake. At 2.4 miles, it reaches the Sebago Dam on Seven Lakes Drive. Crossing to the north end of the dam, it descends the embankment and drops down to the brook level. At this point, the Hillburn-Torne-Sebago Trail (HTS) (orange) starts. T-MI goes right on a wide trail which runs along Stony Brook, crosses a small brook and then the HTS Trail, and starts to climb Diamond Mountain. At 2.8 miles, the trail crosses Diamond Creek. The ridge top, where the Seven Hills Trail crosses, is reached at 3.35 miles.

Here, on Diamond Mountain, we can stop to reflect on the history of the T-MI. It was a favorite project of Major Welch, the Park's first General Manager. It was he who persuaded the Tuxedo Park Association to let the Trail Conference blaze the trail in the spring of 1923 (*N.Y. Post*, 5/11/23). He provided copper markers for the trail crew: Place, Holt, Lewis and Torrey. The route from Tuxedo was joint with T-TJ until T-MI turned right, up a woods road, towards Claudius Smith Rock (see p. 109). There were no Blue Disc or White Cross Trails then, and it was not until 1951 that Claudius Smith Rock became "ours." Going past the Dutch Doctor's clearing, and over the ridge to Burnt Sawmill Bridge (there was no dam or lake there then), the trail went up Halfway Mountain (named Diamond Mountain in 1927) on the old Woodtown Road (West). That road, a narrow overgrown trail, was used in 1933 by the Civilian Conservation Corps to get their trucks and machines over the mountain to build Pine Meadow, Wanoksink and Minsi Lakes. The road became so muddy and eroded that T-MI was relocated in the spring of 1935 to its present route up Diamond Mountain by Ernest Dench and W.P. Bottomley of the Interstate Hiking Club (*N.Y. Post*, 3/16/35).

After crossing the Seven Hills Trail, T-MI crosses old Woodtown Road (West) and, at 4.3 miles, reaches Pine Meadow Road West. It then goes over a rocky knob and passes by a swamp. Pine Meadow Road East crosses at 5.1 miles. In another 400 feet, the Breakneck Mountain Trail (white) starts to the left. Shortly afterward, T-MI joins an ancient woods road that crosses the north end of Big Green Swamp. At 6.0 miles, T-MI reaches Woodtown Road, which it follows to the right. It crosses a little brook that connects Big Green Swamp (on the right) with Squirrel Swamp (on the left).

In 1923, there was a little bridge across the brook, called Tim's Bridge. In 1927, Frank Place nailed a sign on a tree there: "Tim's Bridge," in memory of a faded sign that hikers remembered. Frank's sign, and the bridge too, were gone by 1930. The present bridge was built in 1986.

About 250 feet beyond the bridge, T-MI turns left on what was once known as the Two Bridges Road. It passes through a fairly level swampy area and reaches a fireplace at 6.65 miles, where the Suffern-Bear Mountain Trail (yellow) crosses. Going down gradually, T-MI passes the start of the Red Arrow Trail at 7.25 miles. Soon afterwards, T-MI turns off to the right onto another woods road, and continues to descend more steeply. As the trail descends, Limekiln Mountain is on the left and Eagle Rock is on the right. At 7.8 miles, T-MI reaches a power line and, turns left briefly, then right again, along a gas pipeline. After another 0.25 mile, the trail goes down left on a dirt road to a paved road which leads to a power company substation. This road starts at Mountain Road in Ladentown.

In December 1974, Art Beach, for the Trail Conference, and Tim Sullivan, for the Park, arranged with officials of Orange and Rockland Utilities to allow parking on their land for access to the T-MI Trail (*Trail Walker*, Jan./Feb. 1975). Do not block the road and do not park on the land near the private home on the hill.

The route down the Two Bridges Trail is the same as the one blazed in 1923. From Ladentown the trail was marked along Route 62 (now Route 202) northeast for 1.5 miles to the Erie Railroad station at Mt. Ivy. In 1936, the Interstate Hiking Club, which maintained the trail, rerouted it to avoid the long walk on the highway; instead of taking the Two Bridges Trail from Tim's Bridge, the blazes went north 0.7 mile on Woodtown Road and turned right on the File Factory Hollow Trail. This led downhill 1.0 mile to Calls Hollow Road at Krucker's Farm. The trail then turned right on Camp Hill Road, which it followed to Quaker Road, which led to Mt. Ivy. After some years, Mr. Krucker asked the hikers not to go through his farm. So, in 1944, T-MI was sent from Woodtown Road down the S-BM/Red Arrow Trail to rejoin the Two Bridges route. In 1946, some inexperienced trail worker blazed T-MI down the Two Bridges Trail again and blacked out the "real" route (Trail Conference Minutes, 10/2/46). The Trail Conference decided to let the new route remain (Trail Conference Minutes, 4/2/47). In the fall of 1965, the Park widened T-MI to a 20-foot fire road for 2.5 miles, from Ladentown to Pine Meadow Road East. This accounts somewhat for the appearance of the trail today. In 1951, when the Erie Railroad stopped service to Mt. Ivy, T-MI was made to end at Ladentown. Then, in 1961, it was again marked to Mt. Ivy to join the Hook Mountain/ Tors Trail, in expectation that the latter trail would become part of the new Long Path. In October 1961, the Long Path was started from the George Washington Bridge, and in 1964 the Conference determined its route through Harriman Park. It joined the T-MI at Mt. Ivy and both trails coincided to the Dutch Doctor Shelter where the Long Path took over the White Bar Trail. This route remained until 1981, when the Long Path was routed from Mt. Ivy over Cheesecote Mountain.

Across the road from the parking place in Ladentown is a grove of small trees. This grove shades an old cemetery of several graves, dating to 1858: Eliza Secor, James and Fannie Haring, one stone with the initials "E.S.," and one stone with a weathered, illegible inscription. Eliza Secor was the daughter of Isaac and Mary Secor who in 1836 had bought the land of Michael Laden. In 1865 they donated land for the Methodist Church. The road from the little cemetery to Mountain Road was called Dilts' Lane; it led to farmer Dilts' place, where the Orange & Rockland substation is now.

VICTORY TRAIL

Length: 3.4 miles
Blazes: blue V on white

Miles

0.0	Tri-Trail Corner.
0.2	Telephone line crosses.
0.3	Detour left if wet.
0.4	Old Park boundary.
0.7	White Cross and White Bar Trails cross.
0.8	Rectangle Trail, right.
1.25	Triangle Trail crosses.
1.95	Left on camp service road.
2.15	Hemlock Hill Road, left.
2.25	Turn left off road.
2.65	Join Hemlock Hill Road.
2.85	Trail, right, to Tom Jones Mountain.
3.15	Fireplace; R-D Trail crosses.
3.4	End at Route 106.

The Victory Trail starts at the rock dam on Black Ash Brook, at Tri-Trail Corner, where the Victory, Blue Disc and Ramapo-Dunderberg Trails meet. The trail is rather level for its first 2.25 miles. It follows an old road along the western side of Black Ash Swamp, and generally parallels a telephone line. At 0.3 mile, the trail is on the very edge of the swamp; in wet weather, it might be better to stay on the road higher up. The original boundary between Harriman Park and lands of the Tuxedo Park Association is crossed about ten minutes from the start.

At 0.7 mile, the White Cross Trail crosses. In another 300 feet, the White Bar Trail joins Victory for 100 feet, then departs up right. At 0.8 mile, the Rectangle Trail (recently revived) starts to the right. (It ends near the Dutch Doctor Shelter.) Then, at 1.25 miles, the Victory Trail reaches Lake Skenonto where the Triangle Trail (yellow) crosses. Along the lake shore there are several good lunch spots. At 1.95 miles, Victory joins a paved camp road.

At 2.15 miles, the old Hemlock Hill Road (Continental Road) goes left. Victory continues on the paved road a little farther, then turns left and starts a climb to the foot of Tom Jones Mountain. In another 0.4 mile, it joins the old Hemlock Hill Road. At 2.85 miles, an unmarked trail enters right from Tom Jones Mountain. Soon afterwards, the Ramapo-Dunderberg Trail (R-D) crosses at a fireplace. Victory continues along Hemlock Hill Road another 0.25 mile to end at Route 106 (Old Route 210), 0.5 mile west of the point where the R-D Trail crosses Route 106.

Before 1930, hikes from Tuxedo often went north on an old woods road, known as the Black Ash Swamp Road, that ran along the east side of the Ramapo River. After 0.3 mile, the road turned right and went up the south side of Black Ash Brook. It crossed to the north side just below the rock dam that backs up Black Ash Swamp. The road followed the same route it does now, ending at Sebago Beach on Johnstown Road, except that it crossed over Big Swamp, the predecessor of Lake Skenonto (which was not built until 1935). For one of their hikes, the ADK planned "to take the Black Ash Swamp Trail from Tuxedo to Sebago, thence to Allis' Trail of Seven Hills, etc." (*N.Y. Post*, 1/16/31).

In 1942, J.A. Allis, then Chairman of the Conference Trails Committee, proposed to make Black Ash Swamp Road a Conference trail (Trail Conference Minutes, 6/3/42). In October 1942, Bernard Landau, President of the C.C.N.Y. Hiking Club, volunteered to blaze the trail, but he was recruited into the Army. On April 4, 1943 the trail was cleared and marked with blue V's by a group led by Abe Shechter.

At first, the trail went up Hemlock Hill Road from the camp road and ended at the junction with the R-D Trail. Hemlock Hill Road once was used by the American Continental troops to go from the Ramapo Valley to Johnsontown and points east. It was replaced in 1824 by the Monroe-Haverstraw Turnpike (now Route 106).

In 1949, the trail was extended from the fireplace at the foot of Tom Jones Mountain out to Route 210 (now Route 106). In 1960, the Park created a dump on the old Hemlock Hill Road and, to avoid the dump, the Victory Trail was routed around it in 1964. As of 1999, the dump is still used to dispose of tree limbs. Ignore the dump and enjoy a walk up that old road for 0.15 mile to rejoin the Victory Trail.

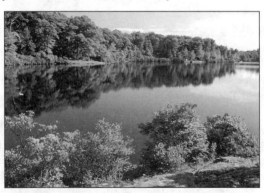

Lake Skenonto

WHITE BAR TRAIL

Length: 7.4 miles
Blazes: horizontal white bars

Miles

0.0	Start from A-SB/LP.
0.3	Join Crooked Road.
0.9	Dunning Trail joins, left.
1.15	Dunning Trail leaves, right.
1.7	Nurian Trail joins, right.
1.75	Site of Camp Deerslayer.
1.8	Nurian Trail leaves, left.
2.0	Island Pond Road joins.
2.05	Route 106 crosses.
2.3	Hilltop Shelter, right.
2.7	Car Pond Mountain (second summit).
3.1	Brook crosses.
3.55	Triangle Trail joins, right.
3.7	Triangle Trail leaves, left.
3.9	R-D Trail crosses.
4.4	White Cross and Victory Trails cross.
5.5	Woods road from Lake Skenonto, left.
5.65	Triangle Trail ends, left; join old Sloatsburg Road.
5.8	Dutch Doctor Shelter, left.
5.85	T-MI Trail joins from right.
5.95	T-MI Trail leaves, left.
6.0	Homestead site of "Old Dutch Doctor," right.
6.3	Unmarked Springbrook Trail begins, right.
6.75	Reach gate; White Bar goes down, right.
6.9	Old Johnsontown Road joins, left.
7.05	Kakiat Trail joins, left.
7.1	Kakiat Trail leaves, right.
7.4	End at Johnsontown Circle.

The White Bar Trail starts from the Arden-Surebridge Trail (A-SB) (red triangle on white), about 0.2 mile from the Lemon Squeezer, at the point where the Long Path (turquoise) comes from the north to join the A-SB. After a fairly level 0.3 mile, White Bar joins a woods road that comes from the east side of Island Pond (the "Crooked Road") for 0.6 mile. At 0.9 mile, the Dunning Trail (yellow) comes in from the left, and both trails run together for a quarter of a mile. Dunning then departs to the right, while White Bar continues southwest, going gently upward through a wide valley that is dotted with straight, tall trees.

At 1.7 miles, the Nurian Trail (white) comes in from the right. In 1922, this area was the site of the Boy Scouts' Camp Deerslayer, a part of their White Bar Trail system. In 1926, Camp Deerslayer was moved to Parker Cabin Hollow. After 0.1 mile, the Nurian Trail leaves to the left. In another 0.2 mile, White Bar joins Island Pond Road and, at 2.05 miles, crosses Route 106. The trail now climbs more steeply. On the first 1,080-foot summit there is a shelter made of corrugated iron, off the trail on the right (but not visible from the trail). White Bar then goes steeply down into a notch and up again to the second 1,100-foot summit, which it reaches at 2.7 miles.

On the current USGS topographic map (Sloatsburg Quadrangle), these two summits, as well as the two summits to the west, are unnamed. On the Park's 1927 topo map, the peak just to the west (which is south of Lake Stahahe, *i.e.*, Car Pond), is named Hemlock Hill. Bill Hoeferlin in his 1944 handbook called our second summit "Car Pond Mountain," call the second summit "Carr although his maps named it Pond Mountain." So be it (al- "Hemlock Hill." All editions though the proper spelling is of the Trail Conference map "Car," not "Carr").

White Bar now goes steeply down into Parker Cabin Hollow, where it crosses a brook at 3.1 miles. A long steady climb up a shoulder of Parker Cabin Mountain follows. At 3.55 miles, the Triangle Trail (yellow) joins from the right, then soon leaves to the left. After another 0.2 mile, the Ramapo-Dunderberg Trail (red on white) crosses in the saddle between Parker Cabin and Black Ash Mountains. Dropping gently down, White Bar crosses the White Cross Trail and briefly joins the Victory Trail (blue V on white). It then climbs over Blauvelt Mountain. At 5.5 miles, a woods road from Lake Skenonto comes in from the left. White Bar passes the end of the Triangle Trail, then passes the Dutch Doctor Shelter (on a rise to the left of the trail) and, at 5.85 miles, joins the Tuxedo-Mt. Ivy Trail (T-MI). T-MI leaves at 5.95 miles, and immediately afterwards one sees on the right an old cellar hole, with a hundred-year-old tree growing from the center.

The cellar hole is all that remains from the homestead of John Frederick Helms, the "Old Dutch Doctor," who lived here from 1874 to about 1892. He bought six marshy acres from David Demarest and built a cabin. He made a living by raising medicinal herbs, such as ginseng. His son, John Wilbur, born in 1866, was brain-damaged at birth. Both father and son were illiterate. The son became the owner of the property in 1884. When the "Old Dutch Doctor" died, the son was taken in and cared for by

John Waldron, whose farm-house was on the hillside where Johnsontown Circle is now. A grove of tall pines marks the site where the farmhouse once stood. Waldron's blacksmith shop was across the road, above Spring Brook. In 1927, John Wilbur, then 61 years old, was committed to the County Home by Dr. Gillette, and he died there in 1950. He is buried near the entrance to the Sloatsburg cemetery, beside a mortuary which once belonged to Warren Waldron (John Waldron's son).

Continuing southward, the beginning of the unblazed Springbrook Trail, an old woods road, is visible to the right at 6.3 miles. That trail goes northwest and, at 0.3 mile, meets the Fox Trail, which goes toward Almost Perpendicular. The Springbrook Trail then bends southward and soon rejoins the White Bar Trail.

Soon White Bar comes to a gate, where it turns down, right. At 6.8 miles, it reaches the end of the Springbrook Trail and then joins old Johnsontown Road, which comes in from the left. (To the left, Johnsontown Road is cut off by the Seven Lakes Drive.) In this vicinity was the 64-acre farm of William Lewis Becraft.

At 7.05 miles, the Kakiat Trail goes up left to cross the Seven Lakes Drive. Shortly thereafter, Kakiat leaves to the right. Our White Bar Trail ends at 7.4 miles, at the Johnsontown Road circle. From the circle, the paved Johnsontown Road continues another 2.2 miles to Route 17 in Sloatsburg.

The White Bar Trail was first marked in 1921-22 by the Boy Scouts from the 17 camps on Kanawauke Lakes, led by Archibald T. Shorey of Brooklyn. Their marker was a red metal disc which had a white bar across it. They used mostly old roads, making a 35-mile circle around the Kanawauke Lakes with five spokes radiating from the center. On those spokes were six camps where Scouts could stay overnight: Camp Forest Ranger, where Lake Skannatati was later built, Camp Leatherstocking at the Old Dutch Doctor's place (until 1926), Camp Hawkeye at the western foot of Jackie Jones Mountain, Camp Pathfinder at the junction of Tiorati and Stillwater Brooks (moved to Hasenclever Mine in 1926), Camp Prairie at Youman Flats near Tiorati Circle, and Camp Deerslayer in the wooded valley north of Car Pond Mountain (moved to Parker Cabin Hollow in 1926). Meals at the camps were thirty-five cents (fifty cents for guests). The camps were connected with headquarters by wireless (Shorey, *N.Y. Post*, 8/12/22).

The piece of the White Bar system that is still known today by that name started on the Crooked Road at the north end of Island Pond. From there, a branch went uphill to the east to join the A-SB Trail. The Appalachian Trail, marked through there in 1922, used the White Bar route up to the Lemon Squeezer. (From the Lemon Squeezer, this branch of White Bar followed A-SB to "Times Square," and then continued on the R-D Trail.)

Going south on Crooked Road past Island Pond, White Bar departed when the road turned left uphill (now the route of the Dunning Trail). It continued south, as it does today, to the Old Dutch Doctor's place and beyond.

Sometime during the next twenty years, the markers were changed to a white blaze with two green stripes. The trail apparently was neglected because in 1943, the Conference minutes state that "an effort is being made by Mr. George Goldthwaite to locate the old White Bar Trail north of Island Pond" (Trail Conference Minutes, 12/1/43). He apparently succeeded because, in 1944, the trail was restored and maintained by H.F. Hamm of the ADK.

This continued until 1964, when the Trail Conference routed the new Long Path along the White Bar route from the Dutch Doctor Shelter to Island Pond. For the next 17 years, only hints of the older blazes could be seen under the new turquoise color. Then in 1981 the white bars were seen again! The Long Path was rerouted and the White Bar Trail was restored (*Trail Walker*, Oct./Nov. 1981, p. 9).

In January 1995, the White Bar Trail was extended south for 1.55 miles from the Dutch Doctor Shelter to the Johnsontown Circle. This extension facilitated access to the park trails from the end of Johnsontown Road, where parking is available.

White Cross Trail

Length: 2.15 miles
Blazes: white cross

Miles

0.0   Claudius Smith Rock.
0.85 Black Ash Swamp, left.
1.0   Old Park boundary.
1.45 White Bar and Victory Trails cross.
1.6   Parker Swamp, down right.
2.15 End at R-D Trail.

The White Cross Trail connects the Tuxedo-Mt. Ivy Trail (T-MI) (red dash on white) at Claudius Smith Rock with the Ramapo-Dunderberg Trail (R-D) (red dot on white) on Parker Cabin Mountain. It starts by going north, downhill from T-MI (in icy weather, it is safer than the parallel Blue Disc Trail), and soon passes to the left of a swampy area. At 0.85 mile, the trail goes along the east side of Black Ash Swamp and soon crosses the old Park boundary. At 1.45 miles, the White Bar and Victory Trails cross. White Cross then ascends gently, with Parker Swamp visible down to the right. At 2.15 miles, White Cross ends at the R-D Trail, just below the steep ascent to Parker Cabin Mountain.

The first mention of this trail appears in the *New York Post* of January 31, 1936, which announced that the Interstate Hiking Club planned to hike on February 2nd on the White Cross Trail, "new to most Interstaters." It had been blazed earlier by Kerson Nurian, the builder of several other trails (HTS in 1928, Nurian in 1929, and Triangle in 1939). In 1939, he asked the Trail Conference to take over the maintenance of this trail. The Adirondack Mountain Club (to which Nurian belonged) was assigned the task, and they have continued to maintain it since then.

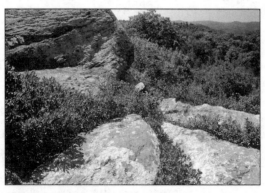

On top of Claudius Smith Rock

THE
REVOLUTIONARY
TRAILS

1777 TRAIL

Length: 2.95 miles (joint section)
Blazes: red 1777 on white diamond

Miles

0.0	Route 9W; Jones Trail.
0.05	Cross grade of spiral railway.
0.4	Cross footbridge.
0.65	Turn left, leaving Jones Trail.
0.7	Second Jones leg goes right.
1.1	Turn up, right.
1.35	Timp-Torne Trail crosses.
1.4	R-D Trail crosses.
1.7	Bockberg Trail joins, right.
2.0	Timp Pass Road, left.
2.05	Cross brook; begin Pleasant Valley Road.
2.35	Cross Timp Brook.
2.65	Bridle Path crosses.
2.9	Road, right, to Herbert Cemetery.
2.95	Trails divide.

The 1777 Trail marks the route taken by British troops under Sir Henry Clinton on October 6, 1777 from Stony Point to attack the American forces at Fort Clinton and Fort Montgomery. To avoid private property, the present-day trail starts from Route 9W, 0.75 mile south of the intersection of the road leading to Jones Point. There is a small parking area about 200 feet south of the trailhead.

At first, the trail follows an old road known as the Jones Trail, which was built about 1890 to take workmen up to the various levels of the Dunderberg Spiral Railway. In 300 feet, it crosses the lowest grade of the railway. Then, at 0.4 mile, the trail crosses a stream on a wooden footbridge, built in 1987 as an Eagle Scout project by Enoch Namenson (note the wide stone abutments from the original bridge).

At 0.65 mile, the trail has been rerouted to the left to avoid an eroded section of the original road. Then, in 150 feet, the 1777 Trail turns left, while the Jones Trail continues straight ahead (on the old road to the right). In another 150 feet, a branch of the Jones Trail comes in from the right. Now the 1777 Trail runs close to the Park boundary, with homes visible to the left. At 1.1 miles, after passing a small wet area to the left, the 1777 Trail turns right and goes steeply up an old road to a saddle on the ridge between The Timp (on the left) and Dunderberg Mountain (on the right). At 1.35 miles, the Timp-Torne Trail (blue) crosses.

This is a good place to look back down the trail towards the valley below. About 0.4 mile to the south is Tomkins Lake (you can glimpse it on the way up), and beyond is Buckberg Mountain. The route taken from Stony Point by the British troops in 1777 went over Buckberg, past the lake and up this road over the ridge. In those days it was called the King's Road. In later years it has been known as Steep Street or the Lumberjack Trail.

In 1900, the lake and the surrounding land belonged to Laura E. Woods, a relative of the local Tomkins family. Her daughter married James Fowler, who was president of Scott and Bowne Co., makers of "Scott's Emulsion." In 1912, Fowler built a house on Bird Hill Road (the old King's Road). The house burned in

1928. Then in 1952 the ruin was bought by Vladimir Sunguroff, who began to restore it. He died before he had finished the restoration, but his wife still lives there in the part of the house that was rebuilt.

In 1947, Mrs. Fowler sold the land around the lake (including Bird Hill Road) to a private developer (Tomkins Lake Colony), and in 1951 she sold the land west of the lake to the Rockland County Girl Scouts. Until then, many hikes started from Tomkins Cove, going up either "Steep Street" or the old Timp Trail from Bulsontown Road.

Now the 1777 Trail continues north, soon crossing the Ramapo-Dunderberg Trail (red on white), and then heading down into Doodletown Valley. At 1.7 miles, the Bockberg Trail joins from the right. (Bockberg is another name for Bald Mountain.) Near the bottom of the slope, the faint Timp Pass Road joins from the left. The trail crosses a little brook on a wooden bridge, and the blazes continue along Pleasant Valley Road through the abandoned settlement of Doodletown. Just past the brook crossing, an old dam and a shelter are visible to the right. This is all that remains of a camp that was maintained there until the 1950s by Riverside Church of New York City. (For more information on this history of this area, see the section on Doodletown, pp. 319-36.)

At 2.35 miles, Timp Brook crosses, and at 2.65 miles the Bridle Path crosses. Then at 2.95 miles the trail reaches the point where the British forces divided into two columns. The east column turned to the right to attack Fort Clinton (where the Trailside Museum is located now). The west column went northwest, up an old road which brought them to Queensboro and the road there to Fort Montgomery.

1777E Trail to Fort Clinton

Length: 2.35 miles

Miles

0.0	Trails divide; continue straight ahead.
0.1	Turn right on Doodletown Road.
0.3	Reservoir on right.
0.35	Lemmon Road, left.
0.5	Go left, off road.
0.6	Join Bridle Path.
0.95	Cornell Mine Trail, right.
1.35	Tunnel under South Entrance Road.
1.4	Tunnel under Seven Lakes Drive.
1.65	Pass Bear Mountain Inn.
1.8	AT joins, left.
1.95	Tunnel under Route 9W.
2.35	Trailside Historical Museum.

From the point where the 1777 Trail divides, the 1777E Trail continues along Pleasant Valley Road. After 0.1 mile, it turns right on Doodletown Road and passes a new (1975) reservoir and Lemmon Road (which goes up left to Seven Lakes Drive). At 0.5 mile, the trail leaves Doodletown Road (which goes downhill to Route 9W) and goes up to join the Bridle Path. Soon the Cornell Mine Trail (blue) comes in from the right, and then the trails go through two tunnels (under the South Entrance Road and the Seven Lakes Drive). After passing the south parking lot and restrooms, the Cornell Mine Trail goes off to the left, while 1777E continues straight ahead on a paved path. It passes to the left of the Bear Mountain Inn, and follows a path above Hessian Lake. At 1.8 miles, the AT (white) joins from the left, and both trails go through a tunnel beneath Route 9W into the museum grounds. 1777E ends at the Trailside Historical Museum. The remains of old Fort Clinton are visible down a side trail.

1777W Trail to Fort Montgomery

Length: 5.3 miles

Miles

0.0	Trails divide.
0.05	Cross Doodlekill.
0.5	S-BM Trail crosses.
1.0	AT joins briefly.
1.05	Go left, leaving AT.
1.3	Cross parking area.
1.95	T-T Trail joins.
2.05	Cross Parkway on overpass.
2.25	Go right, leaving road.
2.45	Rejoin road; PG/1779 comes in.
2.55	Turn right, off road.
2.9	Cross Queensboro Brook.
3.6	Go down left with T-T/1779.
3.65	Cross Popolopen Brook; go right on West Point Aqueduct.
3.75	T-T Trail leaves, left.
3.95	T-T Trail rejoins from left.
4.6	Turn right on Mine Road.
4.95	1777W/1779/T-T turns right.
5.1	Turn right onto residential street.
5.3	End on Route 9W at Popolopen Viaduct.

After the 1777 Trail divides, the 1777W Trail goes through a small clearing, crosses a little brook (the Doodlekill) and goes gently uphill on an old road, past the ruins of some Doodletown homes. At 0.5 mile, an intersection with the Suffern-Bear Mountain Trail (yellow) and Doodletown Road is reached. Here, 1777W turns left onto Doodletown Road, which it follows gently uphill towards the Seven Lakes Drive. At 1.0 mile, the Appalachian Trail joins from the left, and the two trails briefly follow the same route. Just before reaching the Seven Lakes Drive, 1777W leaves the old road and goes left into the woods. Soon a parking area is reached. The trail continues to run roughly parallel to the Seven Lakes Drive until, at 1.95 miles, it joins the Timp-Torne Trail (blue), and both cross the Palisades Interstate Parkway on an overpass. The trails then pass the Queensboro Dam (1915) and a water treatment plant (1929). They then turn right, off the gravel road, to avoid a pistol range. At 2.45 miles, PG/1779 joins, and all four trails continue north along the road for 0.1 mile. The trails then turn right, leaving the Fort Montgomery Road. The road beyond this point is on land of West Point Military Academy, where hiking is allowed only with written permission. In another 0.35 mile, Queensboro Brook is crossed on a footbridge, and the trails turn left and continue along the brook. At 3.6 miles, the Popolopen Gorge Trail continues straight ahead while 1777W/1779/T-T turns left and goes down across Popolopen Brook. Up the bank on the north side, the trails turn right onto the West Point "Patrick" Aqueduct. This 20-inch pipeline was opened on August 31, 1906. It is 33,000 feet long and carries water from Queensboro Brook and Popolopen Brook to the Lusk Reservoir on the Academy grounds.

In another 500 feet, the Timp-Torne Trail turns left and goes up to the Popolopen Torne, while the 1777W/1779 Trails continue along the aqueduct path. The Timp-Torne Trail rejoins from the left in 0.2 mile.

All of the trails continue on the aqueduct path until it crosses Mine Road at 4.6 miles. The trails turn right and follow the paved road for 0.35 mile. They then turn right, leaving the road, and follow an old woods road downhill. At 5.1 miles, the trails climb an embankment and turn right onto a paved residential street. They follow the street for about 600 feet, and then turn right onto a footpath. At 5.3 miles, the trails end on Route 9W, at the north end of the Popolopen Viaduct.

In 1975, when these trails were first marked, they all went to the Trailside Museum, where there was a Dan Beard exhibit. Medals and patches were awarded for hiking either trail.

The Revolutionary trails were first scouted and blazed in 1974-75 as a joint project of the Rockland County Boy Scout and Girl Scout Councils, the Palisades Interstate Park, the Cooperative Extension Association of Rockland County, and the NY/NJ Trail Conference. The routes were determined by Jack Mead, Director of the Trailside Museum. He used information from military records in London and maps drawn by Robert Erskine, Surveyor General of the American army in 1778-79.

For the first hike on the 1777 Trail, a ceremony was held on March 27, 1975. Leading the hike were Brad Bobb, Captain of Shore Guard, Orange County Militia, and John Walker of the 42nd British Regiment Foot "Black Watch." Also present were Jack Focht, who had put up the blazes (he used a stepladder), Tim Sullivan, representing the Park, and representatives of the Scouts and the Trail Conference. This first hike started at the junction of the Buckberg and Mott Farm Roads. It went over Bird Hill, to the right of Tomkins Lake, and up over Dunderberg — the actual route the British troops had taken in 1777. Musket fire was heard again, on Dunderberg and in Doodletown.

A second ceremony, with the same participants, was held on April 12, 1975 for the 1779 Trail. This one started at the Cliff House near the Bear Mountain Viaduct. It proceeded along the Forest of Dean Mine Road and Fort Montgomery Road, past the ruins of the Queensboro Furnace, to Queensboro, and ended at the Bullowa Scout Camp (the old Springsteel farm).

In the years since 1975, the trails have been maintained by the Boy Scouts' Order of the Arrow, and most recently by the Trail Conference. The trails have been rerouted in places to avoid private or West Point property. In some places, they depart from the original route to avoid dangerous highway crossings.

1779 TRAIL

Length: 8.5 miles
Blazes: blue 1779 on white diamond

Miles

0.0	Popolopen viaduct, north end.
0.35	Turn left onto Mine Road.
0.7	Turn left, with T-T/1777W, onto West Point Aqueduct.
1.35	Continue straight ahead; T-T turns right.
1.55	T-T rejoins.
1.65	Turn down left and cross Popolopen Brook.
1.7	Go right with Popolopen Gorge Trail.
2.4	Cross Queensboro Brook.
2.75	Go left on Fort Montgomery Road.
2.85	Turn right, with PG Trail.
3.1	Pass Queensboro Lake.
3.55	Go left (leave PG).
3.7	Left again, onto Summer Hill Road.
4.2	Cross Route 6.
4.3	Cross Seven Lakes Drive.
4.55	Cross Anthony Wayne Trail.
5.7	Orange/Rockland county line.
6.0	Cross AT/R-D.
6.5	Cross Owl Lake Road.
6.95	Cross Palisades Interstate Parkway.
7.05	Join Beechy Bottom Road.
7.15	Go right, off Beechy Bottom Road.
7.5	Join old Black Mountain Trail.
7.6	Go left on Red Cross Trail.
7.7	S-BM joins, briefly.

7.8	Red Cross leaves, left.
8.3	Pines Trail joins from right.
8.45	Beechy Bottom Road joins from left.
8.5	Bulsontown.

The 1779 Trail starts on the west side of Route 9W at the north end of the Popolopen Viaduct, 0.8 mile north of the Bear Mountain Inn. For the first 1.35 miles, it runs jointly with the Timp-Torne Trail (blue) and with the 1777W Trail. The trails soon turn left onto a paved residential street, then go down and continue along an old woods road.

At 0.35 mile, the joint trails turn left onto Mine Road. They follow the road for 0.35 mile and then turn left onto the West Point Aqueduct, which crosses the road at this point.

Of course, the aqueduct was built 127 years after General Wayne passed this way. The scouts who originally blazed this trail followed Wayne's route — along the Mine Road to its junction with the Fort Montgomery Road. Those early blazes can still be seen on the telephone poles along Mine Road, beyond the aqueduct crossing, but the newer blazes turn left with the blue Timp-Torne Trail and follow the aqueduct path.

At 1.35 miles, the Timp-Torne Trail turns up, to the right, to cross Fort Montgomery Road and Mine Road and ascend Popolopen Torne. Our 1779 Trail (along with the 1777W Trail) goes straight ahead along the aqueduct path. After 0.2 mile, our trails meet Timp-Torne again and, in a few hundred feet, all turn left, going down to cross Popolopen Brook. After passing a fireplace, they go up and join the Popolopen Gorge Trail

(P-G) (red dot on white), and all four trails go west on the Bear Mountain Aqueduct (built in 1929-30). In another 300 feet, the trails leave the Aqueduct (it is walkable and can be followed to rejoin the trail 0.4 mile further up the brook). At 2.4 miles, the trails cross Queensboro Brook on a wood-covered concrete bridge, and in another 0.35 mile they turn left on Fort Montgomery Road.

Two years after Forts Clinton and Montgomery had been destroyed by British troops, General George Washington instructed General Anthony Wayne to drive the British from the fort at Stony Point. Starting from several camps north of Fort Montgomery, Wayne led about 1,150 men in four regiments around Bear Mountain by way of the Fort Montgomery Road.

They stopped for lunch on July 15, 1779 near where our present trail joins the old Fort Montgomery Road. They continued south through the valley now called Beechy Bottom and took an old road down to Springsteel's farm (now the Boy Scouts' Camp Bullowa). At midnight, Wayne's troops attacked the fort from three directions and quickly subdued its defenders.

At 2.85 miles, 1779/PG turns right, off the road, while 1777/T-T goes straight ahead towards West Mountain. Now following an old woods road, the trail approaches Queensboro Lake, a pretty spot to stop for lunch. At 3.55 miles, our 1779 Trail turns left from the PG route, and soon joins a wide fire road that goes through a Park work area to Route 6. This fire road, known as the Summer Hill Road, was built by the Civilian Conservation Corps in the spring of 1933. It goes around the foot of Summer Hill to the site of a dam in Curtis Hollow.

After crossing Route 6 (Long Mountain Parkway) near Long Mountain Circle, the trail also crosses the Seven Lakes Drive. Easily seen on the opposite side of the traffic circle is a cemetery of perhaps 100 graves, where the residents of Queensboro hamlet — the Weyants, Brooks and Coons — lie buried. The most recent burial there was in 1993.

Going uphill now toward Black Mountain, the 1779 Trail crosses the Anthony Wayne Trail (white) and joins an old woods road (the Leisure Trail) which goes along the west side of a low ridge.

This ridge was designated DeGaffles' Ridge on a map of the area drawn by Robert Erskine for General Washington in 1778. On his map, a road appears to run along the crest of the ridge. In fact, in those days there was no road on the ridge. There was a well-used road, known as Beechy Bottom Road, on the east side of the ridge. Most of that road was destroyed when the Palisades Interstate Parkway was built in 1953. Since, from the Seven Lakes Drive south, it was no longer possible for the trail to follow the historical route used in 1779, the blazers of our historical trail chose the Leisure Trail on the west side of DeGaffles' Ridge.

At 5.7 miles on the 1779 Trail (1.4 miles south of Seven Lakes Drive), the old Leisure Trail departs down to the left. This point (marked by cairns on both sides of the trail) is on the Orange/Rockland county line. The Leisure Trail continues for another 0.25 mile until it ends at the Appalachian/Ramapo-Dunderberg Trail (AT/R-D), 75 yards above Beechy Bottom West Road.

From the junction, our 1779 Trail proceeds straight ahead. At 6.0 miles, it crosses the AT/R-D, which comes down from Black Mountain. Soon afterward the ridge ends abruptly, and our trail descends to the Owl Lake Road. It crosses this road and picks up another woods road (once named the Black Mountain Trail) which passes through a swampy region. At 6.95 miles, it reaches the Palisades Interstate Parkway.

After crossing the Parkway, the 1779 Trail briefly joins the Beechy Bottom Road, then turns right, off that road, and crosses a little stone viaduct. Continuing through a rocky region (where General Wayne certainly never went), it soon joins a woods road (the Black Mountain Trail), and 0.1 mile further joins the Red Cross Trail. Red Cross and 1779 here follow a well-worn old road which was known as the Dean Trail when the Park was formed in 1910.

At 7.7 miles, the Suffern-Bear Mountain Trail joins for about 400 feet and leaves again. Red Cross then departs to the left, while 1779 continues downhill. At 8.3 miles, the unmarked Pines Trail (the trail along the brook between Pingyp and The Pines) joins from the right. Then, at 8.45 miles, 1779 meets Beechy Bottom Road on the left, and all reach a paved road at 8.5 miles. This is Bulsontown. The houses in this area are mostly owned by Bulson families who have lived here for generations. Just ahead is Cedar Flats Road, where a street sign says that the road we have just left (Beechy Bottom Road) is called Queensboro Road.

Wayne's route went briefly left on Cedar Flats Road, and then continued on Bulsontown Road. After 0.7

mile, it turned left onto Franck Road past the Boy Scouts' Camp Bullowa (where the American troops rested at Springsteel's farm to prepare for their midnight assault on the fort at Stony Point). To reach the Stony Point Battlefield Park, go left on Wayne Avenue 0.7 mile to Route 9W. Turn right on Route 9W for 0.3 mile, then turn left onto Park Road, which goes downhill to the battlefield park. Old 1779 blazes may be occasionally found along these roads.

The Unmarked Trails

ANTHONY WAYNE SOUTH SKI TRAIL

Length: 1.05 miles

Miles

0.0	South end of parking area.
0.2	Fenced enclosure, right; cross first bridge.
0.4	Sharp left over second bridge.
0.45	Cross third bridge.
0.5	Cross fourth bridge.
0.6	AT crosses.
0.7	R-D comes in, left.
0.75	R-D leaves, right.
1.05	End at Beechy Bottom East Road.

The Anthony Wayne South Ski Trail, marked with red plastic plaques as a cross-country ski trail (and with blue-on-white markers as a bike trail), starts from the southeast corner of the southern parking area at the Anthony Wayne Recreation Area. It soon enters a pine forest where, at 0.2 mile, a fenced-in enclosure can be seen on the right (the fence has been broken by a fallen tree). That was a demonstration area, built to show how the vegetation looks where browsing deer are excluded.

At 0.4 mile, the trail turns sharply left, across Beechy Bottom Brook. Here, there is a little dam across a stream that comes down from the right. Two more bridges are crossed, and the trail passes to the right of a small knoll. Just beyond, where the ski trail joins another old road, the Appalachian Trail (AT) crosses.

Then, at 0.7 mile, the Ramapo-Dunderberg Trail (R-D) comes down from the left.

After crossing two culverts, the R-D leaves to the right. Soon, the ski road turns up to the left, with Beechy Bottom Brook to the right of the trail. At 1.0 mile, the trail bears right, and at 1.05 miles it ends at Beechy Bottom East Road. The North "Ski Trail" is 0.1 mile to the left.

Across Beechy Bottom Road from the end of the Anthony Wayne South Ski Trail is another unfinished road. Judging from the piles of stone along the way, it, too, was a CCC project. After 0.1 mile, it goes down and crosses Beechy Bottom Road, to end 100 feet beyond at a "T." Here another unfinished road begins to run parallel to Beechy Bottom Road. It ends 0.1 mile to the south, where it has been cut by the Palisades Parkway. The continuation of that intended road can still be seen, on a knoll west of the Parkway (see p. 217).

Before the Park was started in 1910, the south parking area was part of a farm that had belonged to John Wesley Van Wart. He died in 1891, and his wife Elizabeth died in 1911. In 1916, the heirs sold their 630 acres in Beechy Bottom to the Park. Our Anthony Wayne South Ski Trail was one of John Wesley's farm roads. The little dam we see at 0.35 mile probably provided a pool where his cattle could drink.

ARDEN ROAD

Length: 2.8 miles (Elk Pen to Route 106)

The Arden Road (also known as the Old Arden Road) is the dirt road that hikers take from the Elk Pen parking area (along Arden Valley Road) south to the Nurian bridge across the Thruway.

About 1894, Edward Harriman requested permission from Orange County to close a road through his estate. That road went south from Florence Mountain (east of Central Valley) past Forest Lake to join the road from Twin Lakes (Baileytown Road). Despite some protests from local residents, permission was granted. In order to show his gratitude to his neighbors, Harriman built a new road from Arden to Southfields. A plaque erected later by the County (0.3 mile north of the Nurian Bridge) explained that the road had been made "to show the value of level roads in hilly country." The road started from the Greenwood Furnace at Arden and went south above Arden Brook and the Erie Railroad. After 0.65 mile, it reached the site of Arden Valley Road (built 1934). This section of the road has been partly obliterated by the Thruway, which was built in 1954.

At the Elk Pen (built 1919), Harriman's road turned up to the foot of the mountain (where a branch went up the valley and across some meadows to Echo Lake) and then continued south. The Appalachian Trail (AT) briefly follows the road, but soon turns left and starts up the hill. Just before the AT turns off the road, the

Arden-Surebridge Trail (A-SB) begins, and runs south along the road. At 0.4 mile, the A-SB leaves to the left. Then, at 0.7 mile, the road crosses Stahahe Brook. On the south side of the brook, a faint trail, with old, obliterated blazes, goes up to the left, and soon joins a woods road (the Stahahe Brook Road) that leads in 0.8 mile to Lake Stahahe. (The Stahahe Brook Road continues to Arden Road and ends high up on a cut, 0.1 mile south of the bridge over Stahahe Brook.) The plaque is passed 0.7 mile further south, soon after which the Nurian Trail joins from the left. Finally, 1.8 miles from Arden Valley Road, hikers may cross the Nurian Bridge.

When it was first built, Harriman's "level road" crossed the Ramapo River on a bridge located 0.25 mile north of the bridge that presently carries the Nurian trail over the river. No trace of Harriman's bridge remains. It probably was washed away in the great flood of October 8, 1903. Hoeferlin's older maps indicate a ford at the site of Harriman's bridge.

The road south of the Nurian Bridge was part of the old Haverstraw-Monroe Turnpike (see p. 250). Sometime before 1920 (perhaps after the 1903 flood), a connection was made on the east side of the Ramapo River between the Haverstraw Turnpike and Harriman's "level road." The connecting road was obliterated during the construction of the Thruway, but in 1954 the two roads were again connected, higher on the hillside (Commission Minutes, 12/31/53).

BAILEYTOWN ROAD (TWIN LAKES ROAD)

Length: 2.0 miles

Miles

0.0	Route 6 (Long Mountain Road).
0.2	Lake Te Ata, right; Lower Twin Lake, left.
0.7	Cross brook from Upper Twin Lake.
1.25	Trail, left, to Cave Shelter.
1.5	Cemetery, left.
1.75	Old boundary, right.
1.85	Nawahunta Trail, left.
2.0	Harriman Estate gate.

The Baileytown Road begins as a paved road, starting from Long Mountain Parkway and passing between Lake Te Ata and Lower Twin Lake. At 0.6 mile, a branch goes off to the right and leads to the camps on Upper Twin Lake. A brook from Upper Twin Lake is crossed at 0.7 mile. At 1.25 miles, as the road passes camp buildings on the right, a faint trail on the left goes 0.5 mile up to the Stockbridge Cave Shelter. The pavement ends at the last camp building. A cemetery may be seen on the left at 1.5 miles — the names on the stones are Bailey and Lewis. At 1.75 miles, a stone wall is visible on the right. Until 1942, this was the boundary of the Park. A path along that wall leads down to a brook. More stone walls are above the brook, and beyond is the overgrown farm of William and Mary Bailey. William died in 1924 at the age of 87, and Mary sold the farm to the Park in 1925.

The unmarked Nawahunta Trail comes in on the left at 1.85 miles. The Lewis family lived at the other end of that trail, where Lake Nawahunta is now. There were many marriages between the Baileys and the Lewises, so naturally a road was built to connect their lands.

At 2.0 miles, our road ends at a gate, the entrance to the Harriman estate. The Baileytown Road actually continues for 4.5 more miles through the Harriman Estate to Arden. In the early 1920s, Roland Harriman bought the last Parrott family home on that road, and when the last Bailey farm was sold to the Park in 1930, the County gave permission to close the road to the public. In 1942, Averell Harriman gave to the Park a quarter-mile-wide strip, from the top of Stockbridge Mountain, northwest across Summit Lake, and down nearly to the line of the Thruway.

Standing by the Harriman gate, an old woods road may be seen going to the right. That road leads to the William and Mary Bailey farm. The determined hiker will get through the barberries there and proceed to the northwest corner, where the road will be found again. It goes up over the ridge and down to Summit Lake.

About 0.1 mile up that road from the Harriman gate, an even fainter road goes left. That one, very faint in places, leads to the south end of Summit Lake. On the way up, at the top of a rise about 0.1 mile from the start, a cairn on the right indicates a trail that goes along the ridge on the east side of Summit Lake. It connects with the old road coming up from the Bailey farm.

In the early morning on Friday, October 23, 1942, Lester Bailey, 72 years old, the son of Samuel Bailey, left a note: "I have gone to the fields." Lester still farmed 60 acres of the family farm south of Upper Twin Lake, and tended the family cemetery. When he had not returned a day later, a search was organized. He was found, the following Sunday, November 1st, two miles from home. He had a 16-pound raccoon on his shoulder, a kerosene lantern and a shotgun (*N.Y. Times*, 11/2/42).

Only Lester's cousin Irving remained. He lived as a recluse in a stone veneer cottage near the road. Irving died on Christmas Day 1947 — the last of the Baileys (Commission Minutes, 1/13/48).

BEECHY BOTTOM EAST ROAD

Length: 3.95 miles

Miles

0.0	Seven Lakes Drive (0.3 mile west of overpass).
0.05	Anthony Wayne Trail joins briefly.
0.15	AW Trail rejoins, right, on original B.B. Road.
0.2	Original Beechy Bottom Road leaves, left.
0.45	Anthony Wayne Trail leaves, right.
0.5	Fawn Trail starts, left.
0.8	County line.
0.85	Gravel Park road crosses.
0.9	Mica Mine down, right.
1.6	Appalachian Trail crosses.
1.85	Ramapo-Dunderberg Trail crosses.
2.1	North "Ski Trail" (stone road), left.
2.25	Ski trail comes up, right.
2.45	Beechy Bottom West Road joined, right.
2.65	1779 Trail joins, right.
2.75	1779 Trail leaves, right.
2.85	Suffern-Bear Mountain Trail crosses.
3.0	North-South Connector, left.
3.5	Red Cross Trail crosses.
3.7	Bulsontown-Timp Trail, left.
3.9	1779 Trail joins, right.
3.95	Park boundary; Bulsontown.

When the park was created in 1910, and until 1952, there were two roads going south through Beechy Bottom Valley, on the hillsides above the brook — Beechy Bottom East Road and Beechy Bottom West Road. The easternmost of these roads started just east of Beechy Bottom Brook, 0.25 mile east of the junction of Seven Lakes Drive with Long Mountain Parkway. That road can still be found going south from the Drive. Another route of the eastern road, built in 1933, starts 0.1 mile to the east of the earlier route. We will describe the 1933 road.

The 1933 road starts above a bank on the Drive (now also the route of the Palisades Interstate Parkway). The first part of this road is largely overgrown with barberry and other vegetation. After about 200 feet, the Anthony Wayne Trail (AW) (white) comes in from the left and joins Beechy Bottom East Road. In another 200 feet, AW leaves to the right. The road ahead is now covered with dense barberry, but it is possible to follow a cleared path along the iron pipe. At 0.15 mile, the older route of Beechy Bottom East Road (now followed by AW) comes in from the right, and AW rejoins the newer road (which is now covered with grass and much easier to follow). Immediately afterwards, the road passes two concrete blockhouses. Just before the second blockhouse, the older road leaves the 1933 road and goes up to the left (it joins the Fawn Trail a bit farther south). At 0.45 mile, the Anthony Wayne Trail leaves sharply to the right and goes down to the parking area on a gravel Park service road. Beechy Bottom East Road continues straight ahead along the gravel road (now blazed with blue-on-white plastic markers as a bike trail), and soon afterwards the Fawn Trail (red F on pink) starts up to the left.

At 0.85 mile, a gravel Park road goes off to the left, up to a concrete reservoir (the large pipe along the road also goes to the reservoir). In another 100 feet, this road goes down to the right and leads to the south parking area of the Anthony Wayne Recreation Area. About 300 feet south of that road junction, the Mica Mine may be found, about 50 feet below the level of Beechy Bottom Road.

At 1.6 miles, the Appalachian Trail (AT) crosses. Then, at 1.85 miles, the Ramapo-Dunderberg Trail (R-D) crosses. One of the "stone roads," known as the North "Ski Trail," comes down on the left at 2.1 miles. This "stone road" is an old trail, once part of Horn's Route, which had been blazed with aluminum H's by Jim Horn, who was vice president of the Fresh Air Club in 1921. At 2.25 miles, the Anthony Wayne South Ski Trail comes up on the right, from the R-D and the AT near the brook.

At 2.45 miles, Beechy Bottom West Road once joined, and at 2.65 miles, as the trail rounds the southern end of West Mountain, our modern 1779 Trail comes in on the right (on a path that once was a branch of the Black Mountain Trail). In another 400 feet, the 1779 Trail departs again, to cross a little stone bridge.

Soon the Suffern-Bear Mountain Trail crosses, with Horn Hill to the north. Then, 0.15 mile further, the North-South Connector goes left. Here, the bike trail, with the blue-and-white markers, departs to the left, following the route of the North-South Connector. (100 feet down this trail, the South "Ski Trail" goes right and leads 1.0 mile — on a rather rough route — down to the Red Cross Trail.) At 3.5 miles, the Red Cross Trail crosses. Now we are getting pretty far down the hill, and the road becomes rockier and more difficult to follow. At 3.7 miles, sharp eyes will see the old

Bulsontown-Timp Trail depart on the left. That trail, now marked A-B (Addisone-Boyce), goes past the Girl Scout camp and up to The Timp (following the route of the Red Timp Trail).

The 1779 Trail (the old Dean Trail) comes in on the right at 3.9 miles, and the Beechy Bottom Road ends at the Park boundary at 3.95 miles. Cedar Flats Road is another 0.1 mile ahead.

BEECHY BOTTOM WEST ROAD (TO 1950)

Length: 2.1 miles

Miles

0.0	Junction Seven Lakes Drive and Long Mountain Parkway.
1.0	Parkway cut (0.25 mile north of visitor center).
1.2	County road marker.
1.4	County road marker.
1.55	Site of CCC Camp.
1.6	County road marker.
1.65	AT/R-D crosses.
1.95	Go down, left (trail ahead to Owl Lake).
2.0	Cross Beechy Bottom Brook (and Palisades Interstate Parkway).
2.1	Join Beechy Bottom East Road.

Our Beechy Bottom West Road, known since Revolutionary days as the Queensboro Road, was shown on General Robert Erskine's 1778 map, drawn for General George Washington.

When the Park was created in 1910, this was the most-used road in the Beechy Bottom valley. The several farms along it had been bought out by 1917. The West Road started from Long Mountain Parkway, 0.1 mile southeast of the cemetery, and ran along the hillside. The first mile of the old road was wiped out in 1950 by construction of the Palisades Interstate Parkway. The part which remains begins, on the hillside above the Parkway cut, about 0.25 mile north of the

Park visitor center (former gas station). In the next 0.6 mile, three county road markers can be seen. They were placed there by the WPA in 1934.

At about 1.55 miles (from the original beginning of the road), a Civilian Conservation Corps camp was set up in 1933. The AT/R-D Trail crosses at 1.65 miles. For a short distance south of the AT/R-D, the old road is indistinct, lost in barberry bushes. But then it can be seen again, and at 1.95 miles it turns down left to the Parkway (the newer Owl Lake Road goes straight ahead). Near here, traces of walls are visible in the bushes; this is where George Bulson lived until 1917. A story has it that he moved his house down the road to Bulsontown, but the Bulson families living down there now have not heard that story.

This is where Beechy Bottom West crossed the brook and was joined by Beechy Bottom East.

Beechy Bottom valley is full of history. At the north end, where our two roads start, there was the hamlet of Queensboro — a road center. From here, roads led to the Forest of Dean Mine to the north, and to Kings Ferry (Stony Point) to the south. In 1774, a farm there was owned by Moses Clement. In later years, the Weyant and Brooks families lived there. A cemetery 250 feet north of the road junction (now *on the side of* the Long Mountain Circle) contains the graves of those families. The earliest stone is dated 1868, but many graves are unmarked.

The valley for half a mile south, and the hills to the west, belonged to the Weyant family. Their home was on Beechy Bottom East Road, about 0.3 mile south of Long Mountain Parkway. The home of John Wesley Van Wart, who owned most of the valley south to the junction of the East and West Roads, was a half mile further south.

In 1859, there was a little schoolhouse at the start of the West Road. (The schoolhouse was demolished in 1927.) The next building to the south belonged to T.H. Ferris, and the home of Abraham J. Rose was at 1.55 miles (just north of the AT and just east of the Parkway). His cellar hole and well are still there. Still further south, at 1.85 miles, was the home of William Rose. George Bulson lived at 1.95 miles, and his neighbor George Nickerson was just beyond.

Except for George Bulson's 42 acres, the land in the valley from Nickerson's place north to the Weyant farm (0.1 mile above the county line) was acquired by John Wesley Van Wart between 1869 and 1882. Van Wart died in 1892, and his heirs sold the 680-acre estate (1.1 square miles) to the Park in 1916. It seems possible that the Van Warts were related to Isaac Van Wart who, together with John Paulding and David Williams, had captured the British spy Major André at Tarrytown on September 23, 1780.

The 260 acres of the Nickerson and Rose places were shown as the "Brush Place" on General Robert Erskine's military map of 1778. The 1790 census of Orange County lists the three families of John, Peter and Caleb Brush as living in Haverstraw Town. The 1880 census lists William Brush as a boarder on the Van Wart farm.

There were two farms on the Beechy Bottom East Road — those of Weyant and Van Wart. From the Van Wart home at the county line, a footpath went south along the hillside to join Beechy Bottom West Road (then a county road known as the Queensboro Road). Also, from the Van Wart home a farm road went down across the farm (which is now the south parking area of the Anthony Wayne Recreation Area) and angled uphill to join the West Road about where the

AT/R-D crosses now. Two more Van Wart homes were on that farm road, which can still be followed from the southwest side of the south parking area. After passing two cellar holes, the faint old road vanishes beneath the Parkway, about 0.1 mile south of the visitor center.

In 1933, the first CCC camp was set up on the Van Wart farm (near the location of the present-day south parking area). Their task was to build a road into Curtis Hollow, and to build a reservoir (Turkey Hill Lake) there. A second camp was set up on the West Road just north of the AT/R-D crossing. Their task was to build a road to Owl Swamp, and to construct a lake there. A third camp was set up on the east side of Beechy Bottom Brook where the West Road joined the East Road (this location has been obliterated by the Parkway). Their task was to build fire roads in the region to the south (we call them "stone roads").

One project of the CCC camps was to extend the old Beechy Bottom Roads and transform them into northbound and southbound motor roads which would connect Tiorati Brook Road in the south with Seven Lakes Drive and Long Mountain Parkway at Queensboro. The East Road was to be for northbound traffic, and the West Road for southbound traffic.

The CCC boys widened Beechy Bottom East Road, levelled it, and extended it south of the Van Wart house. The plan was for it to cross the valley and continue to the east side of Owl Lake. From there it was to follow the north side of Stillwater Brook and join the West Road in the notch between the Pingyp and Flaggy Meadow Mountain. The route of this road was cut in 1953 by the construction of the Parkway, but west of the Parkway, evidence of road construction — rock piles gathered for the roadbed, and an "avenue" where trees were cut down — is still visible. Parts of the proposed route along Stillwater Brook were also cleared and can still be followed.

In 1933, the CCC started to improve the old Beechy Bottom Road West. Some of their work near the north end can be seen where the Anthony Wayne Trail crosses it, on the way uphill, west of the Palisades Interstate Parkway overpass. Further south, their new road, as well as the older road, has been destroyed by the Parkway. About a mile south of Route 6, on the hillside west of the Parkway, the CCC road can be seen again, only to be lost in the barberry bushes just south of the AT/R-D crossing. In this region, two roads are visible: the newer, more level road is higher up, while the older Queensboro Road is below it.

At 1.95 miles, where the old road turned southeast (to be cut in 1953 by the Parkway), the new CCC road (now known as the Owl Lake Road) went straight ahead to the west end of the Owl Lake Dam. It was to go down beyond the dam and cross to the south side of Stillwater Brook. There it was to take over the route of the old Burnt House Trail (now known as the Stillwater Trail) and continue east and then south, around the end of Flaggy Meadow Mountain, down to Tiorati Brook Road. Although this section, too, was cut by the Parkway in 1953, its continuation further south, along the side of Flaggy Meadow Mountain, can still be followed.

Neither of the Beechy Bottom Roads was ever opened to general traffic after 1934. Parts of the better-graded East Road are still used by Park vehicles, though.

Bockberg Trail

Length: 2.65 miles

Miles

0.0   End of Pleasant Valley Road.

0.05   Timp Pass Road leaves, right.

0.3   Keep left at fork.

0.7   R-D Trail joins briefly; fireplace to right.

0.8   Go right; R-D continues straight ahead.

1.1   Go right at fork.

1.5   Hairpin turn; R-D is straight ahead.

1.95   R-D; Spiral Railway.

Two Routes from Here:
Left Route:

1.95   Turn down left.

2.0   Keep to left of brook/swamp.

2.35   Trail is in deep gulch.

2.65   Route 9W.

Right Route:

1.95   Follow railway to left.

2.15   At break in rock wall, go left.

2.25   Old workmen's road.

2.65   Route 9W.

Bockberg (Bald Mountain) is the Dutch name for Goat Mountain. The Bockberg Trail starts in Doodletown valley, goes over Dunderberg Mountain and continues down to Route 9W.

The trail starts at the south end of Pleasant Valley Road, where a wooden bridge goes across a brook. Just north of the brook are the remains of a summer camp that once was run by the Riverside Church of New York City. The jeep road which continues south from the bridge and goes uphill is the Bockberg Trail. (It is also marked here as the 1777 Trail.) About 250 feet beyond the bridge, the faint Timp Pass Road begins to the right. The 1777 Trail departs to the right at 0.3 mile, while the Bockberg Trail continues up, parallel to a brook.

At 0.7 mile, just before the Bockberg Trail crosses a brook, the Ramapo-Dunderberg Trail (R-D) joins. The trails run jointly for only a short distance, and the R-D leaves to the left at a fireplace. Soon the trails again join briefly. A bit further up the hill, the Bockberg Trail turns sharp right, while R-D continues straight ahead. At 1.05 miles, a broad path goes up to the left. That is *not* our trail, but a side trail that goes nearly to the R-D on Bald Mountain. The Bockberg Trail turns down to the right, around a swampy area. At 1.6 miles, it makes a hairpin turn (here, the R-D Trail is only 75 feet ahead) and goes steeply down. It then levels off, and meets the R-D once again at 1.95 miles. Just beyond this point, the trail crosses a level of the Dunderberg Spiral Railway. To the right, 0.2 mile down the railway bed, is the Jones Trail.

The Bockberg Trail now divides, as it heads down a gorge between two summits of Dunderberg. One route starts to the left, down from the R-D junction. It is not very distinct, but stays to the left of a little brook and a swamp lower down. It then goes steeply down a gorge, reaching Route 9W at 2.65 miles. Here the hiker may choose to cross the highway and bushwhack down to the older road, 100 feet lower. The older road (which is now part of the Hudson River Trail and is much more pleasant to walk along) can be followed to the left for 0.4 mile until it joins the modern highway.

The other branch of Bockberg Trail goes left along the railway for 0.2 mile, then turns left, through a gap in the stone wall. A faint path leads down with switchbacks toward the brook and swamp mentioned above. Keep to the right this time, and soon a distinct woods road will be seen. That goes down the gorge, fairly high above the brook, and reaches Route 9W at 2.65 miles. This point is 0.25 mile up the road from the first trailhead. Again, it is best to bushwhack down to the lower old road, taking care to avoid a gravel pit there.

The Bockberg Trail is passable for most of its length by Park trucks or jeeps. From 1985 to 1991, it was used to maintain the stations that were erected in several places on Dunderberg Mountain to monitor the air quality around the power plant at Tomkins Cove.

The left-hand trail down the gorge was once the route of an iron pipe that carried water from the spring at the head of the brook down to the old road near the river level. This route was described by William T. Howell, in his diary for May 17, 1908 (*The Hudson Highlands*, vol. II, page 77). The pipe had been laid by John Stalter, a woodcutter who lived in Doodletown, to supply water to the men who were building the new state road there in the summer of 1907. The Stalter Spring, usually leaf-covered, can still be found on the mountain, a short distance below the junction of the Bockberg Trail and the R-D.

BOCKEY SWAMP TRAIL

Length: 3.3 miles

Miles

0.0	Begin at Silvermine ski area.
0.45	Old road comes out of lake.
0.65	Reach end of lake.
0.95	Cross woods road; Menomine Trail leaves, left.
1.0	Pass swamp to left.
1.3	Begin to climb.
1.4	Flat-sided rock to right.
1.55	Cross brook.
1.7	AT/R-D crosses at bridge.
1.8	Turn right near top of rise.
1.95	Blueberry Trail, right.
2.1	Summit of Letterrock Mountain to left.
2.45	Start down.
2.95	Cross Red Cross Trail.
3.25	Cross Tiorati Brook.
3.3	End at Tiorati Brook Road.

The Bockey Swamp Trail starts from the Silvermine Ski Area. Until Silvermine Lake was built in 1934, the big swamp there was called the Bockey Swamp. The name "bockey" refers to the baskets that were woven by the mountain people for carrying charcoal to the local furnaces. For the first 0.95 mile, the Bockey Swamp Trail follows the route of the yellow-blazed Menomine Trail. At 0.45 mile, after rounding a slope, the trail joins an old wagon road coming up out of the lake.

After reaching the end of the lake at 0.65 mile, the

old road follows the foot of the hill, then climbs briefly and comes to a woods road at 0.95 mile. That road starts at Seven Lakes Drive (with the AT) and goes up to the shelter on Letterrock Mountain. Here, the yellow blazes of the Menomine Trail follow the woods road to the left. Our Bockey Swamp Trail crosses the road, and heads south along the foot of a hill. The trail in this section is very faint, but is occasionally marked with white blazes. It passes a small swamp on the left and continues along Bockey Swamp Brook. At about 1.3 miles, it begins to climb and passes through an area with many blowdowns. The Bockey Swamp Trail goes by a very interesting large rock, to the right of the trail, with a smooth, flat side. It then bears left, crosses the brook (which runs under rocks at this point), and soon turns right onto another old road.

At 1.7 miles, the trail approaches the east end of a footbridge that carries the Appalachian Trail and the Ramapo-Dunderberg Trail. The Bockey Swamp Trail continues straight ahead. A little further along, near the top of a rise, our trail turns right (a well-worn path which leads to the Dean Trail continues straight ahead). The Bockey Swamp Trail, now marked by faint yellow and white blazes, goes through a grassy region. Another trail, nearly invisible in the grass, soon joins from the hillside on the right. A bushwhack over that way will lead one to a clearer trail — the Blueberry Trail.

Our trail now climbs up Letterrock Mountain. The summit, which is to the left of the trail, affords limited views through the trees. It then descends, sometimes steeply, and, at 2.95 miles, comes down to the Red Cross

Trail. Here, the Beech Trail is 0.1 mile to the left. The Bockey Swamp Trail continues across the Red Cross Trail and, in another 0.3 mile, crosses Tiorati Brook. There used to be a wooden bridge here, but it was removed in the spring of 1990. The trail ends at Tiorati Brook Road, 3.3 miles from the start. The parking area on the Beech Trail is 0.35 mile to the left, while Tiorati Dam is 0.9 mile to the right.

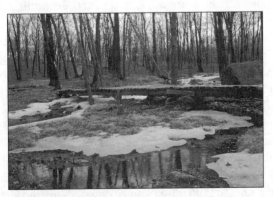

Footbridge over Bockey Swamp Brook

Buck Trail

Length: 1.6 miles

Present-day hikers meet the Buck Trail when they have climbed Conklin Mountain on the Seven Hills Trail from the Sebago parking area. Near the top of the rise there is a cairn. Here the Buck Trail starts to the left. It is a fairly level woods road, marked with some old blazes and maintained (occasionally) as a fire road. At 1.15 miles, the road forks. The lesser used path, which goes off to the left, leads to Pine Meadow Road at 1.6 miles; the right fork goes to the junction of Pine Meadow Road East with Pine Meadow Road West at 1.6 miles.

The approach to the Buck Trail (the Seven Hills Trail) uses an old woods road which was once known as the Monitor Trail. In those days (until 1977) the Buck Trail continued down to the south, to end where Woodtown Road crosses Diamond Creek. This route is now part of the Seven Hills Trail.

Going north along the Buck Trail, a cairn will be seen on the west side of the trail at 1.0 mile. More cairns lead to an old woods road that goes down the mountain to the ski trail below — the Little Doe Trail.

The Buck Trail appears on the 1920 Park trail map. It was then known as the Breakneck Pond Trail. The names Buck and Little Doe were first used in 1943 on Bill Hoeferlin's Map No. 5.

In 1921, the Boy Scouts' White Bar Trail came up Diamond Creek and followed the

Buck Trail over Conklin Mountain. At the north end of the mountain, the scouts followed a woods road (now Pine Meadow Road) down to the Cranberry Mountain Trail, and continued up to Big Hill on the Old Turnpike.

Just northeast of the cairn that marks the junction of the Buck Trail with the Seven Hills Trail, a four-acre parcel was owned from 1885 to 1910 by Enoch Conklin and his sons Roger and Elias. There is no evidence that they ever lived there.

North of the fork in the trail at 1.15 miles, many stone walls and the cellar hole of an old farmhouse are still visible. This 17-acre parcel was given in 1850 by Jonas Wood to Andrews Hill, who had married Susan Wood in 1833. That couple may have built the house beside the road. In 1855, they bought a larger farm on the ridge west of Stony Brook, and in 1862 they sold the 17 acres to Joseph W. Conklin. Joseph sold it three years later to James R. Johnson of Johnsontown.

Conklin Mountain was probably named after Timothy Conklin. His 412 acres, from Stony Brook up to the ridgetop, were bought at auction on December 17, 1850 by Matthew Waldron (1824–1903).

From the mountain ridge down to Seven Lakes Drive, the land through which the Little Doe Trail goes was the property of the Asylum of the Sisters of Saint Dominic (Blauvelt, N.Y.). They had received it as a gift in 1914. To the northeast of this property, the land on both sides of Pine Meadow Road, from the lake edge to the mountain ridge, was home to the Waldron family until 1916.

CROOKED ROAD

Length: 3.3 miles

Miles

0.0	Begin at Arden Valley Road.
0.35	AT joins, right.
0.4	AT leaves, left.
0.55	A-SB joins, left.
0.7	Cross brook draining Dismal Swamp.
0.75	A-SB leaves, right.
0.85	White Bar Trail joins.
1.45	Dunning Trail joins; White Bar Trail leaves.
1.8	R-D Trail crosses.
2.25	Bowling Rocks.
2.4	Abandoned Dunning Trail route goes off, left.
2.8	Turn right, leaving Dunning Trail.
3.3	End at Route 106.

Hikers in 1920 were familiar with the "Crooked Road." On the first Park trail map, it was shown as starting from the Arden Valley Road on the Harriman estate. It skirted Echo Lake and then went southwest to the south side of Island Pond.

The road today starts from the south side of Arden Valley Road, 0.2 mile east of the gravel road leading to Island Pond. At 0.35 mile, near the edge of Island Pond, the Appalachian Trail (AT) joins briefly, on its way down from the Lemon Squeezer.

The old road continues south, high above the pond. The Arden-Surebridge Trail (A-SB) joins from the left at 0.55 mile, and then, at 0.7 mile, the Crooked Road crosses a brook which drains the Dismal Swamp. Soon afterwards, the A-SB departs to the right. At 0.85 mile, the White Bar Trail joins from the left. The clear, wide trail continues south.

At 1.45 miles, the Dunning Trail (yellow) joins, and the White Bar Trail leaves. Here the Crooked Road, now following the route of the Dunning Trail, turns left and soon goes steeply up the slope of Black Rock Mountain. On the way up, it crosses a fairly level region, and then another short, steep climb through laurels brings it to the Ramapo-Dunderberg Trail at 1.8 miles. Now heading gradually down, the road crosses a stream and then goes over a level area of bare rock dotted by boulders (named "Bowling Rocks") at 2.25 miles. The abandoned Dunning route goes off to the left at 2.4 miles, and a junction is reached at 2.8 miles. Straight ahead, the Dunning blazes continue to the Hogencamp Mine. But our Crooked Road turns right and goes south down to Little Long Pond. On the way, it passes through an abandoned Girl Scout camp and reaches Route 106 at 3.3 miles.

When the Park was formed in 1910, Island Pond remained in the Harriman estate. The park boundary followed the Crooked Road from Echo Lake to the point where the Dunning Trail joins it now, at the foot of Black Rock Mountain. In 1921-22, the Boy Scouts marked their White Bar Trail along this road. Their trail came down from the Lemon Squeezer on the route later adopted by the AT trail blazers in 1922. While one leg of the White Bar Trail continued south to the highway, as it does today, another leg followed the Crooked Road to Little Long Pond.

On the hillside above Little Long Pond, the Park, in 1919, built Camp Matinecock for the Boy Scouts. In the winter of 1920-21, when the new Trail Conference was building the R-D Trail, the volunteers were accommodated with bed and board at Camp Matinecock. In 1930, the Queens Council Girl Scouts took over the camp, calling it Camp Quid Nunc (Latin = What Now?). In order to enable the girls safely to cross the road to the lake, a rustic footbridge was built over the road.

The Girl Scouts vacated the camp in 1969, and the camp was demolished in 1976. Its dining hall was moved to "Merritt Bank" (a Park storage area for scrap materials), off Seven Lakes Drive between Silvermine and Tiorati Lakes. The footbridge over the road was demolished in June 1987.

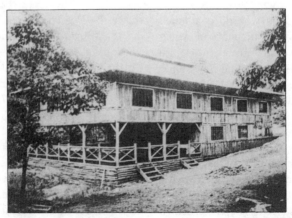

Camp Matinecock – 1920

DEAN TRAIL

Length: 0.85 mile

This is a short trail with a long story. It connects the joint Ramapo-Dunderberg/Appalachian Trail at the William Brien Memorial Shelter with the Red Cross Trail. As it starts down from the shelter, there is a short blue side trail to a spring, which sometimes has water. The Dean Trail bears to the left and follows an old woods road downhill. At first, the route may be a little obscure, but it soon becomes more obvious. At 0.5 mile, another trail, blazed white, joins from the right. (That trail leads to the Bockey Swamp Trail, just south of the junction of the R-D and the AT at the foot of Goshen Mountain.) The Dean Trail, now blazed white, parallels a brook and at 0.85 mile ends at the Red Cross Trail.

This was once a much longer trail, most of which has been incorporated into other trails. The Boy Scouts discovered it in 1922 and included it in their White Bar System, from the Bockey Swamp Trail to Stillwater Brook (*N.Y. Post*, 6/23/33). During the 1930s, George Goldthwaite of the Fresh Air Club researched the trails in this area. His hand-drawn map dated February 22, 1940 shows the Dean Trail passing the "Burnt House" and continuing east to end at Bulsontown (Cedar Flats Road). This is the present route of the Red Cross/1779 Trail.

In 1944, the newly marked Red Cross Trail incorporated the Burnt House Trail from Tiorati Brook Road and then followed the Dean Trail, until it turned off that trail just beyond the S-BM crossing. Then, in 1974, the 1779 Trail was routed down the old Dean Trail all the way to Bulsontown.

There was a local story told by Harvey Bulson, a blacksmith, that a woodcutter named Jonas Lewis lived in the Burnt House beside the trail. One day in 1910, Bulson stopped to visit Jonas.

Opening the door, he found Jonas and his four sons sitting on one side of the room. A spittoon was on the other side. The five tobacco chewers were competing to see who could hit the mark, and a line of tobacco juice crossed the floor from each of them. (Isn't it odd what things go down in history?)

HASENCLEVER ROAD

The Way It Is Now (South of Tiorati Brook Road)

Miles
0.0	Tiorati Brook Road, 0.25 mile below dam.
0.05	Trail, right.
0.45	County line.
0.55	Mine, left; Red Cross Trail departs ahead.
0.6	Vague trail, left, goes to Beech Trail.
0.7	Trail, right, to Red Cross Trail.
1.2	Beech Trail crosses.
1.55	Grape Swamp Mountain Trail, left.
1.6	Trail, right, to Charleston farm.
1.8	End at Lake Welch Drive.

Before 1941
1.95	House, left.
2.0	Road, right.
2.65	Beaver Pond Road (Route 106).

Hasenclever Road begins at Tiorati Brook Road, about 0.25 mile east of the dam at the southeast corner of Lake Tiorati. It proceeds south along the route of the Red Cross Trail. After 275 feet, a trail goes up to the right. This trail (which probably was the route of Hasenclever Road before Tiorati Brook Road was built) goes around the end of the mountain, above and parallel to Tiorati Brook Road, and ends near the camp road just south of the dam. Another trail branches west from this trail and goes up along the ridge of Hasenclever Mountain.

At 0.55 mile, the Hasenclever Mine is seen on the left. It is 100 feet deep, filled with water and mud. Here the Red Cross Trail bears right, while our road goes left around a low knob. On the far side of the knob, a vague trail goes left. If one can follow it, it leads 0.8 mile to the Beech Trail. At 0.7 mile, a clear trail on the right goes 0.2 mile to the Red Cross Trail (for 10 years, 1948-58, that was the route of the Red Cross Trail).

The Beech Trail crosses at 1.2 miles and, just beyond, the road crosses a little concrete bridge — a reminder that until 1910 this was a county road. At 1.6 miles, a fairly clear trail goes down to the right (it leads 0.25 mile to the old Charleston farm on the Beech Trail). Then, at 1.8 miles, the Hasenclever Road ends at a cut, above Lake Welch Drive.

The Hasenclever Road, built in 1760 from Stony Point to Central Valley, is one of the oldest roads in the Park. It was mapped by General Robert Erskine in 1778 for General Washington. It was also described in a press release by Major Welch (Press Release #205, 1/9/30). From Cedar Pond (now Lake Tiorati), it went past Hasenclever Mine to Beaver Pond (now Lake Welch). It followed the brook down *old* Gate Hill Road to Calls Hollow Road, and then continued out to Stony Point.

Going north from Cedar Pond dam (Hasenclever had built the dam about 1765), the road coincided with our Tiorati Brook Road for 0.5 mile, and then went right, away from the lake, around a knob to the north of the lake. It continued to the northwest down a hill, and crossed the Seven Lakes Drive 0.5 mile north of Tiorati Circle. It followed what is now a Park road up past an abandoned girls' camp, and then curved to the south. Just about where it reaches our present Arden Valley Road, the old road turned up sharp right, passing between two peaks of Bradley Mountain. It went gently down past Slaughters Pond (Forest Lake) and north to June's Tavern (Central Valley). The road from Bradley Mountain past Forest Lake is on Harriman land, which is not open to the public. This part of the road is not shown on an 1859 map of Orange County, and probably was abandoned about 1838, when a new road was built to the Greenwood and Bradley Mines.

The Way It Was (North of Tiorati Brook Road)

Miles

0.0	Tiorati Brook Road; go north.
0.3	Trail left to Hasenclever Mountain.
0.35	Tiorati Dam.
0.85	Turn up, right (0.65 mile to Circle).
1.2	Cross R-D Trail.
1.3	Cross original AT route.
1.95	Cross Seven Lakes Drive.
2.35	AT crosses.
2.7	Long Path joins.
2.95	Arden Valley Road; turn right.
3.2	Saddle between Bradley peaks.
3.35	Bending down, right.
3.95	Join Forest Lake Trail.
4.2	Cross Twin Lakes Road.
4.55	Bridge; Forest Lake.
6.45	Route 6.

IRON MOUNTAIN TRAIL

Length: 1.4 miles

Iron Mountain is the southwest end of a ridge labeled Horse Chock Mountain on Conference Map #3. Bill Hoeferlin first called it Iron Mountain on his May 1945 map. On O'Connor's 1845 map, it is called Hasha Hill. It is shown as the property of the Christie Mining Company on an 1876 map. A deep ravine divides the ridge, the portion to the north (to the east of the First Reservoir) being Horse Chock Mountain.

Several trails start up the hill from Woodtown Road. The best of them was described by Bob Marshall in the *Trail Walker* of June/July 1987. It starts from Woodtown Road 500 feet northeast of the point where that road crosses Horse Chock Brook, or 0.85 mile southwest of the dam at the First Reservoir (0.15 mile northeast of the dam at the Second Reservoir). The trail is often used by horse riders, and the hoof marks are the only trail markings.

The trail goes up at a moderate pitch. At 0.5 mile, another horse trail goes right to File Factory Hollow. The trail heads toward the north at 0.6 mile, passing a good viewpoint at 0.8 mile and an equally good one at 0.9 mile. The Hudson River and High Tor above Haverstraw are clearly visible, with the towers of Manhattan in the far distance. The huge white building on the hilltop to the east is the private Shapiro residence. The trail then starts down, still going northeast. At about 1.1 miles, it begins to turn southeast in several switchbacks (a faint road departs to the left here). Then, at 1.4 miles, the trail ends at the Orange and Rockland Utilities power line. The service road, or the wide gas line below, are walkable. File Factory Brook is reached in another 0.45 mile, the Tuxedo-Mt. Ivy Trail joins 0.75 mile beyond the brook, and the parking lot is 0.35 mile further.

ISLAND POND ROAD

Length: 2.35 miles

Miles
0.0   Arden Valley Road.
0.05 Take right branch.
0.25 AT joins, left.
0.35 AT leaves, right.
0.95 A-SB joins, right.
1.15 Road, left, to old cabin.
1.2   A-SB leaves, left.
1.5   Boston Mine, left; Dunning Trail joins.
1.55 Dunning Trail leaves, right.
1.6   Nurian Trail crosses.
1.8   Trail, right, to Stahahe Peak.
2.3   White Bar Trail joins, left.
2.35 Route 106.

The Island Pond Road starts at a gate on Arden Valley Road, 1.1 miles east of the Elk Pen parking area. The wide, graveled road straight ahead is *not* Island Pond Road (it was built in 1963). The older Island Pond Road starts to the right, a short way beyond the gate. It was built in 1934 by the Civilian Conservation Corps as a new approach to the lake. The *original* Island Pond Road comes up from the right 0.25 mile beyond Arden Valley Road.

At 0.25 mile, near the northern end of Island Pond, the Appalachian Trail (AT) joins from the left. The AT leaves to the right at 0.35 mile. Island Pond Road then parallels the lake edge. At 0.95 mile, the Arden-

Surebridge Trail (A-SB) joins from the right. Island Pond Road soon crosses the southern outlet of the pond, and at 1.15 miles a road goes left to a point on the south end of the lake. The stone ruins there are all that remain of a cabin built by the Park for the use of Park rangers.

The road now heads south, and begins to climb. The A-SB soon leaves to the left and, at 1.5 miles, the Dunning Trail joins from the left. The Boston Mine is 200 feet to the left along this trail. The Dunning Trail soon goes off to the right, and shortly afterward the Nurian Trail joins briefly and then leaves to the left. At 1.8 miles an orange-blazed trail leads right to Stahahe High Peak. Going gently down now, the White Bar Trail joins from the left at 2.3 miles, and at 2.35 miles, Island Pond Road ends where it meets Route 106 at a gate.

Island Pond was acquired by Edward Harriman in 1885. It seems likely that he built the original road to Island Pond about 1905. The *Rockland County Times* for February 13, 1908 mentions the road around Island Pond "which Mr. Harriman built two or three years ago." The road came up by switchbacks from the meadows on Harriman's farm. The old road then turned south toward the lake.

After the Park acquired Island Pond in 1927, they widened the road to 20 feet. Then, in 1934, the CCC built a level approach from the new (1930) Arden Valley Road. They widened the road by cutting out the laurels in preparation for enlarging Island Pond. That plan, fortunately, was abandoned. In 1966, the road from Island Pond to Route 210 (now Route 106) was covered with gravel.

JONES TRAIL

Length: 1.55 miles

Miles

0.0	Begin at Route 9W.
0.05	Cross grade of spiral railway.
0.4	Cross wooden bridge.
0.65	1777 Trail departs, left.
1.2	Timp-Torne Trail crosses.
1.55	End at railway bed.

The Jones Trail, which is a woods road, starts at Route 9W, 0.5 mile south of the Anchor Monument. There is a parking area about 200 feet south of the trailhead. At first, the trail is marked with the blazes of the 1777 Trail. About 300 feet from the start, it crosses the lowest grade of the old Dunderberg Spiral Railway. After 0.4 mile, it goes over a wooden bridge. Then, at 0.65 mile, after a brief detour to the left to avoid an eroded section of the old road, the 1777 Trail departs to the left, while the Jones Trail continues straight ahead.

The Jones Trail goes north, up along the face of the eastern Dunderberg cliffs, and soon begins to parallel a little brook. At 1.2 miles from Route 9W (0.55 mile from the 1777 Trail junction), the Timp-Torne Trail (blue) crosses the brook and the Jones Trail. Across the brook, the Timp-Torne Trail leads to the unfinished tunnel of the Spiral Railway.

Uphill beyond the tunnel, the Jones Trail is much eroded. It crosses the brook and ascends through laurels (here the trail is much narrower). At the top of the ascent, it widens again. The Jones Trail ends at 1.55 miles, where it reaches the next-higher level of the railway. It is possible to follow the railbed to the left for 0.2 mile to a junction with the Ramapo-Dunderberg Trail.

The Jones Trail was built about 1890 as a work road to get workmen with their tools and animals up to the several levels of the Spiral Railway. It was named for the family that owned most of the mountain. In 1836, Joshua T. Jones of Westchester County bought 100 acres of the Bradley/Jameson Patent at Caldwell's Landing (later re- named Jones Point). Through the years, the family bought more of the mountain. Then in 1951, with a gift of $25,000 from Laurance S. Rocke- feller, the Park purchased all 640 acres of the Charles H. Jones estate. That tract in- cluded all of the Jones Trail, as well as most of the Spiral Railway.

If one continues on the 1777 Trail for about 200 feet beyond the Jones Trail turn-off, one will notice a woods road (with some old orange blazes) that departs to the right. This road soon rejoins the Jones Trail, but about one minute up this road another faint woods road goes up to the left. This road winds around to the right of a knob, and then becomes an obscure path that continues up toward the cliff. At the cliff face, the path leads to the Escalator, a slanting crack in the cliff. One can climb this steep crack, arriving at a ledge where there is a beautiful view to the east and south. From the Escala- tor, a route has been marked with cairns to the new Timp-Torne Trail.

MANY SWAMP TRAIL

Length: 2.1 miles

Miles

0.0	Ladentown hikers' parking.
0.15	Clearing on power line road; cairn.
0.3	Cross Squirrel Brook.
0.55	Swamp on right; trail bends left.
0.75	S-BM Trail (yellow) crosses; cairns.
0.85	Trail is near swamp edge.
1.05	Trail goes uphill; swamp recedes, left.
1.2	Pass through stone wall.
1.35	Turn left onto well-used trail.
1.8	Cross Many Swamp Brook.
2.1	End at Pine Meadow Road East.

This old trail starts from the hikers' parking area at Ladentown. Follow the Tuxedo-Mt. Ivy Trail blazes up to the buried gas line. Continue straight up, past the power line tower, to the power line service road. Turn right on the road; a small clearing will be seen on the left. At the right end of the clearing there are the remains of an old shack, and much debris.

At the left end of the clearing, look for a cairn in the grass. Go in through the bushes there, and you will see a stone-lined road going uphill. That is the Many Swamp Trail. Ten minutes up the hill, the road crosses Squirrel Brook. It continues uphill, with the brook on the right, until the land begins to level off. The trail then bends left (southwest), with a swamp on the right.

At 0.75 mile, the Suffern-Bear Mountain Trail (S-BM) (yellow) crosses. To the left, it has come down from Panther Mountain; to the right, in 0.35 mile, it will cross Squirrel Swamp Brook and meet the Tuxedo-Mt. Ivy Trail. Watch for cairns at the S-BM crossing, since the Many Swamp Trail here is invisible in the low shrubbery. The trail goes straight ahead towards a low hill, and then bends to the left (southwest).

At 0.85 mile, the trail approaches the laurel-covered edge of a swamp. Here the trail becomes invisible, so it is necessary to watch carefully for cairns. The cairns run fairly near the swamp edge until, at 1.05 miles, they lead uphill, with the swamp receding to the left. Here there is a cairn on the top of a great boulder (left there by Franz Alt), but the main cairn line is to the right of that boulder.

At 1.2 miles, the trail passes through an opening in a stone wall, and then goes straight ahead, with the wall on the left. The area to the right is known as the Starr Clearing. At 1.35 miles, at a cairn, the trail turns left onto a trail frequented by horses. (To the right, this horse trail leads for 0.5 mile to Woodtown Road.) The Pittsboro Trail soon crosses (it can no longer be detected), and Many Swamp Trail continues southwest. At 1.8 miles, the trail crosses Many Swamp Brook. This is the brook that tumbles down the gorge below the Stone Memorial Shelter on the S-BM Trail. At 2.1 miles, our trail arrives at Pine Meadow Road East. The junction is marked with a cairn. The Pine Meadow Trail (red diamond on white) is 0.2 mile to the left.

The ruin of an old shack can be seen where the trail starts, on the power line service road. It was built there about 1936 by Ramsey Conklin and his sons. After they left their cabin at Pine Meadow in 1934, they moved into an abandoned schoolhouse at the corner of Camp Hill and Quaker Roads in Ladentown. Ramsey did not like that new set-up. He complained that seven or eight cars passed his place each day. "Not good for the livestock," he said. So he built two shacks at the foot of Limekiln Mountain, on land that belonged to Ira Hedges of Ladentown. Ramsey paid $1 per month rent. He lived there until 1952, when his body was found near the Second Reservoir. Son Theodore (Dory), who was on the Park payroll, continued to live in the shacks until he was evicted in 1963.

Along the trail, up in the hills at the foot of Squirrel Swamp Mountain, is the Starr Clearing. This was one of many Starr family farms —

another was near the Torne Valley Trail, below the Russian Bear. A third was said to be the site named "Sky Sail Farm" by the men who blazed the S-BM Trail.

Aaron Starr (1862-1956) owned the farm at the junction of the Pittsboro and Many Swamp Trails. He was also a partner in the sawmill that had been built by the grandfather of Joseph E. Christie (of Thiells) at the junction of Woodtown and Pine Meadow Roads.

Aaron also owned the Big Green Swamp where blueberries and cranberries grew in profusion. Each year, mountain folk came from afar to pick the berries there. Then Aaron got the idea to charge a fee to pick berries in his swamp. The neighbors resented this and made veiled threats. Finally, one summer, Aaron's house and barn were set afire. That was in 1919. Aaron's son Daniel sold their 39 acres to the Park, and the family moved to Orangeburg. When he died in 1956, old Aaron Starr was buried in the cemetery at Ladentown. His sister Eliza had married Nicholas Conklin. They are buried in St. John's Cemetery. Her grandson, Ben Jones of Lindbergh Road, Stony Point, a member of St. John's Church, died in 1989. Old Aaron's brother Charlie Starr was for a time the owner of Anderson's file factory at File Factory Hollow. Aaron's grandson James Aaron Starr, Jr. was born in 1916. At the time of this writing, he is in a prison for the criminally insane in Goshen. He remembers as a boy going back up to the Starr Place to pick ginseng.

In the *New York Evening Post* of November 9, 1923, Brooklyn Boy Scout leader Archibald T. Shorey described a hike to the clearing known as the Starr Place, at the foot of Squirrel Swamp Mountain. There was a fine spring and a campsite there. Shorey and his scouts built a cabin on the summit of Squirrel Swamp Mountain. A side trip up from the Starr Clearing will lead to that site. Far over on the north end of the mountain, against a great boulder, are the remains of Shorey's cabin.

The Many Swamp Trail now ends at Pine Meadow Road East. That road, built in 1934, actually followed two branches of the Many Swamp Trail — it followed the left branch of the trail to a junction with another trail that in 1934 was blazed as the Pine Meadow Trail; and it followed the right branch of the Many Swamp Trail to the site of Christie's sawmill, where Woodtown Road comes in.

NAWAHUNTA FIRE ROAD

Length: 1.7 miles

Miles

0.1	Cellar hole, left.
0.15	Menomine Trail leaves, left.
0.3	Dunn Mine, right.
0.5	Trail to Silvermine parking area leaves, right.
1.2	Long Path joins, left.
1.7	End at Route 6.

This wide road starts at a gate on the Seven Lakes Drive near Lake Nawahunta. It goes north 1.7 miles and ends at Route 6, near the Long Path crossing.

For the first 0.15 mile, the yellow-blazed Menomine Trail runs along the fire road. On the left side, 0.1 mile from the gate, is the cellar-hole of the Lewis family home. A minute farther along, the Menomine Trail goes down to the left. At 0.3 mile, the Dunn Mine is on the right, at the foot of the hill. A trail goes up to the right at 0.5 mile, over the ridge and down to the entrance of the Silvermine parking area.

After another 0.7 mile, on the way downhill, the Long Path (turquoise) joins from the left. The fire road ends at 1.7 miles, at the top of a cut on Route 6.

There is an older trail through this valley, parallel to the fire road. Follow the yellow blazes of the Menomine Trail across the brook at the north end of the lake, then look to the right for an old woods road that turns north. This is the Long Mountain Trail; it runs along the hillside above the swamp and the brook. At 0.8 mile, the Long Path comes down from the left, and the two trails go together along the swampy valley for 0.3 mile. They then join the fire road.

Before it was built in 1915, Lake Nawahunta had been the site of "Scobie" Jim Lewis' farm. The family graveyard is across Seven Lakes Drive from the entrance to the fire road. The Lewis family was related by marriage to the Bailey family on the west side of Stockbridge Mountain. That probably accounts for the old road (Nawahunta Trail) that goes between the two places.

Bill Hoeferlin's 1941 trail map shows a road going south 0.75 mile from Long Mountain Parkway (Route 6). The Fingerboard-Storm King Trail (later the Long Path) left that road after 0.5 mile. Things remained that way until 1954 when the present fire road was built from Seven Lakes Drive to Long Mountain Parkway. (Before 1954, the "Lewis Road" ended at the Dunn Mine.) It is interesting to note that this wide, 1.7-mile-long road has never been shown on a trail map published by the Park.

Nawahunta Trail

Length: 1.45 miles

Miles

0.0	Seven Lakes Drive.
0.15	Turn left off fire road.
0.25	Cross brook.
0.7	Trail, right, to Cave Shelter.
1.1	Long Path crosses.
1.2	Trail, right, to Stockbridge Shelter.
1.7	Baileytown Pike.

The Nawahunta Trail starts at a gate on the north side of the Seven Lakes Drive, about 1.8 miles north of Tiorati Circle, and 0.4 mile west of the entrance to the Silvermine parking area. For the first 1.1 miles, it runs concurrently with the yellow-blazed Menomine Trail (see pp. 81-84). The Nawahunta Trail begins by running along the Nawahunta Fire Road. After 0.15 mile, the trail turns left, crosses a brook (the inlet of Lake Nawahunta) on stepping stones and continues through a pine grove. The Nawahunta Trail then crosses a causeway across a swamp and climbs Stockbridge Mountain on an old road. At 0.7 mile, just beyond a bend in the road, a side trail with blacked-out blazes goes off to the right and leads to the Cave Shelter and to the YMCA camp on Baileytown Pike. This junction is marked with a cairn.

The Long Path (turquoise) crosses at 1.1 miles. The Stockbridge Shelter is to the right, while Hippo Rock is to the left. The yellow blazes of the Menomine Trail end at the Long Path crossing, but the continuation of the Nawahunta Trail along the old road is obvious. At 1.2 miles, the trail reaches a junction with a branch road leading right to the shelter, and at 1.7 miles it ends at Baileytown Pike.

It seems likely that this old road over the mountain was made many years before the Park was created in 1910. The Baileys to the west were related to the Lewises to the east, and it would seem that this road might have been used by them to visit each other. The route has always been known to hikers, but it appears to have been first blazed in 1946. "An outlaw trail has been discovered: from Lake Nawahunta to FB-SK, painted white" (Bartha's Trail Committee Minutes, 1/29/47). And to this day, the blazes (now the yellow blazes of the Menomine Trail) go only to the FB-SK (now the Long Path).

OLD TURNPIKE

Length: 3.0 miles

Miles

0.0	Dam of First Reservoir.
0.15	Motorcycle trail, right.
0.6	Long Path crosses.
0.7	Trail, right, to ORAK.
1.25	S-BM crosses.
1.35	Second Reservoir Trail, left.
1.5	Long Path crosses.
2.0	Plane crash site, right.
2.1	Join paved Camp Lanowa Road.
2.4	Cranberry Mountain Trail, left.
3.0	Lake Welch Drive.

At present, the Old Turnpike starts at the northwest end of the First Reservoir, 0.4 mile from Calls Hollow Road. The rather wide road is the route of a buried telephone cable. At 0.6 mile, the Long Path (LP) crosses, and then a path departs to the right — it goes to the paved road which leads from Gate Hill Road to the AT&T microwave relay towers. A trail down right from that path leads to the site of the Buchanan mansion, known as ORAK.

The Suffern-Bear Mountain Trail (S-BM) (yellow) crosses at 1.25 miles, and at 1.35 miles the obscure Second Reservoir Trail goes off to the left (it crosses the LP/S-BM and is more easily followed after that). Soon afterwards, the Long Path comes down from the Big Hill Shelter and crosses the Old Turnpike.

At 2.1 miles, the Old Turnpike joins a paved camp road that comes from Breakneck Pond. The Old Turnpike follows this road to Lake Welch Drive. From this point, St. John's Church is 0.7 mile east, while the Seven Lakes Drive is 0.9 mile west.

The Old Turnpike was a road from Monroe (now known as Southfields) to Haverstraw. It is not known when it was first built, but it became the "old" turnpike in 1824, when a new turnpike (now Gate Hill Road/Route 106) was built. The Old Turnpike was rather overgrown until 1969, when AT&T widened it to 20 feet and buried a coaxial cable along one side.

Originally, the Old Turnpike continued both east and west of the present route. From the vicinity of the present First Reservoir (built in 1912), it continued east (downhill), crossed Horse Chock Brook, and followed Calls Hollow Road to Willow Grove Road (which was then known as Gate Hill Road).

Going west, the Old Turnpike followed the old Johnsontown Road. Beyond Johntown (now the site of Sebago Beach), it may have used the road known as Continental Road or Hemlock Hill Road (part of the route of the Victory Trail) out past Car Pond to the Orange Turnpike.

In 1921, the Boy Scouts used the Old Turnpike as part of their White Bar trail system. This trail followed the Cranberry Mountain Trail to the Old Turnpike, then left it above the First Reservoir to go down to Gate Hill Road where they had their Camp Hawkeye.

PINE MEADOW ROAD

Miles
0.0   Seven Lakes Drive.

0.05   Little Doe Trail, right.

0.4   Ski trail joins, right.

0.8   Cranberry Mountain Trail, straight ahead.

1.0   Buck Trail branch, right.

1.1   Woods road, left, to Breakneck Pond.

1.5   Trail, left (cairn), to lake.

1.7   Road divides:

Pine Meadow Road West
1.7   Buck Trail starts, right.

2.35   T-MI Trail crosses.

3.0   Woodtown Road (West), right.

3.25   Path, left, to Lake Wanoksink.

3.7   Pine Meadow Trail crosses.

3.75   Dam.

4.05   Poached Egg Trail, right.

4.35   Road ends at Torne Valley Road.

Pine Meadow Road East
1.8   T-MI Trail crosses.

1.9   Old woods road, left.

2.45   Woodtown Road joins, left.

2.55   Tri-Trail Junction; take center road.

3.3   Many Swamp Trail, left.

3.45   Pine Meadow Trail crosses.

3.5   Sherwood Path, left.

3.55   Road ends.

Because it is closed to motor traffic, the Pine Meadow Road is a hiking and cross-country ski trail. It starts on the east side of Seven Lakes Drive, 0.35 mile north of the hikers' parking area at Lake Sebago. After 0.4 mile, a ski trail, with red markers, comes in from the right and joins Pine Meadow Road. To the right, this ski trail crosses Seven Lakes Drive 0.15 mile south of the end of Pine Meadow Road.

At 0.8 mile, the Cranberry Mountain Trail continues straight ahead, while Pine Meadow Road turns right and goes up a notch between Cranberry Mountain on the left and Conklin Mountain on the right. On the way up this notch, at 1.0 mile, a branch of the unmarked Buck Trail starts to the right. A little farther, at 1.1 miles, an unmarked woods road goes north, leading to the west side of Breakneck Pond (there are some white blazes, which soon leave the road and lead to the pond). At 1.5 miles, an unmarked trail goes left to the east side of Breakneck Pond (the junction with this trail is marked with a cairn in a tree). Then, at 1.7 miles, the road divides into the east and west branches. On the right side, about 50 feet beyond this junction, look for the unmarked end of the Buck Trail. It goes for 1.6 miles to the Seven Hills Trail above Lake Sebago.

Pine Meadow Road West now heads southwest, crossing the Tuxedo-Mt. Ivy Trail at 2.35 miles. At 3.0 miles, Woodtown Road (West) from Sebago Dam comes in from the right. Here, also, a gravel road goes off to the right, then bears left up Diamond Mountain to the site of the old fire tower.

At 3.25 miles, the road crosses a stone bridge over the outlet of a swamp. In another 150 feet, a path goes left to the top of Lake Wanoksink dam. Then, at 3.7 miles, the Pine Meadow Trail crosses, after which the road goes over a dam (built in 1933-34) and turns eastward around the lake. At 4.05 miles, a trail on the right is marked white with a yellow center. Known as the Poached Egg Trail, it was made about 1985 by Conrad Schaefer as a shortcut to the Raccoon Brook Hills Trail. It was officially adopted by the Trail Conference in 1989. At 4.35 miles, Pine Meadow Road West reaches the unmarked Torne Valley Road, which comes in from the right. This point is actually the end of Pine Meadow Road West. The road ahead, which continues to the edge of the lake, is the continuation of Torne Valley Road. It is a part of the old road from Ramapo to Willow Grove, which crossed Pine Meadow before the lake was built.

Pine Meadow Road East leads south from the junction. At 1.8 miles, the Tuxedo-Mt. Ivy Trail crosses, and 0.1 mile farther an old woods road (the original route of the T-MI) goes left. Woodtown Road joins from the left at 2.45 miles, and about two minutes later the hiker is confronted with a three-trail junction. The trail to the right is Conklin Road, a continuation of Woodtown Road. The middle trail is Pine Meadow Road East. The left trail is a road that goes steeply up, and returns in 0.3 mile to Pine Meadow Road East. It seems to have also been built in 1933, but there is no apparent need for it (it is good for a ski-run, however).

Pine Meadow Road East bears left about 0.1 mile farther, where the road appears to go straight ahead (*that* road leads only to an old CCC campsite). At 2.85 miles, the "No Need" Trail joins to the left, and at 3.05

miles, Pine Meadow Road East turns left. At 3.3 miles, on the way down a gentle slope, if one watches carefully on the left, the Many Swamp Trail can be seen. A pretty woods road, it leads to the Starr Clearing and beyond. The Pine Meadow Trail crosses at 3.45 miles. Soon the Sherwood Path to the Suffern-Bear Mountain Trail at Stone Memorial Shelter goes left, and then Pine Meadow Road East ends.

When it was built in 1933-35, Pine Meadow Road was intended to circle the lake, but the project was suspended before the road was completed. Long planned by Major Welch, construction of Pine Meadow Road was begun in 1933 by workers of the Temporary Emergency Relief Administration. The first trucks and equipment for building the dam were brought over Diamond Mountain from Sebago Dam on old Woodtown Road (West). Because that road was too steep and muddy, a better but longer route was built. They chose a country road called the Cranberry Mountain Trail. That trail started east from Johnsontown Road, at a point opposite the NYU Camp (now Sebago Cabin Camps).

Until 1917, this had been the site of a large white farmhouse, the home of Mary Waldron. On a ski trail through a hemlock grove nearby, one can still read the inscription on a Waldron tombstone:

IN MEMORY
OF
FATHER & MOTHER,
SISTERS &
BROTHERS
WHO WE MISS.
ABRAM WALDRON
BORN 1819
DIED MAY 5, 1897

The Waldron farms extended for 0.5 mile on both sides of the Cranberry Mountain Trail. Beyond, at the foot of the hill, was the farm of Charles Schoonover.

Pine Meadow Road used existing trails until it joined the Woodtown Road. At this junction, where Christie Brook starts from Big Green Swamp, there was once a sawmill operated by the Christie family. In 1865, the beams for the Methodist Church in Ladentown were sawn there. Raymond H. Torrey wrote (*N.Y. Post*, 7/21/33): "There was a sawmill, Christie's, on the Woodtown trail, about two miles north of Pine Meadow, the dam of which still remains. The new road to the CCC camp passes along it."

The TERA workers improved old Woodtown Road. The portion south of our "triplet junction" is now known as Conklin Road, a name which first appeared on Bill Hoeferlin's maps in 1945. It went to the south end of a swamp on Christie Brook (now Lake Wanoksink) where it met the other arm of Woodtown Road which came over the mountain from the Burnt Sawmill Bridge (now Sebago Dam).

Woodtown (Conklin) Road went on south through a notch in Pine Meadow Mountain, crossed swampy Pine Meadow, and continued down the Torne Brook Valley to the hamlet of Ramapo. At the edge of Pine Meadow, a short side road turned east to Ramsey Conklin's cabin.

PITTSBORO TRAIL

Miles

0.0	Ladentown hikers' parking.
0.3	Cross Squirrel Brook.
0.9	Cross Gyascutus Brook.
1.9	Sherwood Path; go right.
2.0	Cross Pittsboro Hollow Brook.
2.1	Turn right on power line road, then left.
2.25	Go around wrecked cars; terraces on left.
2.4	Albert/Gracie Pitt place.
2.5	Gil Pitt/Maggie Gannon place; cross stream.
2.65	Cross stream again.
2.7	Take sharp left uphill at cairn.
2.8	Meet S-BM at "Witness Oak."

This trail is named for the Pitt family, mountain people who lived in the valley until 1947. It was a favorite route for the Boy Scouts in the 1920s. They bought food at Pincus Margulies' store in Ladentown and gave it to the Pitts as they made their way up into the hills.

To reach the Pittsboro Trail from the Tuxedo-Mt. Ivy Trail parking area at Ladentown, it is convenient to follow the buried gas line, going southwest. It is a more level route than the power line service road on the hillside. The route crosses two brooks, and after about 40 minutes arrives at the wide Sherwood Path, with concrete dividers along its sides. Turn right onto the Sherwood Path, which soon crosses Pittsboro Hollow Brook. At 2.1 miles, it reaches the power line service road. Here the Sherwood Path/Pittsboro Trail turns right. It follows the power line road for a short distance, then turns left on an old woods road (do not turn left on the newly-blazed horse trail). After passing a wrecked car, the Sherwood Path bears left, while the Pittsboro Trail continues straight ahead.

A short way up the trail, some more wrecked cars will be encountered. They were left there by several Conklin families who lived along the trail. (There were once eight Conklin cabins along the trail, and they housed 16 adults and 21 children.) One car belonged to Jim Conklin; another pick-up truck was used by Jess Conklin to supply electricity to a washing machine and television set. Jonathan Sherwood, whose father owned the land on which these squatters lived, says that he saw some of them living in the old cars. These Conklin families were described in an article in the *Rockland County Leader* of November 15, 1956.

Find the trail again, beyond the cars. Then, on the left, remains of garden terraces can be seen. At 2.4 miles, just after the road bends to the left, the site of the first Pitt Cabin is reached, with more terraces visible on the hillside. In 1935, former Scout leader A.T. Shorey sent a picture of Maggie Gannon pulling a plow guided by Gil Pitt. The plow was a piece of stove iron, bolted to a piece of oak root (*N.Y. Post*, 1/7/35).

Just a bit uphill, the site of the second Pitt Cabin may be seen. Its stone foundation is clearly visible on the left side of the road. Just beyond here, the road ends, and it is necessary to cross to the other side of the brook and turn left on another road. (To the right, this road leads down 0.3 mile back to the power line service road.) A short way farther up, this road turns left and crosses the brook. Then, at a cairn, it goes sharply left,

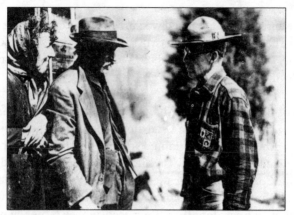
Archibald Shorey talking to Maggie Gannon and Gil Pitt –1925

uphill. After the going becomes more level, cairns lead to a great white oak, known as the Witness Oak. Here the Suffern-Bear Mountain Trail crosses.

This is as far as we can follow the Pittsboro Trail. Old maps show it continuing northeast for 0.55 mile to the Starr Clearing on the Many Swamp Trail and proceeding 0.4 mile further, to end on Woodtown Road. These portions of the old trail are now nearly invisible. The beginning of the trail on Woodtown Road, 250 feet northeast of the junction with Pine Meadow Road East, is marked by a cairn, but the trail is soon lost in the laurels.

The last of the Pitts to live in the valley was Gilbert (Gil) Pitt, 1865-1947. He was a 6-foot 3-inch tall mountaineer who spoke good English with an antique accent. Gil claimed to be descended from Richard Pitt, the son of William Pitt (Lord Pitt of England, first Earl of Chatham, 1708-78). Richard, who remained here after the Revolution, is listed in the 1790 census of Orange County as living in Haverstraw Town. His grandson was Silas Pitt, who settled in Hogencamp Hollow (now known as Sky Meadow Road), where Gil Pitt was born.

When he was 22 years old, Gil Pitt married Mildred Conklin. She left him. At the age of 41, he married again to Amy Pose. She died of pneumonia. After many lonely years, Gil found Maggie Gannon in the county almshouse, and took her to keep house for him. He was about 60 years old then, and she was about 70.

Margaret (Maggie) was born in Southfields and raised in Sandyfield (now Lake Welch). Her mother died in childbirth, and Maggie was raised by her father's aunt, Marg Odell, and by her husband Jacob. On March 22, 1886, she married Bill Gannon, a Civil War veteran. They had a son, Jake, but eventually separated. She married Levi Bulson, a barge captain from Tomkins Cove, after nursing his wife for eleven years. When Levi died, Maggie went back to live with her stepmother. After a brief marriage to Charlie Youmans in 1906 and other mishaps,

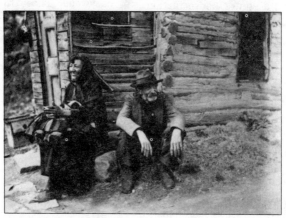

Maggie Gannon and Gil Pitt

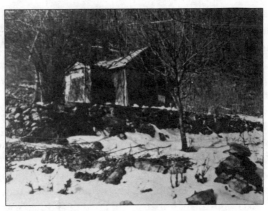

The "Summer House"

Maggie went to live in the county almshouse, where Gil Pitt found her.

Gil and Maggie built two cabins in the hollow — a summer house lower down, and a winter house further uphill. About 1938, Gil's older brother Albert moved into the summer house with his wife Gracie. They said they would stay only until they could build a shack of their own. But the years went by, and Albert and Gracie continued to live there until they died.

To get what money they needed, the Pitt brothers worked for farmers in nearby towns. They were also excel-lent basket makers. Gil made his baskets, which resembled Adirondack pack baskets, from white oak splints which he cut with a spokeshave. He also carved spoons and scoops of basswood. Those things were exchanged at Pincus Margulies' store in Laden-town for various items that the mountain family needed. "Pinky" Margulies extended credit during the winter, but the mountaineers always paid their bills.

During the 1940s, Bill Hoeferlin would lead his group, the Wanderbirds, on hikes to visit Gil and Maggie, bringing canned goods. Usually these hikes were held on Palm Sunday or Easter Sunday, and the notice of the hike in *Walking News* would include a reminder to all participants to bring along a can of food for Gil and Maggie.

Maggie and Gil became seriously ill in March 1946. They were rescued by the Ramapo Police. They stayed for three months in the County Home, then went back to their cabin (*N.Y. Times*, 7/4/46).

Brother Albert died in December 1946, at the age of 82. Gil Pitt died on May 12, 1947, also aged 82. Gracie Pitt died alone in her cabin January 5, 1948, at the age of 80. She was discovered by a neighbor, Norman Conklin, who helped carry her down on his sled. As he passed Maggie Gannon's place, Conklin stopped to ask Maggie to step out and say goodbye to Gracie. Maggie declined, and turned to put more wood on her fire (*N.Y. Times*, 1/6/48). Sometime later, rather than live alone on the mountain, Maggie went to live with friends down in the valley. She died in a Garnerville nursing home on February 9, 1955 at the age of 99.

The Pitts had neighbors on the mountain. Up above the Pitt cabins, where the Pittsboro Trail reaches the S-BM, there is a level region to the left of the trail, below Hawk Cliff. This is probably where Norman Conklin lived with his wife and niece. A half mile west of the S-BM junction was the Starr Place — occupied until 1925.

All the Conklins were evicted by the Park about 1965, after the Park had taken Harold Sherwood's land. Bill Hoeferlin noted the event in his *Walking News* of March 1965.

SHERWOOD PATH

Length: 1.75 miles

Miles
0.0	Pine Meadow Road East.
0.3	Many Swamp Brook crosses.
0.45	S-BM Trail crosses; shelter to right.
1.0	Pittsboro Trail, left.
1.05	Turn right onto power line road.
1.1	Turn left and descend.
1.2	Cross under power line.
1.25	Pittsboro Hollow Brook crosses.
1.3	Gas line crosses.
1.6	Bridge over Mahwah River.
1.75	Route 202.

The Sherwood Path, although no longer an official Conference trail, runs along a woods road for its entire length, and can be easily followed. Most of the hiking trail markers have been obliterated, but a few red markers may still be visible on the lower portion of the trail.

The Sherwood Path begins near where the Pine Meadow Trail (red square on white) crosses Pine Meadow Road East. About 275 feet south of that junction, the Sherwood Path leaves the road, and goes off to the left. It, too, is a wide woods road, and begins on fairly level terrain. At 0.3 mile, Many Swamp Brook crosses, and at 0.45 mile the Suffern-Bear Mountain Trail (yellow) crosses. Just to the right is the Edgar D. Stone Memorial Shelter (built 1935). Soon the trail begins to go down the mountain on a very rocky and eroded road. The Pittsboro Trail goes off to the left at 1.0 mile. At 1.05 miles, after passing a wrecked car in the middle of the trail, the Sherwood Path turns right onto a service road built to maintain the power lines further down the mountain. In another 200 feet you will reach a T-junction. The road going straight ahead (and then curving uphill to the right) is the continuation of the power line service road. Here the Sherwood Path turns left and continues downhill. It goes under the power lines and, at 1.25 miles, crosses Pittsboro Hollow Brook.

Just beyond the brook, the Sherwood Path crosses another open strip of land, the route of a buried gas pipeline. It then descends and turns left along the Mahwah River. At 1.6 miles, the trail turns right and crosses the river on a wide, dilapidated bridge. It then again turns right and runs uphill, between the river and Route 202. At 1.75 miles, the Sherwood Path ends at a cable barrier on Route 202. There is no room for parking at this location.

The Sherwood Path once was a narrow mountain trail. It was first blazed in 1943 by Frank Place of the Tramp and Trail Club. He named it after Judson Sherwood who owned the land through which the trail ran. The Sherwoods are descended from Rev. James Elias Sherwood who owned much land in the vicinity and who, in 1829, founded the Methodist Church known as Wesley Chapel. Many "mountain folk" lived on James Sherwood's land. One of the best known was Silas Pitt, who lived on the Pittsboro Trail. In 1963, the Park acquired the land above the Algonquin pipeline from Harold T.

Sherwood, son of Judson Sherwood. Harold died in 1977, but his son Jonathan, of Pomona, remembers hiking the trail with his father many years ago. In 1965 the Park widened the footpath to a 20-foot fire road, which later became very much eroded.

The land *below* the gas line was bought in 1981 from the Sherwood family by Dr. Charles de Ciutiis, who closed the trail to hikers. In 1988, he sold the land to the Columbia Gas Transmission Company and, in 1991, the Park acquired the 34 acres out to Route 202. Thus, it is once again possible to hike the entire Sherwood Path, although the trail is no longer maintained by the Conference.

SLOATSBURG TRAIL (DEMAREST ROAD)

Length: 2.6 miles

Miles

0.0   Begin at Seven Lakes Drive.
0.75 T-MI Trail joins from right.
0.85 T-MI Trail leaves, left.
0.95 Dutch Doctor Shelter, right.
1.05 White Bar Trail leaves, left; Triangle Trail starts.
1.1   Rectangle Trail starts, left.
1.25 Trail to Camp Nawakwa, right.
1.5   Second trail to Camp Nawakwa, right.
1.6   Triangle Trail leaves, left.
2.4   Rejoin old road.
2.6   End at Sebago Beach parking area.

This trail, a woods road, starts from a gate on Seven Lakes Drive, 1.15 miles northeast of the Reeves Meadow Visitor Center. At first, the Sloatsburg Trail runs concurrently with the white-blazed White Bar Trail. After 0.7 mile, a cellar hole with a large tree in the middle may be seen to the left of the trail. This is where the "Old Dutch Doctor," John Frederick Helms, lived from 1874 to about 1892 (see pp. 177-78). In another 175 feet, the Tuxedo-Mt. Ivy Trail (T-MI) comes down from the right and joins the Sloatsburg/White Bar Trail.

At 0.85 mile, T-MI leaves to the left, and the Sloatsburg Trail continues along the route of the White Bar Trail. Soon afterwards, a path to the right leads to the Dutch Doctor Shelter, up on the hillside. At 1.05 miles, the White Bar Trail goes left, and the Triangle Trail starts. The Sloatsburg Trail now follows the route of the Triangle Trail. At 1.1 miles, the recently revived Rectangle Trail (white blazes and cairns) starts to the left.

At 1.25 miles, a trail goes off to the right, over the hill, to the ADK Camp Nawakwa on the lake. Another trail to the camp starts at 1.5 miles, and then the Sloatsburg Trail (and Triangle Trail) reach the lake edge. They go along together to 1.6 miles, where Triangle departs to the left. Our trail now follows the edge of Lake Sebago. Before the lake was made in 1925, our trail was a road along the edge of Emmetsfield Swamp. The old road here has now been covered by the lake, so the present-day trail is a footpath which parallels the old road.

The footpath rejoins the old road at about 2.4 miles. It then enters a work area and ends at the Sebago Beach parking area, 2.6 miles from Seven Lakes Drive.

STILLWATER TRAIL

Length: 1.8 miles

Miles

0.0	Begin at Red Cross Trail.
0.03	Cross Stillwater Brook.
0.25	CCC road joins, right.
0.7	Meet Palisades Interstate Parkway.
1.0	Turn right from Parkway.
1.1	Rejoin older route.
1.2	Flaggy Meadow Trail, right.
1.8	End at Tiorati Brook Road.

The unmarked Stillwater Trail starts from the Red Cross Trail, 0.3 mile east of its junction with the Dean Trail, and 0.85 mile west of the Palisades Interstate Parkway. This point is 0.2 mile east of the Burnt House site.

The trail crosses Stillwater Brook on a wide wooden bridge. It goes southeast along the hillside, just above the brook. After 0.25 mile, it joins a wider dirt road which comes in from the right. The wide trail is now fairly high above the brook, and at 0.7 mile it reaches the Palisades Interstate Parkway.

The route of the trail was cut when the Parkway was built in 1952. It is possible to bushwhack up along the Parkway cut, or simply follow the Parkway south for 0.3 mile. Then, where the steep hillside comes down to the level of the road, climb over the guard cables and follow a dirt road to the west. That road soon meets the old trail coming down off the hill.

The trail now proceeds south, with Flaggy Meadow Mountain on the right. At 1.2 miles, the Flaggy Meadow Mountain Trail goes up to the right. That trail, which is 1.25 miles long, goes northwest, up to the 970-foot level, then turns south and ends at a gate on Tiorati Brook Road. At times, it is hard to find the trail in the tall grass.

After another 0.6 mile, the Stillwater Trail ends at Tiorati Brook Road, just east of its junction with Lake Welch Drive.

Before the Red Cross Trail was first blazed in April 1944, what is now known as the Stillwater Trail was the southern end of the Burnt House Trail. In 1922, this part of the Burnt House Trail was made a part of the Boy Scouts' White Bar Trail system. Their Camp Pathfinder was located at the junction of the Burnt House Trail and Tiorati Brook Road.

The Burnt House Trail appeared on a New York State Conservation Department map of 1882 and on O'Connor's 1854 map of Rockland County. It was undoubtedly a woodcutters' road.

In 1933-34, Major Welch set the Civilian Conservation Corps workers to building a pair of roads from Tiorati Brook Road north, past the Owl Lake Dam and through the Beechy Bottom valley. An unfinished portion of one of those roads coincided with the Burnt House Trail where it went around Flaggy Meadow Mountain. To reach the beginning of that CCC road, bushwhack south for 0.15 mile from the site of the Burnt House, cross Stillwater Brook and another little brook, and climb a little way up the hillside. The unfinished road starts there and goes east to the Parkway.

STONY BROOK TRAIL

Length: 1.85 miles

Miles

0.0	Begin at HTS Trail.
0.1	Cross Diamond Creek.
1.3	Kakiat Trail joins, left; cross Pine Meadow Brook.
1.4	Kakiat Trail leaves, right.
1.75	Cross gas pipeline.
1.8	Cross Quartz Brook.
1.85	End at Pine Meadow Trail.

To reach the beginning of the Stony Brook Trail, leave Seven Lakes Drive just north of the dam at the south end of Lake Sebago and follow the orange blazes of the Hillburn-Torne-Sebago Trail for 0.25 mile until that trail crosses the Tuxedo-Mt. Ivy Trail and, in another 400 feet, turns a sharp left, uphill. The unblazed Stony Brook Trail starts at this point. It runs along the brook, and for much of the way follows an old woods road. In springtime, the old road is often under water; keep on high ground and it will reappear further along. At 0.1 mile, the trail crosses Diamond Creek, and it continues along the left side of Stony Brook. (If one is hiking *up* Stony Brook, it is important not to follow Diamond Creek.)

At 1.3 miles, the Stony Brook Trail approaches Pine Meadow Brook. Here, the Kakiat Trail, which comes down that brook, joins from the left. Both trails now cross Pine Meadow Brook on a footbridge and turn right on a woods road along Stony Brook. At 1.4 miles, Kakiat goes right and crosses Stony Brook on another footbridge. The Stony Brook Trail stays on the road, crossing a gas pipeline at 1.75 miles and Quartz Brook at 1.8 miles. The Stony Brook Trail ends at 1.85 miles, where the Pine Meadow Trail joins from the left. The Reeves Meadow Visitor Center is 0.4 mile downstream.

At 0.7 mile along the trail, about 20 minutes from the dam, a trail may be seen coming downhill on the west side of the brook. In 1921, this was part of the Boy Scouts' White Bar Trail. It came from their Camp Leatherstocking (where the Dutch Doctor Shelter is now), went up Diamond Creek, crossed Woodtown Road and went over Conklin Mountain on the Buck Trail. The land east of the brook to the top of Halfway Mountain was sold to the Park in 1916 by Miss Julia Siedler of Montclair, N.J. She had inherited it from her father, Charles Siedler, who built a mill at Dater's Crossing in 1882. The land on the west side of the brook, to the top of the ridge, was sold to the Park in 1921 by Fred Snow, a notable citizen of Hillburn.

Surebridge Mine Road

Length: 2.2 miles

Miles

0.0	"Times Square"; R-D/A-SB/LP.
0.1	A-SB leaves, left.
0.15	Surebridge Swamp, left.
0.5	Surebridge Mine, right.
0.6	Bottle Cap Trail crosses.
1.15	AT joins, left.
1.17	Greenwood Mine, right.
1.2	AT leaves, right.
1.45	Long Path crosses.
1.7	Turn right onto paved road.
2.2	End at Arden Valley Road.

"Times Square," the junction of the Ramapo-Dunderberg (R-D) and Arden-Surebridge (A-SB) Trails and the Long Path, is a good place to start on the Surebridge Mine Road. The road is about 20 feet wide, and heads to the northwest. The A-SB soon departs to the left in an evergreen grove and, a little further on, the Mine Road turns north. Soon the Surebridge Swamp is seen on the left. In fact, since the firefighters' bulldozers went that way in 1988 (their scars can still be seen on the rocks), the swamp has invaded the road. In wet seasons, the road may be swampy for quite a distance. The long wet region can be avoided by going up the hillside to the east (there is an old trail up there). That will lead down to the Bottle Cap Trail near the

Surebridge Mine. Many of the highbush blueberries along the Mine Road were uprooted by the bulldozers; perhaps they will recover.

At 0.5 mile, there is a water-filled mine hole on the right — the Surebridge Mine. On the hillside beyond, more impressive mine openings can be found. At 0.6 mile, the Bottle Cap Trail crosses. Then, at 1.15 miles, the Appalachian Trail (AT) joins from the left. Just beyond, the great opening of the Greenwood Mine may be seen on the right, with a large pile of tailings on the left. There is another opening higher up and a little further to the north.

The AT leaves to the right at 1.2 miles. It is necessary to cross Surebridge Brook here (on a pile of mine tailings) and to continue the pleasant walk along the other side of the brook. At about 1.3 miles, a side trip to the left uphill will lead to another fairly large mine opening. Then a swamp is passed, and the Long Path crosses at 1.45 miles. In another 0.25 mile, Upper Lake Cohasset is approached. Before the lake was made in 1922, the Surebridge Mine Road crossed along the edge of a swamp to end at Arden Valley Road. After the lake was completed, a camp road was constructed around the east side of the lake. Turn right on this paved road, and follow it past an abandoned group camp and Camp Ma-Kee-Ya to Arden Valley Road, where the road ends at 2.2 miles.

The Surebridge Mine Road also went 0.25 mile south of Times Square; the Long Path follows that part of the old road. There, where the land begins to dip into a valley, the mineworkers came with their carts from the

Greenwood Furnace (now known as Arden). In the valley beyond was the Hogencamp Mine. The ore from the mine was loaded into buckets on an overhead cable and carried up from the mine, through the valley, to the carts waiting at the hilltop. The stone piers of that cable system may still be seen along the valley, beginning at the cliff above the mine. The overhead cable system was about 0.35 mile long.

In recent years, the Surebridge Mine Road has been called the "Lost Road." This happened because of an error on Bill Hoeferlin's 20th edition of his Hikers Region Map No. 17 (May 1970). That was when he first applied the name "Lost Road" to this well-known road that had never been lost. In fact, Lost Road was the name that had been given by J.A. Allis in 1921 to a section of the Arden-Surebridge Trail, from a brook at the foot of Surebridge Mountain up to the R-D Trail at Times Square (*N.Y. Post*, 11/11/21).

Another branch of the Surebridge Mine Road (now the route of the Arden-Surebridge Trail) went downhill from Times Square 0.5 mile to the Pine Swamp Mine. From that point, in 1936, the Park cut a fire road to Seven Lakes Drive, using the route of the A-SB Trail. In the fall of 1965, the fire road was extended up to Times Square and along the Surebridge Mine Road to Upper Lake Cohasset.

TORNE VALLEY ROAD

Length: 3.9 miles

Miles

0.0	Route 59 (Hillburn Brook, right).
0.25	Site of Fort Ramapough.
1.0	Bridge, left.
1.2	Landfill, right.
1.5	Gate (closes at 5 p.m.).
2.0	Brook (from Russian Bear).
2.2	Park boundary; trail climbs.
2.4	Cobus Trail goes right.
2.7	Brook crosses.
2.8	Gas line crosses.
2.9	Kakiat Trail (white) crosses.
3.6	Pine Meadow Road West, left.
3.9	Edge of lake.

This is a very old road that ran from the factory center at Ramapo to the Monroe-Haverstraw Turnpike at Willow Grove. North of Pine Meadow it was called Woodtown Road, because it passed the sawmills of the Wood family. The road was straighter and drier than the alternate route (now known as Route 202). It was in constant use until about 1854, and is shown on the Cory/Bachman 1859 map of Rockland County.

The road begins on Route 59, 0.85 mile north of the junction of Routes 59 and 202 in Suffern. Hillburn Brook is to the right. For the first two miles, it is a paved road which goes through the private property of the

Ramapo Land Company (the Pierson Estate). At 0.25 mile, it passes the site of Fort Ramapough and continues along Torne Brook. A bridge to the left at 1.0 mile leads to the hamlet of Ramapo. There is a landfill to the right at 1.2 miles, and at 1.5 miles a gate at the Orange and Rockland Utilities power station is reached. This gate may be closed after 5 p.m. and on weekends. Although the road is driveable to this point, parking along the road is not recommended, due to possible vandalism.

An alternative approach is to come down the old (but still blazed) Hillburn-Torne-Sebago Trail (HTS) from the Ramapo Torne. One can follow the fence to the left around the power station until the road is reached at the 1.7-mile point. At 2.0 miles, a little brook crosses. This is the brook that hikers cross on the HTS Trail at the foot of the Russian Bear. Just beyond, below the Russian Bear (formerly Little Torne), a path leads left to the site of a Starr family home. At 2.2 miles, the Park boundary is indicated by gate posts. The Cobus Trail to Cobus Mountain leaves to the right at 2.4 miles. That trail seems clearer on maps than it is in fact. (The Cobus Trail and the mountain are named for Claudius Smith's brother, who was (erroneously) said to have been Jacobus.)

A bit further on, a small brook crosses; the trail climbs, and at 2.7 miles another brook crosses (all this while, Torne Brook has been down on the right). At 2.8 miles, the line of Columbia Gas Transmission Company crosses, and soon afterwards the road crosses the Kakiat Trail (white). Climbing gently, Torne Valley

Road crosses many muddy areas. At 3.6 miles, Pine Meadow Road West comes in from the left. Here, Torne Valley Road turns right and continues on to end at the edge of Pine Meadow Lake.

The end of the road at the edge of the lake was the site of a Civilian Conservation Corps camp, established there in May 1933. (Stone walls and other remains of the camp are still visible.) At that time, the road continued across the meadow, and went north to Willow Grove.

WOODTOWN ROAD

Length: 5.45 miles

Miles

0.0   Start at Calls Hollow Road.
0.35   Letchworth Water Works; paving ends.
0.4   First Reservoir dam.
1.25   Trail, left, over Horsechock Mountain.
1.35   Second Reservoir dam; turn left.
2.2   File Factory Hollow Trail, left.
2.4   S-BM Trail crosses.
3.0   T-MI Trail joins, right; Tim's Bridge.
3.05   T-MI Trail leaves, left.
3.35   Fire road, left, to Starr Place.
3.8   Pittsboro Trail, left.
3.85   Left onto Pine Meadow Road East.
3.95   Tri-Trail Junction:
       right: Conklin (Woodtown) Road.
       center: Pine Meadow Road East.
       left: Crescent Trail.
4.5   Road, right, to site of former Lake Minsi dam.
5.1   Road ends at Lake Wanoksink; continue on
       trail to left.
5.2   Lake Wanoksink dam.
5.45   Pine Meadow Lake.

This old road across the Ramapo Plateau starts from Calls Hollow Road in the hamlet of Willow Grove. There is no convenient parking place near the start.

For many years, the first two miles of the road were maintained by the Letchworth Village State Developmental Center for access to their reservoirs. A few years ago, the Park acquired the land and roads around the reservoirs; however, Letchworth Village retained an easement on the property, and it is not open to the public. Trail Conference members may be permitted to hike on the property upon presentation of identification to the operator at the water treatment plant. Swimming in the reservoirs is strictly prohibited.

The beginning of Woodtown Road is paved. At 0.35 mile, the road passes a water treatment plant. Here the paving ends and the road bears left, past a gate. It soon comes to the east end of the dam of the First Reservoir. Another old road, the Old Turnpike, starts from the west end of the dam.

Woodtown Road goes gently uphill, with Horse Chock Brook to the right. About six minutes from the dam (at 0.65 mile; about 200 feet beyond a broken concrete culvert), a beech tree on the right bears the carving: "J. Christie is coming, Lord." The Christie family owned much land in this region since 1829. It was Joseph E. Christie, who lived in nearby Thiells, who carved the tree. He died on November 28, 1943.

At 1.25 miles, the Iron Mountain Trail up Horse Chock Mountain, used by horse riders, starts to the left. It ends at the power line on the east side of the mountain. (A similar, but completely overgrown and unused trail goes up at 0.9 mile; it should be avoided, since it leads to a dead end.)

The road then crosses Horse Chock Brook. At this point, there is a stone wall along the bank on the right. Above the bank is the site of the Wood family home.

Also on the right is another, older road which follows the wall. This road goes down along the hillside on the left side of the brook, ending at the First Reservoir. It is the original Woodtown Road, abandoned about 1854.

At 1.35 miles, just below the dam of the Second Reservoir, Woodtown Road turns left. (The more obvious route that continues straight ahead and then bears right is a service road which leads to the Third Reservoir.) Beside the brook that runs down from the dam are the foundations of the Wood family sawmill. A little further on, a trench crosses the road. This is part of a sluice that diverts water into the reservoir from a swamp higher up. On the bank, on the south side of the sluice, is a gravestone with the name "Secor." It is flat on the ground, probably covered with leaves. Because the bank was built in 1926, it seems likely that the stone is not in its original position.

Continuing southwest, the reservoir is visible on the right. Shortly afterward, the cellar hole of another Wood home may be seen on a briar-covered bank on the right. The road continues gently up, with stone walls on either side. A brook on the left feeds a swamp which, in turn, drains into the reservoir. Then, at 2.2 miles, the File Factory Hollow Trail departs to the left. At 2.4 miles, the Suffern-Bear Mountain Trail (yellow) crosses, and at 3.0 miles the Tuxedo-Mt. Ivy Trail (T-MI) (red dash on white) comes in from the right.

The T-MI Trail runs along this road for only about 350 feet and soon departs to the left. In that short distance, the road crosses a tiny brook, which connects

Big Green Swamp on the west with Squirrel Swamp on the east. A fairly new footbridge crosses the brook.

Many years ago, before the first *New York Walk Book* was published in 1923, there was a bridge there, big enough to carry wagons. On a nearby tree there was a faded sign: "Tim's Bridge." In 1927, Frank Place, president of the Tramp and Trail Club, put up a new sign (*Mountain Magazine*, Jan. 1928), but by 1930 that sign, too, was gone (*N.Y. Post*, 9/19/30). Nevertheless, for many years the spot was shown on hikers' maps as "Tim's Bridge."

At 3.35 miles, a fire road leaves to the left. It goes to the Starr Clearing, where it meets the Many Swamp Trail. Then, at 3.8 miles, the faint Pittsboro Trail (barely visible here) also goes left to the Starr Clearing (if one does not lose it in the laurels).

Going gently downhill now, Woodtown Road at 3.85 miles turns left onto Pine Meadow Road East. Just beyond the junction, there is a little swampy pond on the left. That was the millpond for Christie's sawmill, which stood there in 1865. In 1933, when the Temporary Emergency Relief workers built Pine Meadow Road, they ran it over Christie's mill dam. No trace of the dam or of the mill remains.

At 3.95 miles, the hiker is faced with a choice of three trails. The center one is Pine Meadow Road; the left one is a crescent-shaped trail that rejoins Pine Meadow Road after 0.3 mile; the right one, called Conklin Road, is the continuation of Woodtown Road. It was much improved by the TERA as an approach to the three lakes the CCC were building (Pine Meadow, Wanoksink and Minsi).

At 4.5 miles, a road to the right leads to the site of the former Lake Minsi dam. That dam was never finished, and after 50 years it was dynamited by the Park in 1984. All that remains is a swamp.

At 5.1 miles, the road approaches the edge of Lake Wanoksink. Here the road presently ends, but a footpath to the left continues south along the shore of the lake and in 0.1 mile reaches one of the dams that make the lake. Before the lake was built, the road divided here: one branch went south through a notch in Pine Meadow Mountain, crossed Pine Meadow, and continued down Torne Valley. The other branch (described on pp. 284-87) went west across the end of the swamp, crossed Christie Brook on a little bridge, then turned north and west over Halfway Mountain (now named Diamond Mountain) to Johnsontown Road at Burnt Sawmill Bridge (now Seven Lakes Drive at Sebago Dam).

Continuing south from the Lake Wanoksink dam, Woodtown Road leads through a notch to Pine Meadow Lake at 5.45 miles. When that was still a swampy meadow, a side road went 0.25 mile east to Ramsey Conklin's cabin.

Woodtown Road is named after a family of woodcutters who had several homes, a sawmill and a barkmill at the site of the Second Reservoir. In the 1800s, much of the land in that area belonged to Ralph Bush. In 1829, he sold several parcels to Henry Christie, who built millponds and sawmills on Horse Chock Brook and also at the source of what was named Christie Brook. He also owned Horse Chock Mountain (sometimes known as Iron Mountain), where he opened several mines. In 1848, Christie sold his sawmill and millpond on Horse Chock Brook to Jonas Wood.

Jonas, who was born in 1801, had two children: Angeline, who married John Secor (remember the name on the gravestone?), and Daniel (born 1845). Daniel left the mountain homestead in 1864 to go to Oneida County, N.Y. In 1870, he returned to Stony Point, where he started a lumber business, and later sold carriages and farm implements. In 1873, he married Mary E. Waldron.

It seems that Jonas was still alive in 1899, when he sold the mills and millpond to Isaac and Mary Bedford. In 1908, they in turn sold a portion of their land south of the millpond to New York State for Letchworth Village.

The Christies continued to own property in the hills east of the millpond. Their last parcel was sold to the Park in 1951 by Lucy Christie of Thiells.

In 1910, the 50-acre Parcel #30, known as the Bedford Pond property (the old Wood millpond), was acquired by Letchworth Village for $538.84 (the pond was 14 acres). During 1912, the dam for the First Reservoir was completed. This served until 1924, when two dry years showed the need for another reservoir. Accordingly, plans were made 1926 for a new dam at the old Wood millpond. Joe Rose, who was living on Calls Hollow Road in 1985, said that he worked on that job in 1927 — the old mill dam was broken down then, and only a muddy little pond was there. In 1928, the new dam and Second Reservoir were complete. Then, in 1951-52, a third reservoir was built on Horse Chock Brook (not on Woodtown Road). This necessitated the relocation of the S-BM Trail by about 400 feet.

Nowadays, with three reservoirs, Letchworth Village still runs out of water in very dry years. When this occurs, a pipe is laid over Breakneck Mountain, and water is pumped out of Breakneck Pond.

Ramsey Conklin, one of the better known Ramapo mountain people, died in 1952 on the bank above Woodtown Road, near the site of the Wood home (see p. 371).

Woodtown Road was used for hauling iron, charcoal and wood to Haverstraw. A hiker, Ruth Gillette Hardy, described the road as she knew it in 1912: "This was a town road until 1854, if not later, straighter and drier than the valley road we now call Route 202, from the iron furnaces in Ramapo Village to Haverstraw" (*Trail Walker*, Sept. 1971).

Raymond Torrey described the road as "rather obscure, the brush being so thick. At one place it crosses an old mill dam (Christie's dam) where the path in summer is quite overgrown with young trees" (*N.Y. Post*, 7/15/21). That overgrown condition was changed when the TERA built Pine Meadow Road, and again in 1957 when Park bulldozers cleared Woodtown Road from the First Reservoir to Pine Meadow Road East (*Trail Conference News*, Feb. 1957). In the fall of 1965, the road was again widened, this time to 20 feet (*Trail Walker*, Mar. 1966).

WOODTOWN ROAD (WEST)

Length: 2.0 miles

Miles

0.0	Leave Seven Lakes Drive at Sebago Dam.
0.1	Cross brook; HTS blazes turn right.
0.4	Turn briefly south.
0.8	Seven Hills Trail joins; cross Diamond Brook.
0.9	Seven Hills Trail leaves, right.
1.0	Land levels; path goes left to incinerator.
1.05	T-MI Trail crosses.
1.3	Pine Meadow Road West ahead. Woodtown Road turns right, parallel to Pine Meadow Road.
1.55	Cross Christie Brook.
1.65	Top of Wanoksink Dam.
1.7	Road, right, to Pine Meadow Lake.
1.9	Cross second dam.
2.0	End at Conklin Road.

This old woods road starts at the foot of Sebago Dam. There it carries the Tuxedo-Mt. Ivy (T-MI) (red dash on white) and Hillburn-Torne-Sebago (HTS) (orange) Trails. Going east, T-MI quickly leaves to the right. Then, after crossing a brook, HTS also leaves to the right. The old road now rises gently, turns briefly south at 0.4 mile, and continues up through a pretty glade, with Diamond Creek to the right.

At 0.8 mile, the trail passes a cascade. Here, the Seven Hills Trail (blue on white) joins from the left, and the road immediately crosses the brook. Seven Hills leaves to the right at 0.9 mile. A white-blazed trail starts left from this point. It goes up a short distance to a large quartz boulder on a ledge, known as Monitor Rock. After a bit the land levels, and a path goes left to an incinerator (built in 1933 by the Civilian Conservation Corps). Just beyond that path, the T-MI Trail crosses. Woodtown Road now goes gently downhill and at 1.3 miles approaches Pine Meadow Road West.

Across Pine Meadow Road here, a path leads through laurels toward Lake Wanoksink. Just beyond the laurels is the foundation of a 1933 Civilian Conservation Corps building. To the right, just before the junction with Pine Meadow Road, another woods road heads back up Diamond Mountain. It goes to the site of the former fire tower (dismantled in 1986).

Woodtown Road was here long before Pine Meadow Road was built. To follow its original route, turn right just before reaching Pine Meadow Road, and head south through the bushes. Soon you will notice a path leading through the laurels. This faint path, which runs parallel to Pine Meadow Road, follows the route of the old Woodtown Road. After 0.25 mile, the path reaches Christie Brook. The little bridge here has long been gone, but the stone abutments are still visible. Raymond Torrey described the road here in 1921: "a fairly open wood road — a wagon width in winter but very narrow in summer . . . . This crosses Christie Brook, a considerable stream in winter, a belt of moss-covered rocks in summer" (*N.Y. Post*, 7/15/21).

After crossing Christie Brook (which drains Lake Wanoksink), Woodtown Road again reaches Pine Meadow Road West. Our old road is now under the dam and in the lake, but a wide path straight ahead leads to a large rock on the shore near the top of the dam. A bit further, a stone-paved road departs to the south — it goes to the Pine Meadow Trail on the north shore of Pine Meadow Lake. Our path, cut through laurels in the 1960s by Jim Stankard of the Westchester Trails Association, continues around the lake edge. In another 0.2 mile, it crosses a second, smaller dam, then turns left and proceeds north. To the right, another trail goes south to Pine Meadow Lake. Our path continues around the southeast corner of the lake and, at 2.0 miles, ends at the old Conklin Road, where it comes up from the lake.

This old road started from the Burnt Sawmill Bridge, which crossed Stony Brook where Sebago Dam was built in 1924. The road went east, up over what was then known as Halfway Mountain. This mountain was designated as Diamond Mountain on the big topographic map published by the Park in 1927.

The road itself had no name until 1943 when, on the seventh edition of his Hikers Region Map No. 5, Bill Hoeferlin labeled it "Deer Trail." On the same map he named for the first time the "Buck Trail" and the "Little Doe Trail." Then, in 1945, Hoeferlin changed the name to Woodtown Road. Maps issued by the Park used this name only after 1966. It can be regarded as having been a leg of the main Woodtown Road which ran south from Willow Grove to Pine Meadow.

In the spring of 1923, when Raymond Torrey and Frank Place first blazed the T-MI Trail, they used this road from Burnt Sawmill Bridge to the top of Halfway Mountain. In the years that followed, the road was used for dragging dead chestnut logs from the Pine Meadow area (*N.Y. Post*, 4/24/28). Then in 1933 the Civilian Conservation Corps used the road to get their machines over the mountain to build Pine Meadow, Wanoksink and Minsi Lakes. The road became so muddy and eroded that the T-MI was rerouted to avoid it.

When they began their work at Pine Meadow, the CCC established an electric generator near Sebago Dam. The power line and telephone line were put on poles erected along Woodtown Road. Some of those poles can still be seen along the road on the west side of the mountain, and several sawed-off pole stumps are still visible on the east side.

When Sebago Dam was built, the road that had crossed Burnt Sawmill Bridge was rerouted across the dam and the nearby wingdam. That work was completed in 1926. Then in 1932 the Park built an area below the dam for overnight motor camping. The ruin of the comfort station there can still be seen on the left at the beginning of Woodtown Road (West). The camp was abandoned when the new Seven Lakes Drive was built in 1961.

Before Lake Wanoksink was built, our Woodtown Road crossed the little bridge on Christie Brook and proceeded east along the foot of Pine Meadow Mountain. It crossed a swampy region (now the south end of Lake Wanoksink), then rose to higher land where it joined the north-south Woodtown Road (now known as Conklin Road).

MORE UNMARKED TRAILS

In this chapter are briefly described twenty more unmarked trails that a hiker will enjoy following. This list by no means includes all the unmarked trails. It is a delightful feature of Bear Mountain / Harriman Park that the number of trails seems endless. It often happens that as one walks again on a well-known trail, a faint side trail will be noticed for the first time. Take the time to follow it — an unexpected pleasure lies ahead.

Brooks Hollow Trail

The Brooks Hollow Trail starts from Route 6, just east of Lake Massawippa. It follows a camp road along the east side of the lake for 0.4 mile, and then heads down into Brooks Hollow. At 0.8 mile, the Long Path crosses, and the trail continues north. The Park boundary is crossed at 1.8 miles. Another 0.4 mile leads to Mine Lake, on the property of the West Point Military Academy (this area is closed to hikers).

Conklin Road

This road, originally part of Woodtown Road, was given its present name by Bill Hoeferlin in 1945. It leaves Pine Meadow Road East about 0.1 mile south of the junction of Woodtown Road and Pine Meadow Road East. It is the road on the right (west). Cisterns on the right (west) side at 0.2 mile were part of the water system for the unfinished Lake Minsi. At 0.55 mile, a road goes off to the right, to the site of the former Lake Minsi dam. The dam was destroyed and the lake drained in 1984. All that remains is a swamp. At 1.15 miles, the road reaches the shore of Lake Wanoksink. Although the old road is now under water here, a path continues south, along the edge of the lake, to the top of the dam. From this point, the old Conklin Road leads another 0.25 mile, through a notch in the hills, to end at the Pine Meadow Trail.

Cranberry Mountain Trail

Pine Meadow Road, from its start at Seven Lakes Drive, follows what was the Cranberry Mountain Trail until 1933. Along the old road lived the Waldrons (near present Seven Lakes Drive) and the Schoonovers (about where the road starts uphill). After 0.8 mile, Pine Meadow Road turns right, uphill. Here the Cranberry Mountain Trail presently starts. It goes straight ahead, along the foot of Cranberry Mountain. A telephone cable was buried in the trail in 1969. After 0.8 mile, orange blazes mark the start of a trail that leaves to the right. This trail goes over Cranberry Mountain and past camp buildings to the northern shore of Breakneck Pond. In another 200 feet, the Cranberry Mountain Trail ends at the paved Camp Lanowa Road.

Deep Hollow Trail

This is *not* the route that the Long Path followed until 1988, down along Deep Hollow Brook. To reach *this* Deep Hollow Trail, go west on the Long Path from Deep Hollow Brook. At 0.4 mile from the second brook crossing, watch for an old road crossing. This is the Deep Hollow Trail. To the north, 0.6 mile on West Point land (closed to the public), it comes down to Deep Hollow Brook, and at 1.5 miles reaches Mine Lake at the same place as the Brooks Hollow Trail.

Going south from the Long Path, Deep Hollow Trail (marked with blacked-out blazes) goes over a hill and reaches Route 6 at 0.8 mile. If one crosses Route 6 and bushwhacks up through a notch in the ridge ahead, a nice trail (also with blacked-out blazes) will be found on the other side. This trail, which starts on an abandoned section of Route 6, skirts a swamp to the west of Stockbridge Mountain and ends on Baileytown Road, at the brook crossing between Upper and Lower Twin Lakes.

File Factory Hollow Trail

The File Factory Hollow Trail starts from Woodtown Road, 0.8 mile north of the Tuxedo-Mt. Ivy Trail at Tim's Bridge (0.2 mile north of the Suffern-Bear Mountain Trail). It goes down to the power line above Calls Hollow Road. At 0.1 mile, the Limekiln Mountain Trail crosses, from the nearby File Factory Brook (which drains Squirrel Swamp). At 0.35 mile, a horse trail goes off to the left, up to Horse Chock Mountain. Other horse trails will be passed — one on the right goes to the top of Limekiln Mountain. Then at 1.0 mile the power line service road is reached. Below is Krucker's picnic grove. The Ladentown hikers' parking area is 1.0 mile west.

Where the trail ends at the power line service road, the remains of an old dam can be seen in the brook. Here, in 1832, a file factory was built by a 21-year-old Englishman named James Slinn and his brother. In 1850, the Slinns sold the factory to John F. Anderson, who had married a local girl named Catherine Secor. Anderson operated the factory until his death in 1883, when it passed to Catherine's brother John H. Secor. *Green's History of Rockland County,* published in 1886, said that Anderson's file factory still employed four or five men.

Flaggy Meadow Mountain Trail

This trail starts at a gate on Tiorati Brook Road, 0.4 mile east of the parking place at the Beech Trail crossing, or 0.3 mile west of another small parking place on the south side of the road. It can be followed uphill to the north for about 1.25 miles, and then it disappears. Bushwhacking north from that point will lead to the Red Cross Trail, near the Dean Trail junction.

On the way up, a trail may be seen on the right at about 0.5 mile. It is marked with a cairn, in a fairly level area. That is another arm of the Flaggy Meadow Mountain Trail. It is much overgrown, but leads in about 0.75 mile to the Stillwater Trail, 0.6 mile north of Tiorati Brook Road, near its junction with the Palisades Interstate Parkway.

Grape Swamp Mountain Trails

Grape Swamp Mountain is on the south side of Tiorati Brook Road, as it heads toward a junction with Lake Welch Drive. The Grape Swamp Mountain Trails lead to the Nickel Mine (see p. 461).

The trails start on the south side of Tiorati Brook Road at the point where the road crosses Tiorati Brook, 0.15 mile below the parking area at the Beech Trail crossing. The main trail begins by running along the right side of the brook. In a few hundred feet, a branch goes off to the right. Continue straight ahead on the trail, which soon leaves the brook and continues east. The trail is often overgrown with mountain laurel, but it can still be followed with care. At 0.5 mile from the start, an old road marked by cairns goes up to the right. Turn right and continue along that road for 0.5 mile, until mine tailings are visible to the left at about the 940-foot contour. Follow these tailings up the hill and you will come to the larger opening of the Nickel Mine. To reach the smaller opening of the mine, bushwhack to the west for about 500 feet.

The mine marks the end of this branch of the trail, despite what some maps may say. Down below, where the leg started, another 0.3 mile east along the main trail brings one to a cut, high above Lake Welch Drive. An old road uphill near there was the route of the Suffern-Bear Mountain Trail until 1969.

One can also reach the Nickel Mine by following the right branch of the trail at the junction a few hundred feet from the beginning. Continue for 0.4 mile from the brook and then, at the 1,020-foot contour, bushwhack 0.1 mile east. Watch for a hill of mine tailings. Next to it is the smaller opening of the Nickel Mine. (The other, larger opening is 0.1 mile to the east and downhill.) This branch of the trail continues on over the mountain, reaching Lake Welch Drive at 1.0 mile.

Hasenclever Mountain Trail

The Hasenclever Mountain Trail starts from Tiorati Brook Road, about 400 feet west of the Red Cross Trail crossing. Follow a dirt road south for about 75 feet, briefly turn left on another dirt road, then immediately turn right (at a cairn) onto a fainter woods road, which begins to ascend gradually. In about 500 feet, as the old road curves to the right, a section of the road is overgrown with barberry. Past this point, however, the road can easily be followed. At 0.2 mile, the road makes a sharp curve to the left and soon reaches the ridge of Hasenclever Mountain, where it narrows to a footpath and levels off. It continues along the ridge until it ends at the Red Cross Trail at 0.85 mile. From this point, on the Red Cross Trail it is 0.9 mile west to Seven Lakes Drive near Lake Askoti, or 0.55 mile east to Hasenclever Mine, and 0.55 mile further to Tiorati Brook Road.

High Hill Trail

This trail, marked by cairns, goes around the south side of High Hill, which is south of Lake Welch Drive and just east of Seven Lakes Drive. An interesting way to approach this trail is to take the old Johnsontown Road north from Baker Camp Road (which goes off Seven Lakes Drive just north of Lake Sebago). About 0.2 mile north, just before old Johnsontown Road ends at a high cut, scramble down and cross Seven Lakes Drive. On the opposite bank, the beginning of the High Hill Trail is marked by a great boulder with a cairn on its top. After 0.1 mile up the hill from the boulder, the trail begins to turn right. At 0.3 mile, on its way around the 950-foot contour, the trail enters an evergreen grove. On the left is the cellar hole of Henrietta Conklin's home. She sold her farm to the Park in 1915.

A bushwhack uphill at 0.4 mile will lead to a trail along the hilltop. The hilltop trail eventually comes down to the Camp Lanowa Road at its junction with Lake Welch Drive. The High Hill Trail, however, leads

downward and vanishes as it nears a swampy region —
regardless of what some maps indicate.

Limekiln Mountain Trail

This trail, as shown on maps made by Bill Hoeferlin,
starts from the Red Arrow Trail and ends at Woodtown
Road. At present, neither end of the trail is visible. It
can be found at other points on its route, however.

One possible approach is from the Red Arrow Trail.
0.15 mile from its start at the T-MI, the Red Arrow Trail
heads northwest, up a fairly steep pitch, with a stone
wall immediately to the right. On a hillside off to the
right, another stone wall, 100 yards away, goes up
north. The Limekiln Mountain Trail is an old woods
road on the east side of that stone wall.

The trail is pretty obvious, at least until it disappears into laurels. Then the hiker must remember that
laurels like to grow on old roads. The road will be seen
again where it emerges from the far side of the laurel
grove.

In this region, the trail is about 0.15 mile to the west
of the summit of Limekiln Mountain. A horse trail goes
to that summit from the File Factory Hollow Trail, and
hikers on that horse trail may prefer to bushwhack
west to this old woods road, instead of retracing their
steps down the mountain.

At 0.25 mile, the trail crosses Squirrel Swamp
Brook, and 50 yards further, the File Factory Hollow
Trail (much used by horse riders) is crossed. Woodtown
Road is 0.1 mile to the left (west). The Limekiln Moun-
tain Trail continues northward, up through a rocky

notch. Somewhere beyond that, the trail vanishes. The hiker will then find Woodtown Road about 100 yards to the west. The point is about 0.25 mile north of the File Factory Hollow Trail and 0.45 mile south of the dam at the Second Reservoir.

Little Doe Trail

Many hikers have looked for this trail, but few have found it. In fact, the Little Doe Trail, an old woods road, starts from Pine Meadow Road, about 375 feet from the gate on Seven Lakes Drive. A cairn is there, on the right side of the road. After 0.15 mile, the old road crosses a Park ski trail (the junction is marked by cairns). At this point, Seven Lakes Drive is 0.2 mile to the right on the ski trail. The Little Doe Trail then crosses a small brook and bears up left, following cairns. After crossing a fairly level region, the road enters a laurel grove, turns right at 0.4 mile, and slabs up the mountain, Where the land becomes more level, the road disappears. From here on, the trail is marked with cairns. At 0.7 mile, it meets the Buck Trail on Conklin Mountain. The fork in the Buck Trail is 0.15 mile to the left.

Owl Lake Road

Owl Lake Road is on the hillside along Beechy Bottom valley, parallel to the Palisades Interstate Parkway. Built in 1933-34 by the Civilian Conservation Corps, it was intended to be the southbound lane of a motor road from Queensboro Circle to Tiorati Brook Road.

We usually encounter this trail as we go up the Appalachian/Ramapo-Dunderberg Trail (AT/R-D) toward Black Mountain. About 125 yards up from the Parkway, the AT/R-D crosses *two* old roads. The lower one is the even older Beechy Bottom West Road that went to Bulsontown. The upper road is the 1933 highway.

A quarter mile north of the AT/R-D, the two roads join, but they soon are cut by the Parkway. To the south of the AT/R-D, the roads are hard to find in a mass of barberry bushes. A short bushwhack will bring one back to the roads — the upper one is Owl Lake Road. At 0.3 mile south of the AT/R-D, a work road goes down to the Parkway, while Owl Lake Road goes straight ahead. The 1779 Trail comes in from the right at 0.4 mile. Then the old Black Mountain Trail crosses (1779 uses that trail, over to the Parkway).

At 0.8 mile, another trail comes steeply down from the mountain. There may be a cairn at the junction. This trail, which goes up to the end of Silvermine Ski Road, was to be one of the "stone roads."

The Owl Lake dam (destroyed in 1988) is reached at 1.2 miles. Here the road ends. Owl Lake Road was originally intended to go down to Stillwater Brook, cross the brook near the Burnt House, and then continue down the right side of the brook to Tiorati Brook Road. Parts of that highway were built, and are waiting for the curious hiker.

Parker Cabin Hollow Trails

There are four trails into Parker Cabin Hollow from Route 106:

Trail #1 begins at a gate on Route 106, 0.3 mile east of the New York Thruway. From the gate, proceed south on the trail for 0.5 mile, until you reach a junction with the Parker Cabin Hollow Trail. Follow the Parker Cabin Hollow Trail up to the east, above a brook. At 0.7 mile, beyond a swamp, a trail leaves to the right to go over Fox Mountain (it ends at the Triangle Trail). From 0.8 to 0.9 mile there is a swamp on the left. At 1.2 miles, Trail #2 comes in from the left. The Hollow Trail now turns right, goes down along an embankment and approaches a swamp. There it veers left and crosses a brook (it does not cross the swamp). On the other side it turns left, and soon meets the White Bar Trail. Our trail goes left with White Bar, then leaves it to the right at 1.3 miles. The trail, rather faint now, continues northeast up the valley, with a brook on the right, to end on Route 106 at 1.65 miles.

Trail #2 begins at a gate at a bend in Route 106, 0.15 mile west of the second Stahahe camps road. From the gate, proceed south on the trail. After 0.35 mile, it joins the Parker Cabin Hollow Trail (see description under Trail #1).

Trail #3: The White Bar Trail, which intersects Route 106 at a point 0.1 mile west of the hikers' parking area, is described earlier in the book (see pp. 175-80). There is another trail that goes uphill through a notch from the hikers' parking area. After a while, it levels off around Car Pond Mountain, to join the White Bar Trail on the south side.

Trail #4: This is the north end of the Parker Cabin Hollow Trail, described under Trail #1. It meets Route 106, 0.4 mile east (actually, south) of the hikers' parking area.

Pines Trail

This trail goes through the valley between the Pingyp and The Pines. Before the Palisades Interstate Parkway was built, the Pines Trail started east from the Stillwater Trail. The old Pines Trail can be seen, as one drives slowly south on the Parkway, just to the right, at the end of a high cut on the mountainside.

The Pines Trail crossed a level region (now filled for the construction of the Parkway), then crossed Stillwater Brook. After crossing the brook (difficult in the spring), the old road will be found. At 0.1 mile from the brook, the road skirts a swamp, then rises to higher ground. The Suffern-Bear Mountain Trail joins from the right at 0.7 mile, and leaves to the left at 0.75 mile. At 0.95 mile, a trail goes right, to the east summit of Pingyp. Another trail leaves to the right at 1.25 miles, and leads down to Cedar Flats Road. Then, at 1.35 miles, the Pines Trail meets the 1779 Trail (the old Dean Trail, once the Red Cross Trail). The paved road at Bulsontown is 0.2 mile ahead.

Pound Swamp Mountain Trail

The main trail on Pound Swamp Mountain is the Suffern-Bear Mountain Trail (S-BM), which goes north from Irish Mountain. It is convenient to describe our trail as starting from the Irish Potato, on the summit of Irish Mountain. From this point, go north on the S-BM Trail for 0.35 mile. Our trail departs to the right there, and begins to descend. At 0.7 mile (from the Irish Potato), it reaches Upper Pound Swamp, which is really a little pond. It crosses the brook at the east end of the pond, and follows a rather good jeep road uphill for 0.25 mile, to join another road that comes up from Gate Hill Road, near its junction with Blanchard Road.

The road now goes up to the ruins of an old mansion. This was the estate of Rose O. Redard, acquired by the Park in April 1961. The mansion was demolished in December 1961.

Quartz Brook Trail

Quartz Brook, which the trail follows, starts from a swamp on Chipmunk Mountain and runs down one mile to Stony Brook, 0.4 mile below its junction with Pine Meadow Brook. Quartz Brook crosses the Pine Meadow Trail a few yards below the gas pipeline crossing. The Quartz Brook *Trail* goes up from the Pine Meadow Trail, along the west side of the brook. At 0.9 mile, it reaches the Seven Hills Trail, about 100 feet south of the gas pipeline (the trail is on the south side of the brook).

This little-used trail became "legal" in 1963, when the Park purchased a large part of the Pierson Estate. It had never been blazed (except by wine bottles stuck on branches by a "Frenchman"). In 1962, it was blazed white by Bob Bloom of the Trail Conference, but it was abandoned again in 1969.

Rockhouse Mountain Trail

The Rockhouse Mountain Trail starts from the north side of Route 106, about 1.1 miles east of the Kanawauke Circle. For the first 0.6 mile, it follows the blue blazes of the Beech Trail. At 0.45 mile, it climbs up along the mountain for a short distance, then begins to descend. Soon, at 0.6 mile, the Rockhouse Mountain Trail leaves to the left on a very faint woods road, while the Beech Trail continues straight ahead. (The junction is marked by a cairn.) The trail was once marked with small 1" x 2" blazes, all of which have been painted out with gray. With care, these old blazes can still be followed by an experienced hiker. After going up gently for about 600 feet, the trail begins to descend until it reaches a shallow brook, which it crosses at 0.9 mile (from Route 106). Here the trail becomes extremely faint, but it is possible to follow the faded gray blazes as the trail climbs to the top of a rise, where it bears right (north) and descends on an old, but clearly evident, woods road. It continues northward, and comes down to a well-worn woods road at 1.2 miles. (This junction is also marked by a cairn.) That old road, followed to the left, goes down to Lake Askoti in 0.6 mile. To the right, it leads in 0.35 mile to the Red Cross Trail (0.25 mile from the Hasenclever Mine).

The "rock house," a cave which gives its name to the mountain, is below (south of) the highway, about 0.2 mile east of the Long Path crossing.

Second Reservoir Trail

This is a short, useful trail between the Second Reservoir and the Old Turnpike near Big Hill Shelter.

From Woodtown Road at the Second Reservoir, go west to the end of the dam, and then follow around the edge of the reservoir for about 0.2 mile. The trail starts up to the right. There used to be a sign there on the roadside, but there is probably just a post there now. The trail is a distinct woods road that goes up to the Suffern-Bear Mountain Trail (S-BM)/Long Path at 0.7 mile (0.5 mile from the reservoir). Beyond that point the trail is overgrown. Never fear — the Old Turnpike is only 0.1 mile farther ahead. To avoid bushwhacking, you can take the S-BM to the right. It reaches the Turnpike in 0.15 mile. Or you can go up left 0.15 mile to the shelter, and then follow the turquoise blazes of the Long Path back to the Old Turnpike.

It probably was the Wood family who made this old road. They had a sawmill at the old millpond (the site of the present-day Second Reservoir), and the road was a shortcut to the Old Turnpike.

Summer Hill Road

The Summer Hill Road was built by the Civilian Conservation Corps in 1933. It starts from the north side of Route 6, 0.1 mile west of the Long Mountain Circle. For the first 0.5 mile, it is the route of the 1779 Trail. At the beginning, it is a Park work road which turns right and goes up into a work area (the road to the left is the old line of Route 6). A sign near the work area says "Brooks Place." This was the site of a large house which formerly belonged to the Brooks family and subsequently became Camp Quannacut (see pp. 373-74).

The Summer Hill Road goes on beyond the work area, along the east side of Summer Hill. At 0.5 mile, the 1779 Trail leaves to the right. Then, at 0.55 mile, an old woods road comes up from the right (it goes down along a brook and runs into Queensboro Lake). At 0.65 mile, the Popolopen Gorge Trail comes in from the left and leaves to the right after 50 yards. The road then rises to the north end of the dam at Turkey Hill Lake. It continues along the lake, with Turkey Hill on the right, and, at 1.4 miles, vanishes near the end of the lake.

Before the lake was built, an old road continued up the valley another 1.6 miles, to the Mine Road near the Forest of Dean. In those days, that was Park property.

Summit Lake Road

The road to Summit Lake begins on Route 6, 3.3 miles west of Long Mountain Circle. At times, the road is closed by a gate, because occasionally the camp dining hall is used as an assembly place for prisoners from the county jail, when they are assigned to work in the Park.

When the road is open, it leads south 0.5 mile to the lake. It then goes uphill, past camp buildings, and heads north. At 1.05 miles, a broad unpaved road goes up to the left. That was the entrance to a big hotel — Stockbridge's Mountain House. Only the foundation remains (see p. 385).

Summit Lake Road goes on down, to end at the fence along Route 6. Hikers can get back to the entrance road by taking a path through the rhododendrons, just before reaching the fence. It leads to the big white house at the entrance road, which is rented to Park employees.

THE STONE ROADS

In 1933-36, the Temporary Emergency Relief Administration and the Civilian Conservation Corps built a number of fire roads for the Park. Mostly, they followed already-existing woods roads. The TERA and CCC workers laid a base of broken stone (Telford base) on the old roads, in preparation for a final coat of gravel. With certain exceptions, the final gravel surface was never finished, so the roads became known as the "stone roads." These roads are described below in two groups:

Stone Roads West of the Palisades Parkway:

1. Deep Hollow Road
2. Silvermine Ski Road
3. Black Mountain Trail
4. Black Mountain II

Stone Roads East of the Palisades Parkway:

5. North "Ski Trail" (and its branch to Timp Pass)
6. Timp Pass Road

Closely related to the latter two roads are several others which were not paved with stone:

7. North-South Connector
8. South "Ski Trail"
9. Horn's Route

The two roads which we have designated as "ski trails," and Timp Pass Road, were marked with red plaques by the Youth Conservation Corps in 1980. It turned out that they were too long and, in places, too dangerous. In 1987, these ski trails were officially de-marked, but many of the red plaques can still be seen. So, although these trails are no longer maintained for skiing, it is still convenient to call them "ski trails."

Deep Hollow Road

This trail is approached from the hikers' parking area off Route 6, where the Long Path crosses. At 0.3 mile (from the parking area), the Long Path departs to the right and goes up Long Mountain (the Popolopen Gorge Trail starts here). Here the stone road begins. It goes down to the site of the old shelter at 0.7 mile (from the parking area), where the Long Path comes down from the ridge and crosses the brook. This may be the first "stone road" new hikers encounter; they will wonder why it was made that way.

Silvermine Ski Road

We usually meet this road at the east side of the dam at Silvermine Lake. The road and dam were both built in 1934. The Silvermine Ski Road actually starts from Seven Lakes Drive, at a comfort station where a motor camp had been built in 1926 (0.5 mile from the present Parkway entrance). The road (which is no longer maintained as a ski trail) goes up along the brook for 0.25 mile, crosses it, and continues up through the notch between Black and Letterrock Mountains, crossing the

Appalachian/Ramapo-Dunderberg Trail (AT/R-D). 0.2 mile above the AT/R-D crossing, another "stone road" (the Black Mountain Trail) leaves to the left, while the Silvermine Ski Road bends right, around a knob. At 0.45 mile from AT/R-D, the "paved" road goes down a steep slope, where the "paving" ends. The remains of a TERA work shed may still be seen here. To the left, a faint "stone road" (which we designate as "Black Mountain II") starts down to Owl Lake Road.

The continuation of the road, now an old footpath, can still be followed. At 0.7 mile, the old trail crosses the AT/R-D on the Letterrock ridge (the junction is 0.3 mile from the Brien Memorial Shelter). Actually, at this junction with the AT/R-D, the trail is hardly visible, and on the other side it is quite invisible. Have faith! Go straight ahead, across a level area, and a clear road will be found, going down off the mountain. 0.4 mile from the AT/R-D, the ski trail joins another stone road which comes down from the shelter. This road is now the route of the yellow-blazed Menomine Trail. After crossing a brook, the Menomine Trail leaves to the right. In another 0.25 mile, a trail on the right leads over the back side of the Silvermine ski hill. Finally, 0.4 mile further, the road ends at Seven Lakes Drive.

Black Mountain Trail

Before the TERA improved it, this old trail started from the Seven Lakes Drive, 0.3 mile east of the present Silvermine parking entrance. It went down to the edge of Bockey Swamp, and crossed Queensboro Brook there. From there it followed the route of the present-day Silvermine Ski Road up the notch. 0.2 mile beyond the

AT/R-D crossing, the Black Mountain Trail departs down left, following a stream. Here and there along the way the beginnings of the TERA "paving" can be seen. They give the hiker confidence that he is on the trail. For much of the way, the trail is at the foot of a high cliff; the AT/R-D is on the top of that cliff. At 0.4 mile down from the ski road, the trail crosses the brook, and it ends on the Owl Lake Road at 0.5 mile.

This old trail continued east along Owl Lake Road and turned right, onto the route of the modern 1779 Trail. Part of its original route has been obliterated by the Palisades Interstate Parkway. But east of the Parkway, the original route is used again by the 1779 Trail for about 0.15 mile, until it ends at the Red Cross Trail (the old Dean Trail).

Black Mountain II

This stone road never had a name. The 1989 Conference map shows it as a dashed red line, leaving the Silvermine Ski Road 0.25 mile from the Black Mountain Trail junction, *i.e.*, 0.45 mile beyond the AT/R-D crossing. (It is not shown on the 1995 edition of the Conference map.) It starts at the end of the "paved" section, near the remains of a TERA work shed. Here and there along the way the TERA workers began to lay their stone base. For 0.3 mile, the trail practically tumbles down the mountainside along a brook. It ends at Owl Lake Road, about 0.4 mile west of the 1779 Trail crossing.

North "Ski Trail"

This "stone road" starts up (east) from the Beechy Bottom Road, 0.25 mile south of the Ramapo-Dunderberg Trail crossing. It was formerly designated as a ski trail, but it is no longer maintained, and most of the red ski markers have been removed (especially at both ends of the trail). The "pavement" of broken stone, laid on the trail by the CCC in 1934, was largely bulldozed to the edges of the trail by the firefighters in 1988.

At first, the trail is marked as a bike trail, with blue-on-white plastic blazes. After 0.15 mile, a trail, formerly marked as a ski trail, can be seen going up to the right. This trail, now the continuation of the bike trail, is known as the North-South Connector Trail. At 0.2 mile, the Suffern-Bear Mountain Trail (yellow) crosses. At 0.3 mile, two cairns on the right show the faint beginning of Horn's Route. Soon the North "Ski Trail" begins to go down, and it curves to the southeast.

At 0.85 mile, in a fairly level wet region, a faint trail departs to the right. This pretty "no-name" trail leads in 0.25 mile to the Red Cross Trail, coming up from the valley below, at a stream crossing.

Continuing down the North "Ski Trail," now more steeply, there is a fork at 1.0 mile. To the right, the Red Cross Trail comes up from below and joins the left fork — another stone road which goes up 0.45 mile to Timp Pass. The North "Ski Trail" follows the right fork. At 1.05 miles, the Red Cross Trail leaves abruptly to the right, and the North "Ski Trail" continues steeply downward. The trail levels off and, soon after a steep S-curve, it ends at the old Bulsontown-Timp Road, marked with A-B blazes. Directly ahead, beyond a stone wall, are buildings of Girl Scout Camp Addisone Boyce. 0.3 mile to the right, the old road leads to the start of the South "Ski Trail."

North-South Connector

This trail — which is not a "stone road" — was formerly marked as a ski trail, and is now blazed with blue-and-white plastic markers as a bike trail. The Connector starts up to the right from the North Ski Trail, 0.15 mile east of Beechy Bottom Road. It goes steeply up Horn Hill, then levels off near the top at 0.15 mile. Going gently down, it crosses the Suffern-Bear Mountain Trail at 0.2 mile. It then levels off, and for a while goes gently up. After going down more steeply at 0.6 mile, it levels off, and it ends at Beechy Bottom Road at 0.75 mile. At the junction, there is a Rockland County highway monument— a reminder that Beechy Bottom Road was once a county road from Bulsontown to Queensboro.

South "Ski Trail"

Beechy Bottom Road, after it leaves the vicinity of the Palisades Interstate Parkway, continues around Horn Hill. The 1779 Trail soon departs to the right, and shortly thereafter the Suffern-Bear Mountain Trail crosses. 0.15 mile east of the S-BM crossing, the North-South Connector comes in on the left (at a highway monument). Go just over 100 feet along the Connector (blazed with blue-and-white markers as a bike trail), and you will see a tree on the right with an old pink ski plaque. This marks the start of the South "Ski Trail." The trail is actually invisible here, being covered with low blueberry bushes. But another old ski marker may be seen on a tree in the near distance. The trail soon becomes visible (although it is often overgrown with brush), and crosses a little brook at 0.15 mile. It then curves to the left and goes uphill, where it turns right on an old road. (This turn may be hard to find when proceeding in the reverse direction.) It heads east, down a valley with a steep hillside on the left. Now an old, eroded road, many blowdowns prevent skiers from enjoying the route (although the ski markers continue). At times it may be difficult to discern the old road, but a marker can usually be found to indicate the correct route. At 0.65 mile, the trail turns right and soon crosses the brook — now pretty wide — at a place where there must once have been a bridge. The ski markers seem to disappear around the brook crossing, but the route can again be found on the other side of the brook. At 0.85 mile, the trail begins to descend, and it ends at the old Bulsontown-Timp Road (which is the route of the Red Cross Trail) at 1.0 mile. To the left, in another 0.15 mile, there is a T-junction. Here, the Red Cross Trail goes left on Horn's Route. To reach the North "Ski Trail," turn right at the T-junction and continue for another 0.15 mile until you see the trail start up on the left.

Horn's Route

On the North "Ski Trail," about 0.1 mile east of where the Suffern-Bear Mountain Trail crosses, a cairn will be seen on the right. Here, at a very gentle angle, a faint woods road departs toward the slope on the right. The faint old road is marked with an occasional cairn as it crosses a fairly level area to the southeast. A big boulder, with a cairn on its top, will be seen on the left at 0.1 mile. The trail goes down a valley and at 0.2 mile reaches the lip of a swampy hollow. Follow cairns along the left edge of the swamp, and cross the brook at 0.25 mile. The trail now is a perfectly visible old road going down the right side of the brook. At 0.65 mile, a side trail goes right, down to a branch of the South "Ski Trail." Further downhill, Horn's Route approaches the brook, where it meets the Red Cross Trail. Red Cross crosses the brook here, on its way up to Timp Pass. Horn's Route turns right onto the route of the Red Cross Trail. In another 0.2 mile, it passes the sites of two old cabins. Here, the branch of the South "Ski Trail" joins from between two stone walls on the right. Then, at 1.15 miles, Horn's Route ends at the Bulsontown-Timp Road (A-B Trail), while Red Cross turns right (southwest). Horn's Route once went left here, and continued another 0.15 mile to a road that went south (through the Scout camp) to a farm road leading to Tomkins Cove (named Mott Farm Road after it was paved about 1935).

This trail was first marked about 1920 by James T. Horn, the vice president of the Fresh Air Club and a founding member of the New York-New Jersey Trail Conference. Horn lived at 15 East 53rd Street, New York City.

Jim Horn's personal trail — marked with a metallic letter H, stamped from sheet aluminum — started at the Tomkins Cove railroad station and followed the route we have described. Continuing on the North "Ski Trail" to Beechy Bottom Road, Horn's Route followed Beechy Bottom Road west around Horn Hill to the point where the 1779 Trail now comes up from the Parkway. (That bit of road, up from the Parkway, was part of the Beechy Bottom West Road, where it crossed over to join Beechy Bottom East.) Horn then followed the woods road, once known as the Black Mountain Trail, that went over toward Owl Swamp. Of course, there was no Owl Lake Road then (it was built in 1933), but Horn's trail can still be seen in the bushes below Owl Lake Road. Perhaps, now that the dam has been removed, Horn's trail can again be followed further around the swamp. If one climbs the hill from the west end of the dam, the continuation of Horn's Route will be found on an old woods road that goes over the hillside and comes down at the Burnt House. Horn then went up the Dean Trail for 0.35 mile to a left fork (lately blazed white). That led to the foot of Goshen Mountain, where the Appalachian Trail and the R-D separate. Then it continued over Goshen Mountain to Seven Lakes Drive at Tiorati Circle on a path later adopted by the R-D and (for a time) the AT.

Jim Horn's Route was taken by hikers who were in a hurry to catch the train at Tomkins Cove (*N.Y. Post*, 11/16/28). Horn died in the mid-1930s on a hike in the Hudson Highlands. He was over 80 years old.

Timp Pass Road

Timp Pass Road really is an ankle breaker! It starts just beyond the little brook at the end of Pleasant Valley Road in Doodletown. A jeep trail (the 1777 Trail) crosses the brook on a bridge and continues straight ahead. In another 275 feet, Timp Pass Road begins to the right. It goes up the valley for 0.7 mile to the pass. In 0.2 mile, a cairn may be seen on a rock to the right.

This marks the start of an old road which leads to the Herbert Mine (see p. 458). Timp Pass Road now begins to ascend more steeply. Near the top of the climb, at 0.55 mile, the Timp-Torne Trail (T-T) joins from the left and runs along Timp Pass Road for 300 feet, then leaves to the right. Timp Pass Road officially ends at the pass, 0.7 mile from its start, at a junction with the Red Cross and Ramapo-Dunderberg Trails.

Of course, the old road continues south from Timp Pass. To continue along this road, follow the red-on-white blazes of the Ramapo-Dunderberg Trail to the left for 175 feet, then continue ahead on the road where the red-on-white blazes turn left. This was formerly the route of the T-T Trail. Although T-T was relocated in 1987, the old blue-on-white blazes of the trail are still clearly visible. At 0.55 mile below the pass, the old road reaches a junction with the Red Timp Trail. To the right, the road soon passes an elevation known as the Boulderberg, or Little Timp. The road (and markers) go down the west side of the Boulderberg about 0.5 mile to the Girl Scouts' Camp Addisone Boyce (private property). Mott Farm Road is just beyond.

In a letter dated October 2, 1935 to C.H. Halevy, Secretary of the New York Mountain Club, Raymond H. Torrey said: "The road through Timp Pass is intended, I am told by the Park officials, as a fireroad only." It used to be a farmers' road. When the cows on the farms in Doodletown stopped giving milk, they were driven up over Timp Pass and down to the farm in Tomkins Cove (the Springsteel farm, now the Boy Scouts' Camp Bullowa). There the bulls "freshened" them, and they went back over the pass with a new outlook on life.

It is interesting to note that, at one time (in January 1950), the Evergreen Outdoor Club blazed the Torger Tokle Memorial Ski Trail, which extended 7.5 miles from the Silvermine Ski Tow to the Bear Mountain Inn. The trail was marked with 2" x 6" red blazes. It went up the Silvermine Ski Road, down the Black Mountain Trail, and across Beechy Bottom Brook, where the new Parkway was being built. It then followed the North "Ski Trail" (Horn Trail) and the leg to Timp Pass, which was described as very dangerous. It continued down Timp Pass Road, through Doodletown, to the Bridle Path and up to the Inn.

Torger Tokle was a young skier from Trondheim, Norway. In 1941, he won the National Ski Jumping championship with a 181-foot leap at

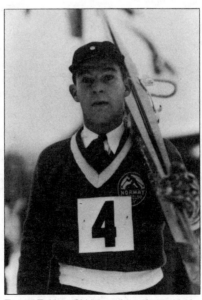

Torger Tokle – Ski jump champion – 1941

Bear Mountain. He served during World War II in the 10th Mountain Division, and was killed in Italy. In 1947, the Torger Tokle Memorial Ski Jump was won by Torger's younger brother, Arthur.

The Tokle Memorial Trail was abandoned in 1960 *(Walking News,* June 1960).

DOODLETOWN AND IONA ISLAND

Doodletown is the site of a former hamlet just south of Bear Mountain and north of Dunderberg Mountain. The picturesque valley was inhabited at least since 1762, when Ithiel June arrived from Connecticut. The Junes (or Jouvins) were descended from the French Huguenots, a group who arrived here about 1700.

Iona Island, originally named Salisbury Island, lies in the Hudson River, connected to the mainland by a road across a marsh. On July 13, 1683, in the reign of Charles II, Salisbury Island, the valley later named Doodletown, and all of Bear Hill (as Bear Mountain was then known) were sold to Stephanus van Cortlandt, Mayor of New York City, by Sakaghkemerk, sachem of the Haverstraw Indian tribe. The same land was sold in 1685 to Thomas Dongan, Governor of New York, by the Haverstraw chief Werekepes.

Not to be outdone by mere savages, King George II granted Bear Hill on July 30, 1743 to Richard Bradley, then Attorney General of the colony. Salisbury Island and the lower part of what was to be Doodletown, a total of 500 acres, was granted to Bradley's children, Sarah, Catherine, George, Elizabeth and Mary. The 500 acres in the upper end of the valley were granted to Thomas Ellison and Lawrence Roome on November 12, 1750.

The Junes and other settlers in the valley were aware that a fort had been built in the summer of 1776 at the foot of Bear Hill. They were taken by surprise on October 6, 1777, when 900 British soldiers marched over Dunderberg and down Pleasant Valley Road through Doodletown. The soldiers turned up Doodletown Road toward Queensboro. Twelve hundred more troops arrived and waited in Doodletown until the first division approached Fort Montgomery. Then the second division marched to attack Fort Clinton. (Today, the 1777 Trail follows the route of the British march of October 6, 1777.)

A romantic story, repeated many times, tells us that the British derided the settlers by playing the tune "Yankee Doodle" as they marched through, giving rise to the name Doodletown. Actually, records show that the hamlet was already called Doodletown when the British arrived. Another possible derivation of the name has been suggested by C.C. Vermeule of East Orange, N.J. He thought that "Dood" may refer to the Dutch word for dead timber, etc., and that "Del" means valley (*N.Y.Post*, 11/4/27).

Until World War I, only about 75 people lived in Doodletown. One of these was John Stalter, a woodcutter. William Thompson Howell, in his diary, *The Hudson Highlands*, tells how John Stalter worked on the new road being built in 1908 around Dunderberg to Jones Point. John Stalter (1852-1920) is buried in the Herbert Cemetery in Doodletown. His grave is marked by a large stone in a fenced-off portion of the cemetery.

Of course, the June family also lived there. In 1860, Caleb A. June (a bachelor) was the preacher in the first church, built in 1851, near the old (1809) road to Jones Point. Others who lived in Doodletown probably worked on Iona Island, or perhaps were employed by the Knickerbocker Ice Company at Hessian Lake.

Iona Island, originally called Salisbury Island, then Weygant's Island, was bought in 1847 by John Beveridge for his son-in-law Dr. E.W. Grant. Dr. Grant planted 20 acres to Iona grapes imported from Hebrides, and several thousand fruit trees. He went bankrupt in 1868, and the island was taken over by his creditor, the Bowery Savings Bank. The bank built an amusement park, a hotel and picnic grounds to entertain thousands of visitors who arrived on the West Shore Railroad (built in 1882) and by boat from New York City. It was probably at that time that a dam was built on lower Doodletown Brook, and a pipeline was installed to carry fresh water out to the island.

In 1900, the U.S. Navy bought the island for $160,000 for use as a naval ammunition depot. This provided employment for the Doodletown wage earners. In the 1930s, the dam on the brook was supplemented by a deep cistern further upstream (where the reservoir is now). A pipeline took the water to the island; our Cornell Mine Trail follows that aqueduct for a short distance. Between 1917 and 1945, the population of Doodletown increased. During those years, the Park gradually bought many of the homes. Some were demolished, others rented. The Navy abandoned Iona Island in 1947. On September 16, 1965, the Park acquired it for $290,000. The plans were to develop the island as a recreation area, and Doodletown was intended to become a ski center.

In 1962, the remaining private holdings in Doodletown were condemned, and by 1965 the hamlet was completely vacated. The last to leave, on January 16, 1965, was Clarence June, Jr. The old road down to Route 9W was blocked off in 1966.

For a comprehensive history of Doodletown, including a detailed hiking guide to Doodletown today, see *Doodletown: Hiking Through History in a Vanished Hamlet on the Hudson*, by Elizabeth "Perk" Stalter, published by the Palisades Interstate Park Commission.

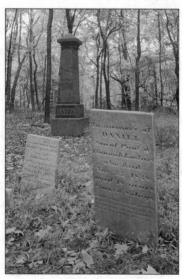

Herbert Cemetery – Doodletown

A Guided Tour of Doodletown

The various sites in Doodletown are indicated by numbers on the accompanying map.

#1.　Somewhat off the beaten track, on a hill looking east toward the Hudson River, is the site of the first Doodletown church. It was built in 1851 by John Beveridge of Newburgh, who had bought Salisbury (Iona) Island in 1847. He also supplied a Presbyterian pastor, but the local people were mostly Methodists. As a result, attendance at services was poor. For a time, the church was used during the week as Schoolhouse #11 of the Haverstraw School District (it later became Schoolhouse #7 of the Stony Point School District, when that town was incorporated in 1865). About 1860, Beveridge gave the church to the parish, who installed Caleb A. June as their "exhorter." After a new church was built on Doodletown Road (see #13), the old church became a private dwelling and was eventually destroyed. The site of the church, which is about 0.1 mile northwest of the point where the Old Turnpike crosses a stream, is now surrounded by barberry bushes, but the impressive stone foundation is still visible.

#2.　To the north of the church, a building was erected in the 1850s as a parsonage. By 1859, it had become a private residence. In the early part of the twentieth century, it was the home of Joseph and Julia Jerminario. The building was acquired by the Park about 1930 and soon demolished. All that can be seen now are the cellar walls and a cement walk.

#3.　Old Doodletown Road, closed since 1966, starts uphill from Route 9W just north of the bridge that crosses

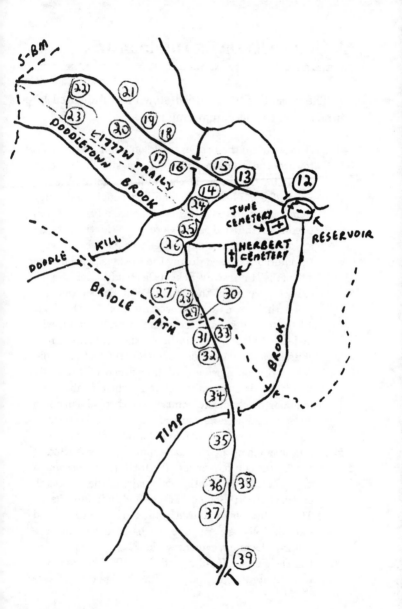

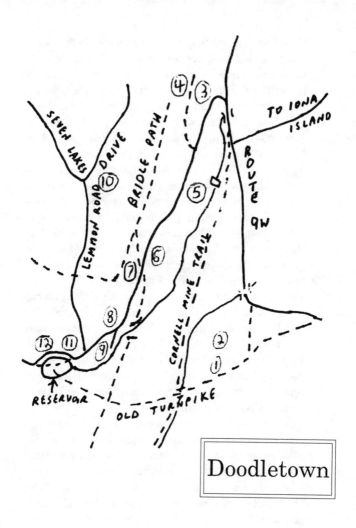

SEVEN LAKES

TO IONA ISLAND

LEMMON ROAD DRIVE

BRIDLE PATH

ROUTE 9W

CORNELL MINE TRAIL

RESERVOIR

OLD TURNPIKE

Doodletown

Doodletown Brook leading into the marsh. (At present, it begins as a grass-covered road, blocked off by boulders, and marked with a Park sign giving the background of Doodletown.) On the right side, just up where the road bends sharply to the left, there was once a small hotel, operated until 1921 by Antonio Manglass. A branch of Doodletown Road passed in front of the hotel and ended on the South Entrance Road that goes up to the Bear Mountain Inn. On the right side of the old Doodletown Road, at the sharp bend in the road and for some distance beyond, there is a low stone retaining wall. The first home on the right belonged to Knut and Alma Magnell. A bit further up the road, where a boulder barrier has been made, was the home (right) and garage (left, on a flat area) of the Horace Herbert family.

#4. The Cornell Mine Trail comes down here along an old road. A little way up that road was the five-room home of John Magnell, Knut's son, built in 1935. It was sold in 1950 to Angelo and Ruth Donato, who worked for the Park. The Park acquired it in 1962. A driveway which goes off the Cornell Mine Trail parallels Doodletown Road, then soon joins it. The home of Mr. Wamble was up to the right of the driveway.

#5. To the left of Doodletown Road, as it goes uphill, the land falls steeply down to the brook. Down there is an old dam, known as Gray's Dam, now filled with gravel and mud. The hillside down to the brook was once the terraced garden of Dr. and Mrs. Thomas Gray. The Grays, who were from New York City, had adopted a girl named Millicent Eady. Sometime in 1899, Millicent came up the Hudson in a motorboat, and discovered Doodletown. She decided to buy the house and land of Amelia Thomas so that her adoptive parents could live there. During the next ten years, Millicent (who

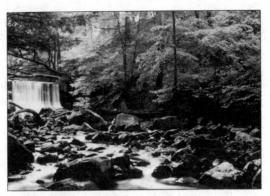
Gray's Dam on Doodletown Brook

later married a musician named Phillip James) acquired much of the land on both sides of Doodletown Brook, including the first church, which was still standing in 1903.

After the Grays died, Millicent James rented the Gray home to Harold and Hilda Herbert. Harold was a plumber who worked for the Navy at Iona Island. In 1930, the Park acquired part of Millicent's property for $55,000, and it obtained the remainder of the property for $20,000 in 1941.

#6.   Next on the left was the home of William and Olivia Herbert. Their home, on an 0.7-acre parcel, was a wedding gift to them in 1910 from Mrs. Gray. Olivia, a Swedish girl, was Mrs. Gray's cook and housekeeper. William worked as a blacksmith on Iona Island and had a shop on the hillside below his house.

#7.   The Bridle Path crosses, and then on the right, above a low rock wall (partially obscured by barberry), was the home of Eddie Steinman, who worked for the Park. On the roadside is the foundation of a garage built for the Park by the WPA in 1934.

#8. A little further along, on the right side, was a home that Harold Herbert built in 1923. It was sold to the Park in 1958.

#9. A work road leads to the left, down to the water plant below the reservoir. A home to the left of that road was the birthplace of retired Park employee Denzel Livingston (of the June family). It was called "The Beehive" because of a swarm of bees in the attic.

#10. A wide road enters from the right — Lemmon Road, which goes for 0.3 mile up to the Seven Lakes Drive. It was named for Newton and Rebecca June Lemmon, who owned 107 acres in the area. Their home was on the east side of Lemmon Road, 125 yards south of Seven Lakes Drive. Rebecca sold the house to the Park in 1917. Later, it was occupied by Raymond Adolph, Park Forester and subsequently Park Superintendent. Adolph retired in 1947, and the house was demolished in 1952. The land below the house was devoted to the Park nursery, the lower edge of which was marked by a stone wall. Near that wall, on the east

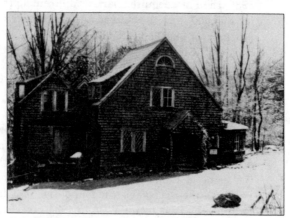

"The Beehive"

side of Lemmon Road, was the first cemetery of the June family. The graves were marked with simple fieldstones. The first to be buried there was Charity Baxter June, wife of Ithiel June. The flat gravestones were taken by the TERA workers in 1933 to line the ditches of the new Bridle Path. A possible location for this long-lost cemetery has recently been established, and a commemorative monument has been placed there.

#11. Back on Doodletown Road, just west of Lemmon Road, a large tree with broken macadam paving and a few large rocks around its base may be seen on the right. Just beyond that tree was the second Doodletown school, built in the late 1800s as Schoolhouse #7 of the Stony Point School District. After 1926, the old school was used for square dances and community events. It was demolished in 1960.

#12. Recently paved, Doodletown Road now sweeps around the reservoir and crosses Doodletown Brook on a culvert. Before the reservoir was built, the road went straight down to the water and crossed the brook on a low cement bridge. The old road can still be seen, and the surface of the bridge (known as "The Riding Bridge") is just below the surface of the reservoir. The old Dunderberg Turnpike also crossed this low region, and a branch rose from it to the June cemetery on the knoll.

#13. At the end of the reservoir, the road straight ahead goes to the June Cemetery. Doodletown Road turns right and goes uphill for about 500 feet to a junction with Pleasant Valley Road, which departs to the left and goes uphill, while Doodletown Road continues straight ahead. Near the junction, on the right side, was the Montville Community Church (Montville was another name for Doodletown). Although it was a Methodist Church, it was not a member of the Method-

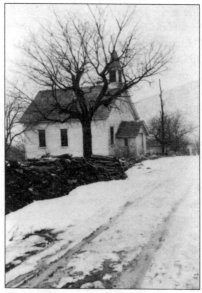

Montville Community Church – 1910

ist Conference. This was Doodletown's second church, built in 1889. There were five rows of pews in the church, but no stained glass. When the church was demolished in 1965, the pews and the bell were given to the Episcopal Church of Jones Point.

#14. Across from the church was the home of Mildred Stember, who married Mr. Seigel. She sold it to Schoenfeld, who in turn sold it to the Park in 1962. The driveway and the clearing for the house may still be seen.

#15. Up the road from the church there is a clearing on the right — the site of the new (1926) school, near a great hickory tree. It was a substantial fieldstone building. Up the front steps, a hallway led to two classrooms. There was a coal furnace for hot-air heat in the basement. In 1938, an electric generator was installed to light the classrooms. Two teachers taught the six grades. After acquiring the school in the early 1960s, the Park kept it for use as part of the ski center that was dreamed of by Superintendent McManus. In time it was vandalized, and it was demolished in 1984.

#16. Doodletown Brook now crosses the road, and just beyond on the left is a driveway. The home of Joseph and Estelle June was on the drive under spruce trees. Remains of the cow barn, hen house, and apple and pear orchard can still be seen in the clearings behind the site of the house. The last to live there were Luther Stalter, Jr. and his wife Caroline.

#17. Next up the road on the left is a great pine tree and a driveway which led to the home of May Brown, the school nurse, and her artist son Eugene.

#18. A little further, just off the road on the right, is a great willow tree. There stood the 100-year-old home of Clarence and Irene June.

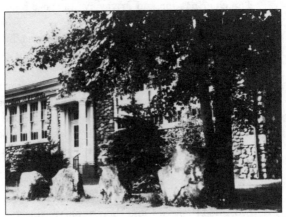

New Doodletown School – 1961

#19. Next on the right, a low concrete retaining wall is visible. It marks the site of the McLean home, built in the 1950s and sold to the Park in 1962.

#20. Two hundred feet up the road, on the left, there is a stone wall high up on the hill, and a flight of concrete steps going up. A driveway just beyond led to the home of Roland Bambino. He sold out in 1959.

#21. A driveway on the right side of the road, opposite the Bambino steps, marks the site of the home of Belding Rose, sold in 1963. This was once the home of Caleb M. June and his daughter Gertrude Barrie. Their barn was down to the right; wild roses are there now.

#22. About 500 feet further uphill, a side road may be seen on the left. On that side road, the first house on the left was the bungalow of Frank and Dora (June) Seely, sold in 1961. Next on the left was the home of Wilbur and Violet Lauber (to 1962). To the right was the last home of Caleb A. and Ida June (to 1961). On a lane to the left was the home of Charles and Dorothy Lauber (to 1962). The clearings for and driveways to these homes are still visible.

#23. At the end of the side road, on the hilltop, was the home of John and Elaine (June) Decoteau. It was sold in 1961.

#24. Go back now, down to the junction of Doodletown and Pleasant Valley Roads, and turn right onto Pleasant Valley Road. On the right, about 300 feet up the road, there is a large hemlock and a driveway that led to the house of Oscar and Minnie Herbert. Just before the hemlock, there are steps in the wall along the road. These led to the store which the Herberts kept on their lower floor. Oscar also had a blacksmith shop. A fence protected their cow and their apple trees.

#25. The 1777W Trail now leaves on the right. Then, between a horse chestnut and a maple tree, was the home, around the turn of the century, of Isaac "Ike" and Elizabeth (Welch) Scandell. It was the residence of Howard and Naomi (June) Urnaz Lewis from the 1940s until its acquisition by the Park in 1964.

#26. About 250 feet further along, a road goes left to the Herbert Cemetery. Opposite the cemetery road there is a stone wall, and a driveway which led to one of the homes of Caleb A. and Ida June, located south of a large ash tree. In later years, this was the home of Grace and Denzel Livingston and their children. Denzel is Caleb A. June's grandson.

#27. In another 400 feet, on the right, is a paved driveway that led to the home of Jacob Newell. He sold it to the Park in 1928. After that it was rented to Joseph Savignac. Also living there was his son-in-law, Art Pohl, who was a road supervisor for the Park. He paved his drive with macadam left over at the end of his day's work. Last to live there was Clarence June, Jr. His family was the last to leave Doodletown—on January 16, 1965. The house was set back rather far from the road, and it was close to the Bridle Path that was built later in 1934-35. One of Clarence's clothes poles (with pulleys still attached) may be seen on the west side of the Bridle Path. And just east of the Path, the stone foundation of a spring house is still visible.

#28. Another 125 feet up the road, on the right, a driveway leads uphill to a house near a blue spruce tree that was owned by Mr. King. After he sold it, the Park rented it to John Rose, and then to the Bowers. A small bungalow was next door.

#29. The next house on the right was high on a knoll, with two foundations below on the road—one, of a garage, and the other of a shop. It belonged to Mr. Thomas, a watchmaker at the Iona Island arsenal, whose daughter worked at the Trailside Zoo. He sold out in the 1950s and moved to California. The stone foundation of the house may be seen on top of the knoll, and two iron pipes are visible along the hillside.

#30. On the right side of the road, about 150 feet before the Bridle Path crossing, a highway monument is visible, surrounded by tree roots. This monument was put there by the WPA in 1933.

#31. Just beyond the Bridle Path, on the right, a low stone wall and a clearing mark the site of the home of the retired New York City Dr. W. Robinson. His large two-story house, which had a stone chimney, was just west of a big sugar maple. Nearby was a large barn. Dr. Robinson's son Lee, who worked for the Park, was the last owner.

#32. Dr. Robinson's son George lived next door. A great rhododendron bush is there now.

#33. Across the road from the Robinson estate (#31), a driveway next to a stone wall goes uphill to the Howard and Anna Scandell site. Their house was one of the oldest homes in Doodletown. After their heirs sold it in 1927, it was demolished. The foundation is still there, and it is worth a visit.

#34. Next up the road on the right, after descending briefly, is a row of spruce trees. Here was a home once owned by Lee Robinson. He sold the house to Luther Stalter, Sr., a stone mason, who added a fieldstone veneer and porches. "Luke" also built a barn by the brook, which was used for square dancing. Chauncey Pease was the last owner, holding out until 1962.

#35. Pleasant Valley Road now crosses Timp Brook on a concrete bridge. Just beyond the brook crossing, on the right, was the home of James Hurley, Sr. and his wife

Edna. Edna was one of the eight children of John and Elmira Stalter (they had three sons: John, Luke and Gerald). Son John was a carpenter; Gerald was the foreman at Lake Kanawauke. John and Elmira had bought the place in 1918 from Calvin Tomkins. When John, Sr. died in 1920, Elmira continued to live here with her daughter and son-in-law.

#36. Just at the top of the rise, before two huge spruce trees, a driveway goes right. Here, to the right of the driveway, Nelson and Elizabeth Rose built their home on an 0.3-acre parcel purchased from Elizabeth's mother, Elmira Stalter, in 1946. In 1950, they sold the home to their nephew Gerald Stalter, Jr. (Ed) and his wife Elizabeth (Perk). For a time, Gerald, Jr. ran an auto wrecking business there. When the Stalters sold their home to the Park and left Doodletown in 1959, they took with them many of the useful materials they had recently used to remodel the house. The stone foundation is still there, close to the road.

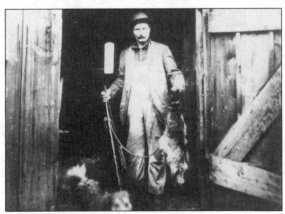

John Stalter – 1908

#37. Next on the west side of the road was a large 58-acre parcel which once was the site of the home of John and Elmira Stalter. They sold to Charles Oakley in 1915 and later moved nearby to #35, which they bought in 1918. Elmira was a Bulson, born at Beechy Bottom. John was a woodcutter who came over from Verplancks about 1887. He was mentioned several times by William Thompson Howell in his diary *The Hudson Highlands* (Walking News, 1982). Elmira (1862-1948) and John (1852-1920) are buried in the Herbert Cemetery. John and Elmira had eight children. The Stalter family is still represented on the Park work force by James Hurley, Jr.

#38. Across the road from Gerald Stalter, Jr.'s driveway was the two-story frame dwelling of Jeremiah Bailey. He raised chickens which ran around everywhere nearby. About 1940, the place was bought by Louis Salit of New York City. It was due to his persistent efforts that Rockland Light and Power Co. brought electricity to Doodletown in 1949. He sold his place to the Park in 1961.

#39. 0.35 mile south of Timp Brook, at the very end of Pleasant Valley Road, another brook crosses. Here, to the left of the road, are the remains of a small bungalow and the walls of a garage (now a shelter) on 1.7 acres. The remains of a pond and dam are also visible. The bungalow had been the home of Mary Moore, who sold it to the Park in 1928. The Park rented it to a Mr. Chandler of New York City; then, about 1932, it was rented to the Riverside Church of New York City for use as a summer camp until 1953. The bungalow was demolished in 1954, and its stone chimney was knocked down in 1991.

THE DOODLETOWN BRIDLE PATH

Length: 6.35 miles round trip

Miles

0.0	Tunnel under Seven Lakes Drive.
0.05	Tunnel under South Entrance Road.
0.5	Cornell Mine Trail leaves, left.
0.8	1777E Trail (returning loop of Path), left.
0.95	Covered reservoir, right.
1.0	Cross Lemmon Road.
1.75	S-BM joins.
2.25	Turn right on Doodletown Road; S-BM leaves; 1777W joins.
2.8	Turn left; 1777W leaves; AT parallels Path.
3.0	Fawn Trail, right.
3.05	AT goes up, right.
3.7	S-BM joins, left.
3.85	S-BM leaves, right.
4.0	Cross Doodlekill.
4.35	Cross Pleasant Valley Road (1777 Trail).
4.65	Cross Timp Brook.
5.2	Old Turnpike goes right.
5.35	Cross bridge.
5.45	Cross Doodletown Road; go up with 1777E Trail.
5.55	Rejoin north loop.

The Bridle Path starts at the south edge of the South Parking Area at Bear Mountain, near the Administration Building. It is a Park ski trail, marked with red plaques. At first, it runs jointly with the Cornell Mine (blue) and 1777E Trails. It goes through a tunnel under Seven Lakes Drive, then turns right from the paved path and goes through another tunnel under the South Entrance Road. It then passes above a field where old cars are "stored." In the 1920s, that field was used for pony rides; it later became a police pistol range. After 0.5 mile, the Cornell Mine Trail leaves to the left, and in another 0.3 mile the 1777E Trail (which is also the returning loop of the Bridle Path) departs to the left. Soon a large covered reservoir — part of the Doodletown water system — may be seen on the right. In another 150 feet, the Bridle Path crosses Lemmon Road. The Path now swings north and parallels the Seven Lakes Drive. At 1.75 miles, the Suffern-Bear Mountain Trail (S-BM) enters from the hillside on the right. This section of the S-BM was scouted and blazed in 1926 by Raymond Torrey. His route was later incorporated into the Bridle Path.

At 2.25 miles, the Path turns right on old Doodletown Road. Just beyond this point, as the road curves to the right, the S-BM departs to the left, while the 1777W Trail comes in from the left and joins the Path. The Path continues along the road, reaching the Appalachian Trail (AT) at 2.8 miles. Here, the Path turns left, while 1777W continues straight ahead. The AT, built in 1923, used an old woods road here. The Bridle Path builders chose to avoid that rocky old road and built a parallel route to the left, but after a short distance the two trails rejoin. Soon the Fawn Trail (red F on pink) leaves to the right; then the AT leaves to the right and goes up to West Mountain.

The Path, now at an altitude of about 650 feet, starts a mile-long descent to elevation 400 feet, where it crosses Pleasant Valley Road. On the way, it runs jointly with the S-BM for 0.15 mile, then crosses the Doodlekill. After crossing Pleasant Valley Road (the route of the 1777 Trail), the Path drops more steeply to cross Timp Brook. It then climbs again and descends to cross Doodletown Brook below the dam on a pretty stone bridge. The Path now joins Doodletown Road for a bit, then (jointly with the 1777E Trail) goes up an old road to rejoin the outgoing loop.

The Bridle Path was built during 1934-35 by workmen from New York City supplied by the Temporary Emergency Relief Administration (TERA). It was opened to the public on Sunday, May 5, 1935. It was intended for use as a ski trail as well as for horses.

On May 7, 1937, permission was granted to a Highland Falls stable to furnish and maintain riding horses at Bear Mountain State Park for rental to the public. Fourteen saddle horses were supplied and rented for $1.50 per hour.

The *Bergen Evening Record* of January 10, 1961 stated that 40 horses were stabled at Bear Mountain. They served 25,000 riders per year. At the end of 1961, it was determined that conditions at the stable were not fit for horses. The operation was discontinued, and the stable demolished.

THE DOODLETOWN WATERWORKS

There are two reservoirs in Doodletown: an open pond behind the dam (1975) on Doodletown Brook, and a covered reservoir near the junction of the Bridle Path with Lemmon Road. Below the dam is a filtration plant — the source of water to the installations on Iona Island.

The covered reservoir on the Bridle Path has a capacity of 660,000 gallons. It is connected by a six-inch pipe under the Bridle Path to another reservoir on Bear Mountain above Hessian Lake. The latter has a capacity of 500,000 gallons. Those two tanks are both at 350 feet altitude and can fill one another. Normally, the water is sent by gravity from Queensboro Reservoir through the Popolopen Aqueduct to the reservoir above Hessian Lake, and from there to the Doodletown covered reservoir.

A pipe was also laid from Queensboro Lake down Doodletown Road to deliver water into Doodletown Brook, which leads to the open reservoir. If necessary, water from the water plant at the open reservoir can be pumped up to the covered reservoir on the Bridle Path, and thence to the reservoir on Bear Mountain.

Water from the reservoir on Bear Mountain is pumped to the Perkins Memorial Tower, to the Bear Mountain Inn and to the other buildings at Bear Mountain. Overlook Lodge has a separate reservoir, also supplied from Queensboro Lake.

THE DUNDERBERG
SPIRAL RAILWAY

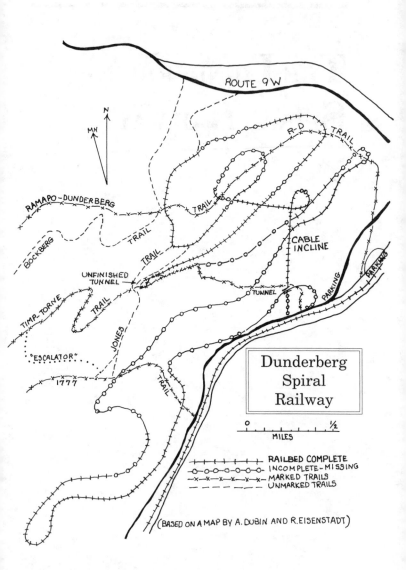

ROUTE 9 W

N

MN

RAMAPO - DUNDERBERG

BOCKBERG

TRAIL

R - D   TRAIL

TRAIL

TRAIL

CABLE
INCLINE

UNFINISHED
TUNNEL

TIMP-TORNE

TRAIL

TUNNEL

PARKING

PARKING

"ESCALATOR"

JONES

1777

TRAIL

Dunderberg
Spiral
Railway

0   ½

MILES

RAILBED COMPLETE
INCOMPLETE-MISSING
MARKED TRAILS
UNMARKED TRAILS

(BASED ON A MAP BY A. DUBIN AND R. EISENSTADT)

342

This railway was a project started in 1890 and abandoned, unfinished, in 1891. Only parts of the railway bed had been graded, and it is these parts that hikers see as they explore the mountain.

The easiest approach to the railway is the Timp-Torne Trail (T-T). 0.2 mile from its start on Route 9W near Jones Point, the trail goes up stone steps and passes above a 100-foot-long masonry tunnel. The railway cars were to be drawn up by cable from the river level, over that tunnel. The final descending leg of the railway was to pass through the tunnel.

From the tunnel, the cars were to have been drawn up by cable to a loop at the 500-foot level. There the route changed to a westerly direction, and continued up to the 900-foot summit. The prepared grade can be followed almost to the top of the mountain. When the obvious grade ends, hikers can climb over the top. The Ramapo-Dunderberg Trail (R-D) is just beyond.

Follow the R-D west for about five minutes — it will meet another level of the graded railway bed. Followed left (south), that level will arrive in 0.2 mile at the upper end of the Jones Trail, a woods road which descends to the right. Go down on the Jones Trail, which is pretty clear for a short way because until 1991 it was used to maintain an air-sensing station of Orange and Rockland Utilities. The trail gets rougher as it goes down along a brook. In 0.35 mile, the Timp-Torne Trail crosses. Turn left on the T-T and cross a brook. On the other side of the brook, to the left, is one end of another great, unfinished tunnel. Continue east on the T-T — it leads to the other end of the tunnel. On the way around, there is a beautiful view of the Haverstraw Bay to the south.

One can attempt to hike the entire 10-mile route of the railway or incorporate parts of the route in a day's outing. It is always astonishing to see how much work was accomplished in that one year, only to be abandoned to Mother Nature.

The Spiral Railway project was promoted in 1889 by Henry J. Mumford of Mauch Chunk (now Jim Thorpe), Pa. In 1870, he and his brother leased from the Central Railroad of New Jersey the abandoned Mauch Chunk, Summit Hill and Switchback Railroad. It had been built in 1826 to haul coal from Summit Hill to the Lehigh River at Mauch Chunk. Mumford operated it successfully as a pleasure ride for visitors from New York City and Philadelphia. The passenger cars were pulled by cable up the mountain and returned to the base by gravity.

Mumford and his associates chose to build a spiral railway on Dunderberg Mountain, realizing that it was easily accessible from New York City by the Hudson River steamships and the recently completed West Shore Railroad. The Dunderberg Spiral Railway was incorporated on November 9, 1889. 7,500 shares of stock, worth $100 each, were issued. Mumford bought 200 shares.

Work on the mountain started in the spring of 1890. About ten gangs of laborers began in various places to create the railbed. One of the first parts to near completion was the lower tunnel — a beautiful example of stonemason work. Bids were prepared by the Wright Steam Engine Works of Newburgh for the engines which were to haul the cars up the mountain. After a year, the enterprise faltered for lack of funds. A series of questionable deals by the Holland Trust Company — which was financing the Spiral Railway — came to light in 1890, and investors became more reluctant to risk their money. Mumford could not meet his bills or pay his workers. After about $1,000,000 had been spent, work ended in the spring of 1891, and the workers rioted. The project was completely abandoned, and soon grass and trees were growing where rails had never been laid.

The story of the Dunderberg Spiral Railway was related by George E. Goldthwaite of AMC (*Appalachia,* November 1935), by Priscilla Chipman (*In the Hudson Highlands*, AMC, 1945, pp. 196-201), and most recently by John Scott ("South of the Mountains," *Journal of the Rockland County Historical Society*, Jan. 1989).

Dunderberg Mountain itself has an interesting history. In 1791, Joshua Cholwill bought land from Caleb Seaman at the tip of Dunderberg Mountain. Cholwill (later changed to Caldwell) kept a tavern and ran a ferry across the river to Peekskill. A town named Gibraltar was laid out

there in 1833. Then in 1836 Joshua T. Jones bought 100 acres of the Bradley/Jamison Patent on the east side of Dunderberg, including a hotel and dock on the waterfront. Eventually, the Jones family bought most of Dunderberg Mountain.

In 1883, when the West Shore Railroad was completed from Weehawken, N.J. to Albany, a station and post office were established at the foot of Dunderberg Mountain. Two years later, the Jones family managed to get the name of the locality changed from Caldwell's Landing to Jones Point, in memory of Charles H. Jones (brother of Joshua T. Jones), a major landowner on Dunderberg, who had recently died. The name change was not well received by many local residents.

The Jones family sold land on the mountaintop to the Spiral Railway company. When the railway went bankrupt, the mountaintop became the property of Rockland County, which sold it to the Park in 1913. The rest of the railway right-of-way was acquired by the Park on December 31, 1938. Then in 1951 the remaining 640 acres of the Mary E. Jones estate were bought by the Park for $25,000 — a gift of Laurance S. Rockefeller. This last purchase included most of the land on the east side of the mountain, below the railway loop at the 500-foot level, and the sand quarries where the Timp-Torne Trail now starts and where the R-D ends.

As the railway bed became increasingly hidden in new growth, hikers occasionally stumbled across it and enjoyed following the route. One such hiker was William Thompson Howell (1873-1916), son of Charles Howell of Newburgh who had prepared bids for the cable engines. William Howell was a hiker and photographer who worked for the New York Telephone Company. He often hiked with the Fresh Air Club, a branch of the New York Athletic Club. His diary, first published privately by Frederick Delano Weekes in 1933-34, was reprinted in 1982 by Walking News, Inc. (Weekes, who was one of the oldest members of the Fresh Air Club, died on May 24, 1936, aged 84 years.)

Howell's diary entry for May 30, 1906 describes a climb up the north side of Dunderberg on a woods road (our Bockberg Trail). A flume-like slide had been built along the road, down which cordwood was slid to the river level. At the top, Howell met John Stalter, the woodcutter, whom he had previously met on April 2. (Stalter, who lived in Doodletown, was given a contract in 1908 to build part of an improved State road — since abandoned — around Dunderberg to Jones Point.)

In March 1908, Howell was picking his way down another old road, now called the Jones Trail, when he discovered the "pretentious" upper tunnel and a magnificent view south to Haverstraw Bay.

THE LAKES IN
BEAR MOUNTAIN /
HARRIMAN PARK

There are thirty-six lakes and ponds in the Park. Fourteen of these are natural water bodies, some of which have been enlarged by the construction of dams. The others are entirely man-made. Some information about these lakes is shown in the adjacent table.

Soon after he began his duties in 1912 as General Manager and Chief Engineer, Major William A. Welch began the construction of many lakes in the Park. At first the lakes were given numbers — Hessian Lake was Lake No. 1, Tiorati was Lake No. 2, and so on. In 1918, Major Welch sought the advice of Dr. E.H. Hall, secretary of the American Scenic and Historic Preservation Society, for help in naming the Park lakes. Dr. Hall made numerous suggestions, few of which were accepted by Major Welch. Instead, Welch favored names from the Mohegan Indian tongue: TIORATEE meant "blue like the sky"; KANAWAHKEE meant "place of much water"; STAHAHE meant "stones in the water." The Major's wife Camille was also interested in Indian lore, and offered suggestions.

THE LAKES

NAME OF LAKE	Dam No.	Date of Dam
Askoti	22	1935
Barnes		1913
Breakneck Pond		1888
Brooks		
Cohasset, Upper	9	1922
Cohasset, Lower	8	1919
Green Pond		
Hessian	1	1914
Island Pond		
Kanawauke, Upper		
Kanawauke, Middle	6	1916
Kanawauke, Lower	3	1915
Letchworth Reservoirs		
First Reservoir		1912
Second Reservoir		1927
Third Reservoir		1951
Lily Pond		
Massawippa	15	1934
Nawahunta	4	1915
Pine Meadow	13	1934
Queensboro	5	1915
Reynolds Pond		
Sebago	10	1925
Silvermine	20	1934
Skannatati	23	1938
Skenonto	18	1935
Spring Pond		1919
Spruce Pond		
Stahahe	7	1918
Summit		1873
Te Ata	11	1927
Tiorati	2	1915
Turkey Hill	14	1934
Twin, Upper		1850
Twin, Lower		1850
Wanoksink	16	1934
Welch	12	1942
Unfinished or Destroyed:		
Minsi	17	1934
Oonotookwa	21	1934
Owl	19	1934

Elevation (Feet)	Size (Acres)	Shore Line (Miles)	Other Names, etc.
914	41.0	1.3	Upper Stillwater Lake
894	14.7	0.7	Acquired 8/27/21
1,083	66.0	2.0	Cranberry Reservoir
139	25.5	0.8	
901	40.0	1.5	
863	13.0	0.7	
		0.2	
156	32.8	1.2	Highland Lake
961	51.4	1.3	
828	46.0		Little Long Pond
828	62.0	5.7	
828	77.5		
690	10.0	0.5	
947	14.0	0.9	
1,076	31.4	1.2	
	3.2		
830	32.4	1.3	Brooks Hollow
781	15.2	0.7	
972	77.5	2.3	
453	35.0	1.5	
772	310.6	6.5	
715	83.9	1.7	Menomine
891	38.3	1.5	second dam built 1947
830	37.0	1.4	Big Swamp
872	2.7	0.3	old dam repaired 1934
728	4.8		
715	88.2	3.2	Car Pond
1,065	33.7	1.3	
859	31.0	1.2	
1,032	291.0	4.8	
610	58.4	1.9	
896	21.6	0.8	
861	22.7	1.1	
1,030	38.0	1.7	Christie Brook No. 1
1,015	216.0	2.9	Beaver Pond
1,070	30.0		destroyed 1984
980	70.5		Pine Meadow No. 2
712	52.0		destroyed 1987

Lake Askoti

Going south from Lake Tiorati, Seven Lakes Drive originally descended a valley called Deep Hollow, and went along the edge of a swamp through which Stillwater Creek ran. In 1935, the Works Progress Administration built a dam across the creek, creating Upper Stillwater Lake. The road was rebuilt to cross the dam. By 1937, when the lake was filled with water, it had been given a new name: Askoti, which means "this side."

An old woods road goes around the south end of the lake and then climbs gradually up Rockhouse Mountain along the east side of the lake. From 1944 to 1947, that road was part of the new Red Cross Trail. The trail joined the Hasenclever Fire Road near the mine. At present, the Red Cross Trail starts on Pine Swamp Mountain, which is west of Lake Askoti. It goes across the north end of Lake Askoti and uses a new route to the Hasenclever Fire Road.

Another woods road, which presently carries the Long Path, goes south from the dam. From 1963 to 1981, this road was part of the Skannatati Trail to Big Hill Shelter.

Barnes Lake

Once known as Lake Miltana, Barnes Lake is on Route 293, about 0.5 mile north of the entrance to Summit Lake on Route 6. The Park acquired it in 1921 from J. Milton Barnes for $15,000. (Also included were

86 acres which extended to the top of the ridge to the east.) During that year, the lake was used for bathing and boating by children from the Central Jewish Institute of New York City. The 120 boys and girls were housed in Stockbridge's Summit Lake House at the entrance to Summit Lake (the YWCA had the use of Summit Lake).

Barnes Lake is fed by Popolopen Creek, which runs north from Summit Lake. It is a natural lake which was somewhat enlarged in 1913, during J. Milton Barnes' time, by a dam at the north end.

There still are eight private cottages near the lake, rented by the Park to the Central Valley Colony Club. Mr. Barnes stipulated in the deed that the members of the club were to have a lifetime right of occupancy. After the original club members had all died, the Park sought to acquire the cottages. But the heirs started a lawsuit, claiming that they had a right to continued occupancy. Rather than fight them in court, the Park has permitted them to remain.

The land across the highway from Barnes Lake was acquired by the Park in 1955. The Long Path is now marked through there.

Breakneck Pond

The *New York Times* reported on April 8, 1928: "Governor Smith last week signed an act transferring title to Breakneck Pond from Rockland Finishing Company of Garnerville to Palisades Interstate Park. It is the source of the north branch of Minisceongo (crooked water) Creek."

Previously called Cranberry Pond or Cranberry Reservoir by the local residents, Breakneck Pond is a natural lake that was enlarged by a dam in 1888. Its outlet is Beaver Pond Brook, which goes into Lake Welch. The Long Path crosses that brook on a pretty wooden footbridge — where a generation of older hikers crossed on a beaver dam.

To the northwest of the pond is Cranberry Mountain, sold to the Park in 1928 by William Huffman. To the southeast is Breakneck Mountain, once called Knapp Mountain, and owned by Emma Knapp until 1917. Two unmarked trails come down from Breakneck Mountain, near the north end of the pond. Another trail goes along the eastern shore and south through laurels, to end at a cairn on Pine Meadow Road (see pp. 33-34).

Camp Winake of the Rockland County Council, Boy Scouts of America, was opened in 1930 at Breakneck Pond. Winake, which means "a pleasant place," was the Algonquin name of the home of William P. Abbott, an active member of the Council's camp committee in 1927. The camp is now known as Camp Lanowa, and it is currently operated by Homes for Homeless Children.

The paved Park road going northeast from the Pond joins the Old Turnpike. That road comes from Willow Grove, meets the old (now abandoned) St. John's Road, and ends at Lake Welch Drive.

Brooks Lake

On the north side of Popolopen Brook, near the village of Fort Montgomery, most of the land between the brook and Mine Road is part of Bear Mountain State Park. The Park also owns a parcel of land on the north side of Mine Road, which includes Brooks Lake. The region around the lake was improved in 1934 for camping, bathing and picnicking. It is used mostly by local residents.

The lake and about 100 acres to the north were acquired by the Park in 1918 from the heirs of Eliza Brooks. At that time, an aerial tramway crossed above the south side of the lake. Iron ore from the Forest of Dean Mine was carried in little railway cars to a point on the eastern slope of Torne Mountain. There it was transferred to the tramway and carried for one mile to boats at the river edge below the town.

The West Point Aqueduct, built in 1906, goes across the hillside north of the lake. In 1925, there were five camps at Brooks Lake.

Upper and Lower Cohasset Lakes

There are two Cohasset Lakes, both on Arden Valley Road. (The name Cohasset means "place of pines.") The lower lake, completed in 1919, was the eighth lake made by the Park. A 1923 map by Camps Director Ruby Jolliffe showed four girls' camps there (*N.Y. Post*, 5/18/23). They were used by the YWCA of the Oranges, by the Hebrew Orphan Asylum, and by the Settlement Houses. (Today, the lower lake is generally known as Lake Cohasset.)

Upper Lake Cohasset — only a short distance from the lower lake — was created in 1922. The construc-

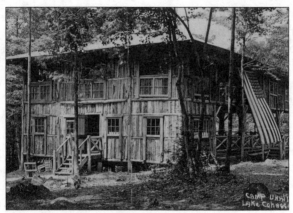
Camp Unaliye on Lake Cohasset – 1928

tion of this lake required realignment of Arden Valley
Road. It also cut off the junction between Surebridge
Mine Road and Arden Valley Road. By 1947, five camps
and a nature museum had been built on Upper Cohasset
Lake. The nature museum has been closed for several
years.

These two lakes were called "Eden without Adams,"
because only girls were seen there. An occasional visitor during the 1930s was Eleanor Roosevelt, wife of
Governor Franklin D. Roosevelt.

Two heights familiar to hikers look down upon
Upper Cohasset Lake: the northeast end of Echo Mountain (the Long Path goes up there from Surebridge
Mine Road), and a rocky summit southeast of the lake,
known as Paradise Rock, which can be reached by
bushwhacking up from the Long Path. A shelter was
built on each of these heights, at private expense, for

the use of the campers. The one on Echo Mountain is still in good condition. In 1937, Camps Director Ruby Jolliffe had pipes installed to send water to the Paradise Rock Shelter. For some reason unknown to the author, that shelter was later removed. All that remains are some pipes and a trash barrel.

Green Pond

Green Pond is familiar to hikers who walk the Dunning Trail. It lies in the hills west of Lake Stahahe and south of Island Pond, and is about 0.1 mile west of Island Pond Road. Green Pond is a tiny pond, whose shoreline is only 0.15 mile, but the marsh on its south side, which drains west into Lake Stahahe, is six or seven times as large. In 1918, during the early years of camping at Lake Stahahe, a pipeline brought fresh water down from Green Pond (PIPC Annual Report, 1/31/19).

Hessian Lake

The pond at the foot of Bear Mountain had been known since 1740 as Lake Sinnipink, from the Indian name of the nearby creek — Assinapink. When the British attacked Fort Clinton on October 6, 1777, there was a wall of sharpened logs between the pond and the edge of the cliff overlooking the Hudson River. After the battle, because many bodies of Hessian chasseurs had been thrown into the pond, it became known as Bloody Pond (Lossing, *Pictorial Field Book of the Revolution*).

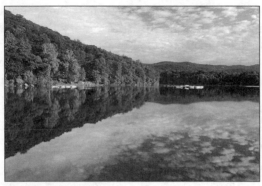
Hessian Lake

In later years, it was given more genteel names —
Highland Lake, then Hessian Lake. Ice was cut there
by the Knickerbocker Ice Company and shipped to New
York City.

In 1911, the year after Bear Mountain State Park
was created, a great playground was cleared near the
lake. In 1913, Boy Scouts were camping on the lakeshore,
and a trail was made to the top of Bear Mountain. In
1914, the lake, which is spring-fed and 40 feet deep, was
slightly enlarged by the construction of three small
dams.

Island Pond

Island Pond is a natural lake with rocky shores at
the north end, and extensive marshes at the south end.
It has two outlets: one drains to the north into Echo
Lake; the other goes south, draining into Stahahe

Brook. About halfway down the pond and 500 feet from shore is the island which gives the pond its name. To the west is a ridge known as Green Pond Mountain. To the northeast is the southern peak of Echo Mountain, which hikers have always called Island Pond Mountain.

The lake and surrounding hills were part of the estate of iron maker Peter Parrott, acquired in 1885 by Edward H. Harriman. At the top of Island Pond Mountain, Harriman built a summer house (the big stones up there were the foundation) and a fire tower of wooden poles.

When Edward Harriman's widow Mary Averell Harriman gave 10,000 acres to the Palisades Interstate Park Commission in 1910, Island Pond was not part of the gift. The family retained the pond for their own use. The Park boundary on the east side of the pond was a road that came south from Echo Lake. After passing Island Pond, this "Crooked Road" turned uphill over Surebridge Mountain (its route is now used by the Dunning Trail). In 1921, the Boy Scouts' White Bar Trail came down from the Lemon Squeezer to that road. Where the road went left and started uphill, White Bar went south on a newly cut trail to Highway 416 (now Route 106). The Boy Scouts' Camp Deerslayer was located along that trail, 0.3 mile north of Route 106.

On the west side of the pond was Island Pond Road, which came up from the Harriman farm by several switchbacks, then went around the south end of the lake and continued on southward to Highway 416. Built by Edward Harriman in 1905, the road originally started at the Greenwood Furnace in Arden.

In 1927, in an exchange of land, Roland Harriman gave Island Pond to the Park. In return, he received a narrow strip of land near Echo Lake that his mother had given to the Park in 1910. When the Park became its owner, plans were made to improve Island Pond. In 1930, the road on the west side was widened to 20 feet, graded, and covered with gravel for three miles from the Harriman farm south to the state highway near Lake Stahahe. In the same year, the new Arden Valley Road, which came closer to Island Pond and avoided entering the Harriman estate, was built.

At the south end of the pond, on a point of land, the Park built a stone cabin for the Park ranger. Major Welch entertained visitors there. A young man from Johnsontown named Muzz Jones worked there as a part-time cook, caretaker and patrolman. Muzz later became a ranger on the Park police force. He was the last resident of Johnsontown, where he lived until the new Sebago Beach was opened. The cabin at the south end of Island Pond was burned by vandals on January 1, 1962.

A short distance from the pond, along the northern outlet, an old unfinished stone dam can be seen. Beyond that is a more modern but also unfinished spillway made of cut stones. Near the spillway is part of a rotary gravel classifier.

About 1905, Edward Harriman started to build that stone dam. He also built a road from the dam to his Island Pond Road (*Rockland County Times*, 2/13/08). However, he abandoned the dam, which was used in

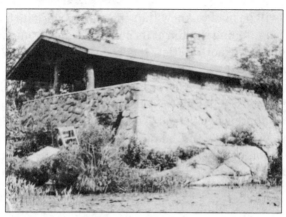
Ranger cabin at Island Pond – 1927

later years by beavers for their own purposes. In 1930, gravel for the new Arden Valley Road was removed from the nearby hillside, by way of the convenient road to the old dam.

In 1934, with the labor force of the Civilian Conservation Corps available, the Park again planned to improve Island Pond. Plans were developed to build two dams, at the north and south ends, which would greatly enlarge the lake by extending it into the southern marshy region. Work was begun by cutting the brush along the lake shores. Also, a new level road to the lake was made from the new Arden Valley Road. It ran south along the hillside to join the older Harriman switchback road. In 1934, too, the Park began to build the northern dam, the spillway of which can still be seen. For some reason, these plans were canceled, and Raymond H. Torrey wrote: "Those who know the beauty of Island Pond . . . with its border of swamp vegetation

. . . will be glad to know that the plan to raise its level by heightening its dam at its north end, and by another dam at its south outlet, has been abandoned" (*N.Y. Post*, 2/8/35).

In November 1957, the Park built the William Brien Memorial Shelter on the ledge where the Appalachian Trail approached the north end of the Pond. The project was funded by the bequest of William Brien, first president of the New York Ramblers, who died on October 12, 1954. A pump was also installed at the shelter.

In the spring of 1963, a new entrance was made to Island Pond from Arden Valley Road. A parking area was constructed near the shelter to accommodate fishermen's cars (they paid $1 a day for parking). In the years that followed, the easily accessible shelter became the scene of midnight parties and excessive littering. As a result, the shelter was dismantled in 1973, and Letterrock Shelter was renamed the William Brien Memorial Shelter. In 1980, the Appalachian Trail was relocated away from the north end of the pond, but the route along the north end of the pond was restored in 1993.

Lower Kanawauke Lake

This lake was created in 1915 by damming Stony Brook about 0.4 mile above Johnsontown (where Sebago Beach was later created). Boy Scout camping began there in 1917, and by 1930 there were fourteen camps around the lake.

During the construction of Lower Kanawauke Lake, old Goodspring Road was relocated. This road had run from St. John's Road, near Lily Pond, to the Turnpike (now Route 106), following Stony Brook. It is now a camp road which ends at a gate on Route 106, 0.1 mile west of the Kanawauke Circle.

The Onondaga name KANAWAHKEE, which means "place of much water," was chosen in 1918 by Major Welch from a book by W.M. Beauchamp, *Indian Names in New York* (Fayetteville, N.Y., 1893).

Middle Kanawauke Lake

This lake was made in 1916 by damming Stillwater Creek where it went under the Monroe-Haverstraw Turnpike (now Route 106). The road was sent across the dam, and the big swamp on the north side became a lake.

Six Boy Scout camps were opened in 1917 on Middle Kanawauke Lake. The decayed, abandoned camp in the woods north of the lake once was K-9 — Camp Leeming.

Middle Kanawauke Lake was the location of the summer camping headquarters of the Brooklyn Boy Scout Council. Harvey A. Gordon was chief camp director. Beginning in 1921, the Scouts built a 35-mile system of hiking trails, known as the White Bar Trail system, with five spokes radiating from the camps on Middle Kanawauke Lake (see pp. 178-79).

Upper Kanawauke Lake: Little Long Pond

This 43-foot-deep natural lake on Route 106 (old Route 210) drains into Middle Kanawauke Lake. At the west end of the lake, the old Johnsontown Road ends at Route 106. The old road now serves as the entrance to the Haverstraw Masons' Camp. One hundred fifty years ago, there were homes near Upper Kanawauke Lake, inhabited by the Johnsons, Conklins, Hills and Joneses.

Boy Scout camps were built at Little Long Pond in 1917. A 1930 Park map shows seven camps there. On the hillside north of the lake, on the old Crooked Road, was the Boy Scouts' Camp Matinecock (which subsequently became a Girl Scout camp, known as Camp Quid Nunc — see p. 229).

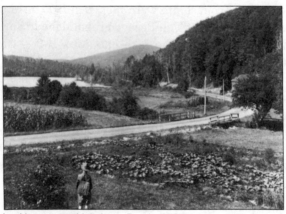

Looking west to Little Long Pond – 1924

Letchworth Reservoirs

Letchworth Village State Developmental Center is a New York State custodial institution on Willow Grove Road, just east of the Palisades Interstate Parkway. It was founded in 1908 by William Pryor Letchworth, and named for him in 1909. He died on December 1, 1910 at the age of 88.

In 1908, the far-sighted planners bought 640 acres in the hills drained by Horse Chock Brook, a branch of Minisceongo Creek. This was to be used for water supply (*Rockland County Times*, 2/13/08).

At present, there are three Letchworth reservoirs. A few years ago, the Park acquired the land and roads around the reservoirs, but Letchworth Village retained an easement on the property, and it is not currently open to the public.

The First Reservoir was built in 1912, where the Old Turnpike comes down near Calls Hollow Road. A high dam was made, and below it a water treatment plant was built.

After two years of water shortage, the Second Reservoir was built in 1927-28, using an old mill pond that belonged to the Wood family (and in 1908 was owned by the Bedford family). There once was a sawmill on the brook below the dam. The Wood home was on high ground across the road from the sawmill.

Woodtown Road, which connects the First and Second Reservoirs, continues south from the Second Reservoir. Another road goes around the west side of the Second Reservoir, upstream to the Third Reservoir, which was built in 1951-52 in the valley where the

Suffern-Bear Mountain Trail comes down off Ladentown Mountain and starts up Big Hill. The trail was moved 400 feet to the west when the reservoir was filled.

For more information regarding the history of these reservoirs, see p. 282.

Lily Pond

Lily Pond is located on Lake Welch Drive, 0.5 mile east of its start near Sebago Beach. To the right of the road, High Hill is visible. Between the Parkway and High Hill is the abandoned Johnsontown Road; just south of the road is a three-acre, 0.2-mile-long natural lake known as Lily Pond.

A Park news release, dated August 29, 1934, states that this pond was the site of an old mill. The brook that drains the pond joins Whitney Brook, which runs into Lake Sebago. The High Hill that looks down on the lake was sold to the Park in 1921 by Ada Carey, who had been the caretaker of St. John's Church until 1914.

Traces of several homes can be found near the pond. Ben Jones who was, until he died recently, the caretaker of St. John's Cemetery, used to live here.

Lake Massawippa

This lake is located in Brooks Hollow, adjacent to Route 6. In 1918, the land for 0.8 mile east of the Barnes property — which included the site of present-day Lake Massawippa — was given to the Park by W. Averell Harriman. In the fall of 1934, Civilian Conservation Corps Camp SP-23 was set up in Brooks Hollow, and work began on Dam #15, now known as Lake Massawippa (meaning "heroine"). At one time, there were Boy Scout camps along the lake. A footpath goes along the west side of the lake, and there is a camp road (the Brooks Hollow Trail) on the east side. If the camp road is followed north in Brooks Hollow, it will intercept the Long Path which comes down from Howell Mountain (see p. 291).

Lake Nawahunta

Lake Nawahunta was created in 1915 by the construction of a dam across Lewis Brook, a tributary of Queensboro Brook. The land did not belong to the Park then, and it was built to be a trout hatchery. It is a small lake, 7 to 10 feet deep, visible from Seven Lakes Drive just south of the Silvermine Ski Area. Beyond the lake is a grove of pines, planted after the lake was made.

The lake bed was formerly a farm cultivated by several generations of the Lewis family. "Scobie" Jim Lewis' grave is on the knoll across Seven Lakes Drive from the entrance to the Nawahunta Fire Road. The Park purchased the land on January 22, 1917 from Isaac Lemmon. At first, the lake was known as Lemmon Lake. The name Nawahunta is Mohegan for "place of trout."

A park fire road, built in 1954 (now the route of the yellow-blazed Menomine Trail), runs north along the east shore of the lake, on a bank above the lake. A cellar hole on that road marks the site of the Lewis farmhouse.

Seven Lakes Drive, where it passes the site of the Lewis farm, was built on the old Greenwood Turnpike. That road came over the hill from the Greenwood Furnace (now Arden), went to Queensboro, and continued on to Fort Montgomery.

Pine Meadow Lake

Pine Meadow Lake, located in the center of the Ramapo Plateau, is a hikers' favorite place. It may be reached from the west by the Pine Meadow Trail and Pine Meadow Road West, from the north by Conklin Road, from the east by the Pine Meadow and Conklins Crossing Trails, and from the south by the Torne Valley Road and by the Poached Egg Trail, which leads to the Raccoon Brook Hills Trail.

The Pine Meadow Trail follows a pipeline along the north side of the lake. That pipeline, which can be followed all around the lake, ends at a never-used septic tank on Christie Brook.

About halfway along the lake, the Pine Meadow Trail passes the ruin of a stone building. It often is supposed that this was the famous Conklin's Cabin. Actually, this building was built in 1936 as a pumphouse. (Palisades Interstate Park News Release, 3/11/36). The pumps there were to fill the reservoir which had been built on the hilltop, north of the lake.

Conklin's Cabin was in a clear, flat area about 0.2 mile east of the pumphouse ruin. It stood next to a black walnut tree which still is growing there, but no trace of the cabin remains. Around the base of the tree, remnants of an old wire fence can still be seen. The fence was put around the cabin in the fall of 1936, to preserve it. In spite of the fence, the cabin had been ruined by 1942 (*Walking News*, Nov. 1942). A small cow barn was behind the cabin, built against a rock. One stone wall of the barn can still be seen.

Across the lake and a little to the west was the James Conklin farm and orchard. A CCC camp was erected there in May 1933 (*N.Y. Post*, 6/23/33). On a knoll above the lake, about 0.1 mile west of the CCC campsite, is the James Conklin cemetery. It has been reported that there are eight known graves there, as well as a number of unmarked ones. Ramsey Conklin was buried there in 1952, but his grave has no head-stone.

In the lake nearby is an island where (it has been said) there is a graveyard of the Starr family. Also in the lake, slightly to the west of Conklin's Cabin site, there was a tiny island. Nowadays, this island is visible only when the water level is low. In 1934, when the dam had been built and the lake began to fill, Ramsey Conklin protested that the water would cover the 19 graves there, including those of his mother and father. So John Tamsen, the Superintendent of the New York Division of the Park, built a pyramid of earth above the grave site, covered the sides of the mound with stone rip-rap, and planted some laurels on the top (*N.Y. Post*, 6/9/37). When the lake had filled with water, the little graveyard island could still be seen. Wind and water, however, have since lowered it to the lake level.

The history of Pine Meadow is the history of the Conklin family. The first Conklin to arrive was Nicholas (1661-1747). Cole's *History of Rockland County* shows Nicholas Conklin owning 200 acres at Pine Meadow in 1724. Those 200 acres (all of Pine Meadow) were granted by the State of New York on December 5, 1800 to Nicholas N. Conklin, by payment of $100 and the improvement of the property. The improvement was Conklin's Cabin, built there in 1779 by Nicholas' brother Matthew.

In 1895, Nicholas N. Conklin's grandson James Conklin (1866-1940) inherited 60 acres on the south side of the meadow. He eventually sold his land to Nicholas Rose for $800 in 1902. Rose in turn sold it in 1906 to Bessie Gillette, wife of a Sloatsburg doctor. (Actually, it was transferred to the doctor in payment for medical bills.) It was James Conklin who persuaded the CCC not to destroy the family cemetery on the knoll. He and his two wives are buried there.

Matthew Conklin, who had the farm on the north side of the meadow, married an American Indian woman named Phebe Jane. Their eighth child, Stephen Conklin (1815-1902), left his farm and cabin to his son Ramsey (1873-1952).

Ramsey became well known to hikers, starting in the 1920s. When the Brooklyn Boy Scouts, led by Archibald Shorey, visited the cabin in 1923, Ramsey's mother Hannah Marie was still living there, although his father had died in 1902 (Adirondack Mountain Club *Cloud Splitter*, Sept. 1973). Ramsey had three sons: Theodore (Dory), Nicholas and Stephen. In 1933, both Nick and Steve were married and had daughters, 14 and 3 years old.

So, when the Park began to build the lake, eight people were living in that two-room cabin. Like his father, Ramsey made what little money he needed by weaving baskets, called "bockeys." These baskets had been much used in times past to carry charcoal out of the hills to the iron furnaces at Greenwood (Arden). Now they were sold to tourists in New York City. Other saleable items were whittled wooden scoops for handling gunpowder in World War I, and boat bailers that floated. The mountain people brought those things down to Pincus Margulies' store in Ladentown, and Pincus sold them in New York City.

As early as 1922, Major Welch had planned a lake at Pine Meadow. A great deal of free labor became available when the Civilian Conservation Corps was formed in 1933. In May of that year, Camp SP-2 was set up in Pine Meadow on the old James Conklin farm. The construction materials were transported by trucks which went over Diamond Mountain on the western branch of Woodtown Road. That road went across the

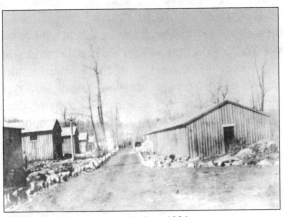

CCC camp at Pine Meadow Lake – 1934

south end of a swamp on Christie Brook (later, Lake Wanoksink) and joined the north-south Woodtown Road which crossed the meadow just west of Ramsey's cabin.

Two hundred men went to work to clear trees and brush from the meadow, and to build a 650-foot core-wall dam. By September 1934, they had built 8.5 miles of roads (Pine Meadow Roads, East and West), eleven buildings, an incinerator on Diamond Mountain, a small camp on Pine Meadow Road East, and the dam.

Camps were also built for Lake Wanoksink (SP-20) and for Lake Minsi (SP-21), and all the crews built the water/sewer system around the three lakes as well as the two concrete reservoirs nearby. That system was to serve 35 camps which were to be built by the Works Progress Administration.

Needless to say, life was pretty hectic for Ramsey Conklin in those days. His sons joined the CCC and worked on the new dams. By 1934, when the lake began to fill with water, Ramsey knew he would have to leave. Major Welch said that he and his family could stay as long as they liked, and that their cabin would be repaired, but, of course, the lake would cover their fields and their spring. Apparently, Ramsey did not have a deed to his land. In 1931, the Park Commission paid New York City lawyer Philip Poger to search for such a deed, but he found none.

On February 15, 1935, the Conklins left their 29 acres and moved their belongings to an abandoned schoolhouse in Ladentown, at the junction of Camp Hill and Quaker Roads. A boy who had played in that schoolyard many years before (about 1830) was Abram S. Hewitt (*N.Y. Times*, 3/24/35). He later married the daughter of industrialist Peter Cooper, became mayor of New York City, and (from 1900 to 1903) served as a Commissioner of the Palisades Interstate Park. Another of those schoolboys was Walter Gurnee, who became mayor of Chicago (in those days, Mt. Ivy was called Gurnee's Corners). The schoolhouse had been abandoned since 1923.

Ramsey and his sons were disturbed by all the traffic going by their door, so after a while they moved to a shack they built on the side of Limekiln Mountain (the remains of that shack can still be seen in a clearing on the road that services the power line, just a little west of the Tuxedo-Mt. Ivy Trail). On Monday morning, May 19, 1952, 80-year-old Ramsey left home to go hunting, and did not return. Eighteen Park rangers searched for him (*N.Y. Times*, 5/22/52). Five months later his body was found by three Babcock boys, near the Second Reservoir. He was buried at Pine Meadow Lake, the last one to be buried there (*N.Y. Times*, 10/31/52). The Reverend Austin Conklin, who had been pastor of the Johnsontown church, officiated. Ramsey's son Theodore continued to live in the shack on Limekiln Mountain until 1963 when the Park acquired all the land along the Ramapo Rampart and evicted the last of the mountain people.

Queensboro Lake

Queensboro Lake was created in 1915 by building a dam on Queensboro Brook, which runs north, parallel to Seven Lakes Drive, from Lake Nawahunta and Silvermine Lake. The lake, which is about 20 feet deep, is also fed by brooks from Beechy Bottom (Anthony Wayne Recreation Area) and from Turkey Hill Lake. Queensboro Lake is a reservoir that serves Bear Mountain (and, formerly, West Point). Just below the dam, on Fort Montgomery Road, is a water filtration and purification plant which was built in 1929. In 1930, an aqueduct was built along Popolopen Brook to carry water from Queensboro Lake to Bear Mountain. Another pipe was laid about 1954 to bring water to the new Anthony Wayne Recreation Area.

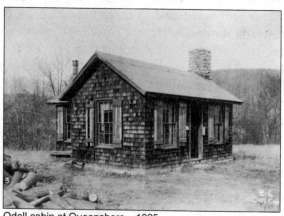

Odell cabin at Queensboro – 1925

Near the lake is a road junction, now known as Long Mountain Circle. At the time of the American Revolution, this was Queensboro, a road center and the site of several farms. On June 2, 1774, Rivington's *New York Gazetteer* advertised for sale "2000 acres, known as Queensberry. Owner Moses Clement. There are a good frame house, large garden, meadows for 50 head of cattle, three tenant houses, landings on the river at Popolopen Kill (the road to the furnace of Dean) or on the west side of Salisbury Island [Iona Island] — a good cart road to Queensberry (the Doodletown Road)."

In 1920, there still was a little red schoolhouse at Queensboro Junction which Major Welch was trying to acquire (Memo of Major Welch to Edmund Brown, 6/15/20). Nearby was the graveyard of the Weyant and Brooks families, who owned much of the land around Queensboro. The little schoolhouse was finally acquired in 1927 (*N.Y. Times*, 11/20/27). The present road interchange was completed in September 1959.

The large home of the Brooks family stood near Long Mountain Circle, not far from the new lake. In 1919, it was made available to organizations, and was called Camp Quannacut. It was occupied in April-May 1924 by the new (1922) Adirondack Mountain Club. The new (1923) Westchester Trails Association also used Camp Quannacut in February 1924 (*N.Y. Post*, 1/14/24). To visit Camp Quannacut, take the Park work road off Long Mountain Circle. Turn right, to a work area where there are sand piles. The very first dirt road on the left goes up to a level area now used as a dump. On the hillside, in the bushes, is all that remains of the

Brooks house, Camp Quannacut. In the brambles just beyond is all that remains of their latrine.

Reynolds Pond

Reynolds Pond is a small pond in the northwest region of the Park. It is just to the northeast of Summit Lake Road, about 0.1 mile before that road ends at the fence on Route 6. (It is shown as a swamp on the 1995 edition of the Conference map.) Until 1964, a 16-acre parcel of land that started down at the highway was owned by Harold G. Reynolds, a heating oil dealer who lived in Central Valley. Sometime before 1945, Reynolds had one of his employees (a young man named Bailey, descended from the residents of Baileytown) build an earthen dam with a backhoe. Reynolds then built a summer bungalow near the lake. The remains of the bungalow can still be seen, near the stone wall above Summit Lake Road. In November 1964, the Park acquired Reynolds' land and pond for $31,500.

Lake Sebago

Lake Sebago was created by the construction of Dam #10 where Johnsontown Road crossed Stony Brook. The dam was begun in 1923 and completed early in 1925. A 1,000-foot wingdam was also built at that time.

Before the lake was built, the great Emmetfield Swamp filled the valley. Stony Brook ran south, through Johnsontown. Whitney Brook, which ran along the east side of Brundige Mountain, joined Stony Brook oppo-

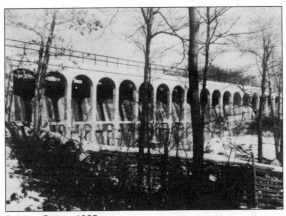
Sebago Dam – 1925

site the present American Canoe Association Camp. At the junction of the two brooks, about 200 feet from either shore of the present-day lake, there was a saw-mill owned by George Blanchard. Scuba divers from the Canoe Association dock can still see that mill on the lake bottom. The bridge across Stony Brook, 1,000 feet downstream from the mill, was named the Burnt Saw-mill Bridge.

When the dam was built, the old bridge was re-moved. At the same time, the Park improved the old Johnsontown Road from Sloatsburg and renamed it Stony Brook Drive. It crossed the top of the new dam, and went along the wingdam. In 1926, the new lake was flooded and named Sebago, which is the Algonquin word for "big water" (*N.Y. Times*, 7/6/26).

In 1925, Ruby Jolliffe, the Director of Park Camps, asked the new Adirondack Mountain Club (formed in November 1922) if they would like to build a camp on the lake. They were enthusiastically in favor and, under chairman Frank Oliver, chose a site on the west side of the lake. The camp was opened on April 10, 1926. About 1930, they named their camp "Nawakwa," which means "in the midst of the wilderness." The Adirondack Mountain Club still occupies Camp Nawakwa.

In 1928, the Park built a camp, not far from the dam, for the Rogers Peet Co. The camp, originally known as Camp ROPECO, was taken over in 1933 by the American Canoe Association, and is still maintained by that group.

In 1927, Baker Camp was built on Lake Sebago for the employees of four New York City banks (First National, Bankers Trust, U.S. Trust and N.Y. Trust). For this purpose, George F. Baker, Sr., President of the First National Bank, donated $100,000 to the Park Commission in 1925. (He had given $50,000 in 1909 and $100,000 more in both 1917 and 1920.) George F. Baker, Sr. died on May 2, 1931, at the age of 91. In 1986, Baker Camp was turned over to a concessionaire, and it is currently operated as a camp open to the public.

In 1927, New York University opened a camp on the east side of Lake Sebago. They used it until 1961. Since 1962, it has been called Sebago Cabin Camps, and cabins can be rented by interested persons.

On the east side of Brundige Mountain, not far from Baker Camp, there is a cave. In the old days, this was called Emmet's Cave, and it was believed to be the home of a witch named Auntie Emmet. She was said to be able to change herself into the form of a toad, and wayfarers were warned not to kick a toad lest it turned out to be Auntie Emmet, who could suitably punish the thoughtless one.

Around 1900, a man named Conklin who was traveling toward Johnsontown was robbed and murdered. His body was hidden in Emmet's Cave. Many years later, a local farmer named Schoonover, who lay dying in the hospital, confessed to the murder. Schoonover's farm was where the present Pine Meadow Road meets the Cranberry Mountain Trail.

In 1928, facilities for motor camping were built in the flat area by Stony Brook below the dam (*N.Y. Times*, 5/15/28). By 1931, there was a comfort station there and space for 250 cars. The remains of that camp can still be seen.

In 1931, a beach area was constructed near the present hikers' parking area. Two rustic buildings were erected, and 70 concrete tables and benches were installed. That "Old Sebago Beach" served until 1952 when "New Sebago Beach" was opened at the north end of the lake, where Johnsontown had once stood. A roller rink was built there in 1957.

When the new Seven Lakes Drive was opened from Sloatsburg in 1962, the road no longer crossed the wingdam at the southern end of the lake. That section of the older road was closed to traffic, but was made available for hiker parking. From there, hikers had access to the Tuxedo-Mt. Ivy, Hillburn-Torne-Sebago and Seven Hills Trails. Unfortunately, vandalism at the Park building there led, in 1977, to the closing of that area for parking. Since then, hikers must park 0.6 mile north of the dam at the fishermen's launching area (next to Old Sebago Beach). The Seven Hills Trail was rerouted by the New York Ramblers in 1977, using the old Monitor Trail down to Old Sebago Beach.

Silvermine Lake

Silvermine Lake is on Seven Lakes Drive, 1.7 miles south of Long Mountain Circle and 2.0 miles north of Tiorati Circle. The Silvermine Ski Area (no longer operated as such) is adjacent to the lake, as are extensive picnic areas with ample room for parking. Swimming in the lake is not permitted. From the lake, hikers can start up Stockbridge, Black and Letterrock Mountains. The yellow-blazed Menomine Trail provides a convenient route north to Stockbridge Mountain or south to Letterrock Mountain. A wide path (the Silvermine Ski Road) goes up from the dam into the notch between Black and Letterrock Mountains, crossing the Appalachian/Ramapo-Dunderberg Trail. In 1989, the Park removed the wooden walkway across the dam. Hikers must now go down and cross the brook on stepping stones, or they may use the bridge just a bit further downstream.

When the Park was first created in 1910, this basket-shaped depression in the hills was called the Bockey Swamp. Bockey — a term peculiar to this mountain region — refers to a wide-splinted woven basket used by charcoal burners. They were made and sold by mountain people, who were themselves sometimes called "bockeys."

As early as 1922, Major Welch planned to create a lake from that swamp (*N.Y. Post*, 1/2/23). In 1926, a 30-acre motor camp was built there, with a well, tables and restrooms. During these years, beavers (which had been introduced in the Park in 1920) built a dam that backed up the water in the swamp. As a result, many trees were killed. Park workers cleared the dead trees and planted rice, which they thought would attract birds. But deer ate the rice.

Then, in the spring of 1934, Civilian Conservation Corps Camp SP-27 was set up at Bockey Swamp. By September, a 600-foot dam had been built and the new reservoir began to fill. The lake was named Menomine, meaning "wild rice." More picnic tables were installed. The old picnic area extended down the road from the present parking area.

In the fall of 1936, a ski slope and rope-tow were built on the hill next to the lake. It was named the Old Silvermine Ski Area because of its proximity to the legendary Spanish silver mine on Black Mountain. R.H. Torrey related the story of the "Lone Tinker Mine" (*N.Y. Post*, 10/6/23): About 1735, a small ship visited Caldwell's Landing (now Jones Point) each year. The

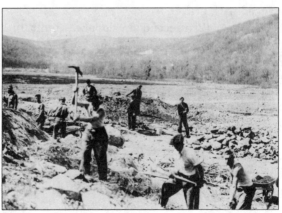

Building Lake Menomine – 1934

crew were Spanish. They made their way to Black Mountain and to a mine on its north side, near some houses of the Conklin family. They came out each time with heavy sacks. Once, in the tavern at the river, they boasted of the silver they were carrying. On their last trip, one of the crew did not return with the others. Local natives, searching for the mine, found his body in a cabin on the mountain. The crew never was seen again, and the silver mine never was found. There are two mine openings on the top of Black Mountain, but only a little iron ore came from them.

In 1934, the TERA used a section of the old Black Mountain Trail to build a fire road past Bockey Swamp up through the notch between Black Mountain and Letterrock Mountain. It was intended to be a one-way loop, but the TERA was disbanded before it was finished. This road was used for cross-country skiing. In 1955, the lower end of the fire road near the lake was surfaced with gravel.

During 1942, a second ski slope was built. In 1951, the lake was renamed Silvermine Lake. A large overflow parking area was created in 1968, but the ski area has been closed since 1986.

Lake Skannatati

After Lake Askoti had been filled with water in 1937, work began on another lake across the road, already named Skannatati, which means "the other side." This second lake needed two dams. The first was finished in 1938; the second in 1947. The lake is fed by the overflow from Lake Askoti (once the Stillwater

Creek, which ran into Lake Kanawauke) and by the brook, further to the west, which runs down from Pine Swamp.

There is a good parking area at the lake edge, much used by fishermen and picnickers. The Arden-Surebridge Trail starts from the parking area and climbs up Pine Swamp Mountain, where there is a beautiful view of the Kanawauke Lakes to the south. The Long Path, too, crosses the parking area and heads west, between the lake and the mountain.

A gentle knoll projects into the north side of the lake, and just beyond is the cascade from Pine Swamp. In 1921, when the Boy Scouts built their White Bar Trail system, their Camp Forest Ranger was located on that knoll (there were six such camps on the 35-mile trail). About 1942, the Boy Scouts marked a path from Lake Skannatati to the Hogencamp Mine. This path was adopted in 1944 by the Trail Conference for their Red Cross Trail. Later it became the Skannatati Trail, and it is now part of the Long Path.

Lake Skenonto

After Lake Sebago was finished in 1924, there was still a "Big Swamp" just over the hill on the western side. This swamp became Lake Skenonto. Available records say very little about the construction of this lake — we know only that the dam was built in 1934 and that the lake was filled with water by 1936. The old Black Ash Swamp Road, marked in 1943 as the Victory Trail, passes along the west side of the lake. The Triangle Trail comes down Parker Cabin Mountain and crosses below the south end of Lake Skenonto. Also at the south end, near a brook that comes in from a swamp, an unmarked woods road goes south for 0.5 mile to join the White Bar Trail near Dutch Doctor Shelter. There is also a trail on the east side which starts from the site of the former Boys' Athletic League camp (demolished 1993), goes over the dam and continues through the laurels to the Triangle Trail. All along the hilly west side are delightful spots for lunch stops.

Spring Pond

This little pond is 0.1 mile east of Kanawauke Circle, on the south side of Route 106. A natural pond, it was enlarged in 1919, and a pumphouse was built there to supply water to the camps on the Kanawauke Lakes. The dam was repaired in 1934.

Just across the road from the pond is a stone wall, the remains of Kiles' harness shop. On the bank above the road is a cement sidewalk — it led to the home of James and John Johnson, which had been built by B.S. Kile. Their property — a 63-acre triangular area at the junction of Seven Lakes Drive and Route 106 — was bought by the Park in 1921.

Jim Johnson worked for the Park as foreman of dam construction for Lakes Nawahunta, Cohasset, Kana-wauke, Sebago and Welch (PIPC News Release #207, 1/23/30). He was a direct descendant of the James Johnson who first settled Johnsontown in 1750. After he sold his home, he continued to live there, paying the Park $4.00 per month rent. Later, the Park rented the house to Paul and Essie Jones. It burned about 1960.

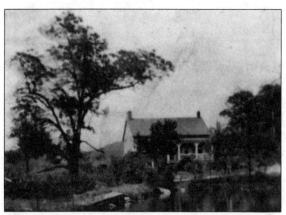
Spring Pond – 1920 (James Johnson home in background)

The county line crosses the tip of Spring Pond. Here, Orange County Route 106 ends and Rockland County Route 106 (also known as Gate Hill Road) begins.

Spruce Pond

This little pond lies in the hills west of Route 17, about 0.5 mile south of the Red Apple Rest in Southfields. A dirt road goes up from the highway, curves around the north side of 875-foot Wildcat Mountain, and leads to the east side of the pond. The pond itself is in a marshy region. There are about 15 leantos near the pond — the remains of an abandoned scout camp. In 1925, the Boy Scouts set up their Rock Oak Forest Ranger Camp here for 60 Scouts. In recent years, the camp was used for short-term camping by the Greater New York Councils of the Boy Scouts, and was known as Spruce Pond Scout Camp. It was abandoned in the early 1980s.

The region around Spruce Pond is part of the original gift of the Harriman family. The parcel starts about 0.25 mile south of the Route 106 overpass. It goes up northwest about 0.75 mile, turns northeast for 1.5 miles, and then continues southeast, coming within 235 feet of Orange Turnpike, 0.15 mile north of its junction with Route 17.

Lake Stahahe

Lake Stahahe, located on Route 106, 1.25 miles east of Route 17, is a natural lake. It is called Car Pond on old maps, but there is no record of the origin of this name. The Mohegan name STAHAHE was adopted as early as 1913 (it means "stones in the water").

Boy Scout camps were established on the lake in 1913 by Assistant Park Superintendent A.M. Herbert, who lived on the Lemmon's place in Doodletown. At that time, the area of the lake was only 17 acres — much smaller than it is now. The lake was enlarged in 1914 by the construction of three small dams (still visible below the surface). In 1918, a larger dam was completed, bringing the lake to its present size of 88 acres. A pipeline brought fresh water to the camps from Green Pond in the hills to the east (PIPC Annual Report, 1/31/19). In 1919, the camps on Lake Stahahe were used by social welfare organizations. Children were weighed when they entered the camp, and again when they left. The Annual Reports of the Commissioners proudly record the weight gains.

The height east of the lake is called Stahahe High Peak. It can be reached by a white-blazed trail that goes up from the road at the southeast end of the camps.

Summit Lake

This natural lake is the source of Popolopen Creek. In 1873, when it was owned by Elisha Stockbridge, it was somewhat enlarged by a low dam. Beers' 1875 map shows Stockbridge owning 263 acres (0.4 sq. mile) in the area. Around that time, two hotels were built near the lake by Isaac Noxon of Central Valley, and they were soon sold to Stockbridge.

The first hotel, known as the Stockbridge Mountain House, was on the mountaintop northwest of the lake. It was a very large three-story building, with verandas on two levels. In 1900, the hotel was leased by New York City doctors Whitmore and Wellwood for use as a convalescent center. The rates were $20 per person per week. After Edward Harriman bought the place in 1905, it was abandoned. Local citizens helped themselves to the contents, and the building was demolished about 1908. Hikers can still visit the spot, which overlooks Central Valley, and see the old foundation (it can be reached from Summit Lake Road; see pp. 305-06).

The second hotel was on the main road (then known as the Dunderberg Road, now Route 6) at the road which led to the lake. In 1903, Mrs. Stockbridge still owned this 30-room hotel and 35 acres, and the hotel was operated by George Weygant as the Summit Lake House. Edward Harriman bought the hotel and the surrounding land about 1905. In 1918, Averell Harriman leased the hotel to the Park. After being used for some years as a children's camp, first by the Central Jewish Institute, and then in 1923 by the Paulist Church, it was demolished about 1930. Only its foundation can be found now, in the barberry bushes across the road from the present white Park building on Route 6. (That building was moved to this site in 1965 from another location a half mile west.)

In 1915, the YWCA of New York City operated Camp Bluefield, the old Blauvelt rifle range which had been bought by the State in 1911 and transferred to the Park in 1913. Governor Charles S. Whitman visited this YWCA camp after a luncheon with George Perkins at the Bear Mountain Inn (*N.Y. Times*, 6/27/15). The camp director at Bluefield was Miss Ruby Jolliffe.

When the United States went to war, Camp Bluefield was requisitioned for army use, and Averell Harriman invited the YWCA to use his Summit Lake. In 1919, the Park built a camp on the lake, and it was occupied by the YWCA from 1920 to 1951. Ruby Jolliffe, who had made a very favorable impression on Major Welch, became Camps Director for the Interstate Park on December 1, 1920, replacing Edward Brown. In 1942, Averell Harriman gave the lake and the surrounding land to the Park.

At the northeast end of the lake, there is a pumphouse that pumps water to a reservoir on the hill above. (An older concrete pumphouse, which looks like a jail cell, can be seen on the opposite side of the lake.) A road which leads up the hill behind the pumphouse goes to the reservoir, which serves both Summit Lake and Upper Twin Lakes. On the way up to the reservoir, a trail diverges to Upper Twin Lake, passing along the way a corrugated metal shelter. Where the road turns north toward the reservoir, another fork leads southeast and goes down to the farm of William and Mary Bailey (abandoned in 1925).

At the south end of Summit Lake, an overgrown carriage road comes over the hill from the Harriman gate on Baileytown Road. Many camp buildings at the north end of the lake have recently been demolished. The entrance road has been repaved, however, and the dining hall repaired for the use of convicts from the Mid-Orange Correctional Facility who are often brought in to work in the Park during the day. For this reason, the north end of the lake may be closed to hikers.

Lake Te Ata

Near Upper and Lower Twin Lakes, a third lake was built in 1927. For want of a name, the Girl Scouts there called it "Triplet Lake." The Park authorities, however, preferred Indian names. They decided that the new lake should be called Te Ata, which in the Chickasaw language means "bearer of the morning," or "the dawn."

During the 1920s, Camps Director Ruby Jolliffe and Park Manager Major Welch became acquainted with a young Indian woman named Te Ata. In 1929, they invited her to tour the children's camps in the Park. She sang Indian songs and related Indian legends. In this way, Te Ata became acquainted with Eleanor Roosevelt, wife of the Governor, who often visited the camps in the Park.

On the evening of July 11, 1932, at Camp Paterson (LT-6), Mrs. Roosevelt dedicated Lake Te Ata with a bottle containing water from each of the lakes in the Park. Several thousand campers were present. Speakers included Major Welch; Frederick Sutro, Park Executive Director; and Miss Ruby Jolliffe, Director of Camps. Te Ata, the Chickasaw princess, came down the lake standing in the front of a canoe (*N.Y. Times*, 7/12/32).

Te Ata was born Mary Thompson in Emet, Oklahoma in 1895 and grew up in nearby Tishomingo, the capital of the Chickasaw nation. After graduating from Oklahoma College for Women, she studied for a year at the Theater School of the Carnegie Institute in Pittsburgh. She appeared on the New York stage as Andromache in *The Trojan Women*, and became proficient at interpreting Indian songs, stories and dances. Through her work in the Harriman Park camps, she became acquainted with Governor and Mrs. Franklin D. Roosevelt, performing for them at the Governor's mansion in Albany. When President Roosevelt gave his first state dinner for British Prime Minister Ramsay McDonald in the spring of 1933, "Princess" Te Ata was on the after-dinner program.

On September 28, 1934, Te Ata married Dr. Clyde Fisher (he was 17 years older than she), who was the curator of the Hayden Planetarium. They lived together until his death on January 7, 1949. Te Ata was invited to appear before King George and Queen Elizabeth on July 1, 1939 (*N.Y. Herald Tribune*, 6/5/39). Her last performance in the Park camps was in 1946. After Dr. Fisher's death, she returned to Oklahoma, where she lived in Moore, a suburb of Oklahoma City. There she continued to lecture and perform. On Statehood Day, November 16, 1958, Te Ata was inducted into the Oklahoma Hall of Fame, and on September 18, 1987 she was proclaimed a "State Treasure" at the Governor's Arts Awards (*Sunday Oklahoman*, 9/13/87). She died on October 26, 1995 at the age of 99.

Despite its auspicious beginning, Lake Te Ata was not used by the Girl Scouts in the years that followed, and no camps were ever built on its shores. The Twin Lakes Regional Museum is situated on the hill overlooking the lake.

Lake Tiorati

Before the Lake Tiorati dam was constructed, there were two ponds at the site of the present-day lake: Cedar Pond, half a mile long, which is the northeast end of the present lake; and Little Cedar Pond, a bogencircled mud hole at the southwest end. When the dam was completed in May 1915, the water level was raised twenty feet, and the two ponds became one.

William Thompson Howell, in his diary *The Hudson Highlands* (Sept. 1910), described Cedar Ponds as originally one glacial lake, which gradually filled with silt and became two lakes. In 1765, when Peter Hasenclever came looking for iron ore, he journeyed up the road from Stony Point that had been made in 1760. He opened a mine not far from Cedar Ponds Brook, and bought 1,000 acres of Great Mountain Lot #3 of the Cheesecocks Patent, which included part of Cedar Ponds. To provide power for an intended furnace, he dammed the outlet of the ponds and created one large lake. After Hasenclever abandoned his project in 1769, the property passed through many hands. An iron furnace was erected on the brook in 1800.

In 1844, William Knight of Stony Point bought the lake. He broke out the dam, restoring the two ponds, and raised vegetables on the mud flats around the edges. (In 1910, the local settlers still remembered the fields of rye, buckwheat, corn and onions which grew in the flats.) Below the site of the dam, Knight built a chemical factory to produce pyroligneous acid — a mixture of acetic acid and wood alcohol, made by the destructive distillation of wood. When added to iron ore, it formed "iron liquor," a mordant used in calico printing by the textile mill in nearby Garnerville.

In 1915, the Park bought the Cedar Ponds from the Rockland County Realty Co. and built a new dam, creating what was then known as Lake No. 2. At that time, Cedar Ponds Brook (Tiorati Brook) was a source of water for the Town of Haverstraw. In 1921, after Haverstraw built a filtration plant on the brook, the Park began to move its youth camps from Hessian Lake to the Cedar Ponds area (PIPC Annual Report, 1/31/22).

When asked about names, the American Scenic and Historic Preservation Society favored "Cedar Lake" as the name for Lake No. 2. Nevertheless, Major Welch's Mohegan name TIORATEE, meaning "blue like the sky," was adopted by the Commissioners.

During 1915, a large double cabin was built at Cedar Ponds to house the Park engineer, forester and laborers. This cabin was made available to Trail Conference volunteers on November 27-28, 1920, when they were building the Ramapo-Dunderberg Trail. On January 1, 1923, the cabin was rented to the New York Section of the Green Mountain Club, which had been formed in 1915. They named their camp "THENDARA," said to mean "Mountain of the Gods." Camp Thendara is still used by this group, now known as the Thendara Mountain Club.

In 1922, another camp was built for the New York Life Insurance Co. on a knoll on the west side of the lake. The company contributed $25,000 for the construction of their Camp NYLIC. In 1932, they gave it up, and it became Camp TERA for unemployed women (Temporary Emergency Relief Administration), sponsored by Eleanor Roosevelt. During 1936-37, the National Youth Administration used the camp; from 1938 to 1944 it was used by the Metropolitan Jewish Center. It was then demolished.

In 1935, the beach and a refreshment stand were built near Tiorati Circle. At present, Lake Tiorati is extensively used for group camping and public recreation.

Turkey Hill Lake

Turkey Hill Lake nestles in a valley bounded by Long Mountain on the west, Summer Hill on the south, and Turkey Hill on the east. The valley was once called Curtis Hollow, and there was a Curtis Hollow Trail which went north from Route 6, passing to the west of Summer Hill and along the west side of the swamp in the hollow. That trail is now part of the Anthony Wayne Trail. The Popolopen Gorge Trail goes along the southern side of the present lake.

In April 1933, Civilian Conservation Corps Camp SP-1 was set up on the Van Wart farm, near the Mica Mine on the Beechy Bottom East Road. Those 200 young men were assigned to build a new reservoir at Turkey Hill. First they built the Summer Hill Road around the east side of Summer Hill to the dam site and beyond, a total of 1.4 miles. By April 1934, they had cleared the swamp and finished the road and the dam.

At first, the new lake was called Curtis Lake (*Paterson Morning Call*, 7/10/36). R.H. Torrey proposed the name "Shikenumpak," which is Lenape for Turkey Hollow (*N.Y. Post*, 4/4/36). The name "Turkey Hill Lake" first appeared on the Park's 1937 trail map.

The water which goes over the dam continues down the brook into the Queensboro Lake reservoir. The pipes that are seen hanging over the dam were installed during a period of low water, to enable water to be siphoned over into the brook.

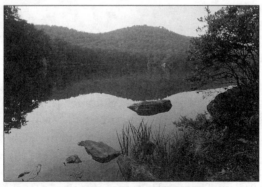

Long Mountain reflected on Turkey Hill Lake

Upper and Lower Twin Lakes

Upper and Lower Twin Lakes are natural bodies of water that were somewhat enlarged by dams built about 1850. They are the headwaters of Popolopen Brook, and drain northward through Brooks Hollow to Mine Lake, a pretty lake visible from Route 293 on the way to West Point.

In 1918, the Park acquired Lower (North) Twin Lake, with two camp buildings and a tenant house. In 1919, the Park purchased Upper (South) Twin Lake and the 30 acres around its shore from William Weygant. That sale included a house and five furnished cottages. In 1924, Charles Bailey sold to the Park 100 acres on the hillside west of Upper Twin Lake, and 73 acres south of that (an old farm, now covered by barberry bushes) was sold to the Park in 1925 by Mary Bailey. In 1930, the Park bought 170 acres on the southwest side of Baileytown Road (adjacent to Stockbridge Mountain) from Samuel Bailey. That parcel included the family cemetery.

The Dunderberg Lodge, owned by Mrs. R.H. Green in 1903, was located where Baileytown Road reached the road from Central Valley (Route 6, then known as the Dunderberg Road). The lodge and the surrounding 250 acres were acquired by Averell Harriman in 1918 and leased by him to the Park.

The region around Upper Twin Lake was called Baileytown. In 1930, when the Park acquired the last Bailey properties, the family was permitted to remain in their homes for the rest of their lives. In 1942, Lester Bailey died while hunting raccoons nearby (*N.Y. Times*,

11/2/42). He was 72 years old. The last surviving member of the family was Lester's cousin Irving Bailey, a recluse. On Christmas Day 1947, he died alone in his home, aged 59.

When the Commission bought the Bailey properties, a search was made of the titles to lands in the area. It was then discovered that the area had once been owned by Peter Hasenclever, the engineer for an English mining company. The first conveyance is entitled: "The Colony of New York, to Peter Hasenclever, Letters Patent, Dated March 25, 1767, Recorded in the Office of the Secretary of State, Book No. 14 of Patents, page 201." This patent covered 1,000 acres lying between the Ludlow patent northwest of Baileytown, toward Popolopen Pond, and 4,000 acres granted to the children of Richard Bradley (who was formerly Attorney General of New York) (Park News Release #261A, 2/9/31).

In the summer of 1924, the recently organized Adirondack Mountain Club rented a two-story farmhouse on Upper Twin Lake — one of the Weygant buildings. They named it Camp Bluebird (UT-10). To get to their camp, those members who didn't have cars had to walk four miles up from Central Valley. They used that camp for two years until the spring of 1926, when they opened Camp Nawakwa on Lake Sebago.

The camps on Upper and Lower Twin Lakes have been in continuous use since 1918. At present, they are used by various Girl Scout councils, by the YMCA and by "Homes for the Homeless."

Lake Wanoksink

Lake Wanoksink is on the Ramapo plateau, 0.2 mile north of Pine Meadow Lake. Wanoksink, and unfinished Lakes Minsi and Oonotookwa, were built on Christie Brook, a tributary of Pine Meadow Brook. Christie Brook is named for the Christie family who had a sawmill in 1850 on the headwaters of the brook, at the junction of Woodtown Road and Pine Meadow Road East.

Before 1933, the brook there ran through a swamp. A wagon road came through the notch between Conklin and Diamond Mountains, turned south down the valley, crossed Christie Brook, and then went across the south end of the swamp. There it met a north-south road called Woodtown Road. From that junction, Woodtown Road went south across Pine Meadow, through the old James Conklin farm, and on down Torne Valley to Ramapo.

In the fall of 1933, Civilian Conservation Corps Camp SP-20 was built where the road came down from Diamond Mountain. Its foundations still can be seen there, in the laurels just east of the road. Two hundred young men started to build an 850-foot dam across the east end of the swamp. At the same time, the men from Camp SP-2 at Pine Meadow built a 300-foot dam across the notch that had carried the Woodtown Road. Camp SP-21 also built a 113,000-cubic-foot concrete reservoir on a hilltop east of the new lake and north of Pine Meadow.

The lake called Christie Brook No. 1 was finished in 1934 and named Lake Wanoksink. According to Major

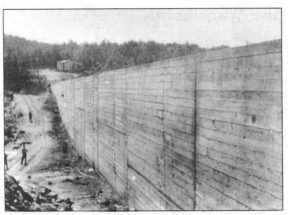
Wanoksink dam – 1934

Welch, this meant "place of sassafras" in the Mohegan language. The mile-long section of Woodtown Road north of the new dam was renamed Conklin Road by Bill Hoeferlin in 1945.

As with Pine Meadow Lake to the south and Lake Minsi to the north, pipelines and reservoirs were installed around the lake to serve the children's camps that were never built. Once the Great Depression ended and World War II had been won, there was no longer a need for more children's camps in Harriman.

Lake Welch

Lake Welch was started in 1928, on a large swampy area which had been dammed by beavers long before. It was then known as Beaver Pond. State Route 210 (now County Route 106) crossed the region over a slightly higher area where there were five homes. The community of Sandyfield, where there were about 25 more homes, was located on high ground to the north and west of the swamp. Sandyfield had been founded about 1760 when the first road through the hills had been built from Stony Point to Central Valley. Hikers now know this road as the Hasenclever Road.

Soon after the Park was created in 1910, the Commissioners notified residents of Sandyfield that the Park wished to acquire their homes. The residents resisted. They had an early supporter in the Reverend Mytton Maury, rector of St. John's Church (*N.Y. Times*, 8/16/14). In 1927, the Park began to plan a lake for the Beaver Pond site. The dam was completed in 1929. Apparently, it was not high enough, because a new dam was started in 1934 using workers from CCC Camp SP-26. Sandyfield residents, who opposed the construction of the dams, petitioned Governor Lehman and President Roosevelt to abolish the Park Commission (*N.Y. Times*, 11/22/34).

In 1939, the Park ordered residents Fred Odell, Albert and Aaron Baisley, and Sarah Benson to move out. The residents finally moved out in 1942. The new road around the lake was completed on October 11, 1942, and the lake began to fill with water. There was a cemetery (about where the beach is now) which would be flooded by the lake. The graves and gravestones were all removed to a cemetery in Stony Point.

On October 6, 1947, the new lake was dedicated in memory of Major William A. Welch, General Manager of the Park, who had died in 1941. In 1953, family camping began on the site of the earlier CCC camp. And on June 15, 1962, a new beach and bathhouses were opened to the public.

Where St. John's Road meets Gate Hill Road (old Route 210), an unused road leads down to the lake. Along that road there is a memorial to Major Welch. From the memorial, a gravel road goes along a hillside above the lake. Near the start of this road, there is a plaque which marks the site of the Sandyfield school. Further along the road, near a refreshment building, is the Odell cemetery. (The Odell home was flooded by the lake.) The road continues past picnic areas to the north end of the lake.

The Unfinished Lakes

Lake Minsi

For many years, hikers visited an unfinished lake, northeast of Lake Wanoksink and near Conklin Road. This was Lake Minsi, called Christie Brook No. 2 when work on it was started in 1934. Civilian Conservation Corps Camp SP-21 was built on the high ground just north of a swamp on Christie Brook. The CCC boys cleared the swamp and built a 500-foot dam, but the dam was never finished by filling both sides with rocks and earth. On a low hill west of the lake, a 141,000-cubic-foot concrete reservoir was built. Around the lake went the water and sewer pipes that were to serve the camps that never were built.

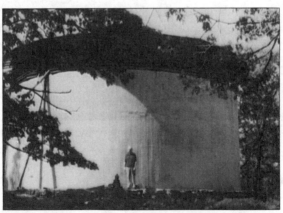

Reservoir at Lake Minsi – 1975 (shows Al Mastrodonato, who helped build it in 1934).

In fact, the men of the three CCC camps built a water and sewage system all around Pine Meadow, Wanoksink and Minsi Lakes. The water was to come from the reservoirs; the sewage was to go to a great septic tank on Christie Brook just above its junction with Pine Meadow Brook.

A letter from Park Manager W.A. Welch, dated March 9, 1935, to Conrad L. Wirth, Assistant Director of the National Park Service, explained why the work was not finished. Major Welch requested the withdrawal of CCC workers from Bear Mountain/Harriman State Park because the State could not supply the funds that would be needed to maintain the camps which were to be built. (Although work here was suspended, some other Park CCC camps were continued until 1942.)

Sometime after the work was suspended, the drainage pipe at the dam became clogged, and the lake actually was partly filled. The dam, however, was always a hazard. In 1984, it was destroyed, and the lake was drained. At the north end of what was formerly the lake, the old road which the CCC boys took to their camp is once again visible.

The name Minsi means "stones piled together." It is also the name of the Indian tribe that inhabited this area until they were driven away by the Dutch, and later by the English.

Lake Oonotookwa

A third lake on Christie Brook was also begun in 1934. At first called Pine Meadow No. 2, it later was named Lake Oonotookwa, meaning "place of cattails." The lake was to be downstream from Lake Wanoksink, in the swamp between Diamond Mountain and Pine Meadow Mountain. An office was built at the foot of Diamond Mountain, where the Pine Meadow Trail meets the Diamond Mountain-Tower Trail. The foundation of the building can still be seen there. A flat region was created below the camp office, bounded by a wall — perhaps for a parking area. The dam which was begun just upstream from that place was left unfinished. The great septic tank was finished but never used.

Owl Lake

In 1934, the Civilian Conservation Corps set up their Camp SP-22 in lower Beechy Bottom. Their task was to transform Owl Swamp into a lake. A concrete dam was built but, like the one at Lake Minsi, it was left unfinished when the CCC camps were withdrawn in 1935 (*N.Y. Post*, 7/12/35). For about 50 years, hikers often sat on the end of the dam and ate their lunches. Then in 1987 the Park opened the dam, and in 1988 the concrete was broken into pieces. Had it been finished, Owl Swamp was to have been named Ookwae ("bear").

Another task assigned to those CCC boys by Major Welch was to build a pair of scenic roads through the

Beechy Bottom valley, approaching each other at the two ends of Owl Lake dam. They would connect Tiorati Brook Road in the south with Seven Lakes Drive and Long Mountain Parkway at Queensboro. Some work was done on these roads, but they were never completed. (For a discussion of these roads and the extent to which they were actually built, see pp. 217-18.)

THE ROADS IN AND
AROUND THE PARK

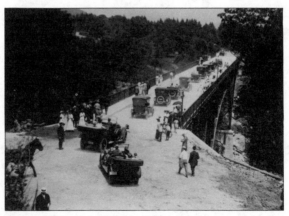

Popolopen Viaduct – July 15, 1916

Route 6 (Long Mountain Parkway)

As we know it today, Route 6 in the Park starts from the Bear Mountain Circle and runs west 8.3 miles to Route 17 at Harriman. Since it was first built, the road has had many changes.

In 1809, the Dunderberg and Clove Turnpike Company was chartered by Orange County, with a capital of $20,000. It built a road from Joshua Caldwell's ferry at the point of Dunderberg Mountain (now Jones Point), around the foot of the mountain and up through Doodletown. That old road can still be seen where it is cut by modern Route 9W, 0.1 mile south of the gate that blocks the 1907 road. The 1809 road is up on the bank, 15 feet above the present-day paved road. Still further south, it can be seen on the hillside *below* Route 9W. Hikers on the Cornell Mine Trail will step across the old road as they approach Bald Mountain. It joined Doodletown Road (where a reservoir was built in 1974), and used that road to Long Mountain Circle (Queensboro). From there, it went west to Smith's Clove (now Central Valley).

The road was improved in 1919, when Major Welch made it a 16-foot-wide gravel-surfaced road from Queensboro to Summit Lake. The line of the road was changed, too. It followed a sweeping arc up along the side of Cranberry Hill, went around a knob (where our present hikers' pull-out is now), and then made another sweeping arc south of a swamp (this arc is visible from the Long Path).

The road still was not very good, as evidenced by a letter, dated August 8, 1926, from George C. Myer,

Postmaster at Highland Falls, to Major Welch: "Sir: It is my duty to report to you that the condition of the Long Mountain Highway makes it unsafe to travel in safety with the United States mails." The postmaster mentioned stretches of bare rock, 31 ditches, and visibility obscured by high brush.

In 1930, the road was designated as U.S. Route 6, and in 1936 it was made 30 feet wide (*N.Y. Times*, 4/26/36). The 1919 line can be compared with the 1936 line on the sweeping arc west of the Long Mountain pull-out. The older route uses a little bridge at the southern edge of that wide curve, where it crosses a brook.

As one starts up towards Long Mountain from the Queensboro Circle, a Park road departs to the right. That was the old Route 6 until 1967. A quarter-mile up that road there is an abandoned motor camp on the left. Beyond there, the 1919 and 1936 roads made a big arc, crossing the present highway and rejoining it higher up.

Near the old motor camp, a woods road comes in from the right. That woods road was the original 1809 Dunderberg-Clove Turnpike. It comes down from the hikers' pull-out on Long Mountain. From there, the old road went west, approximately on the line of the present road.

The present route was built in 1965-67, and was opened to traffic on September 24, 1967. It goes up toward Long Mountain on a less sweeping curve, and cuts through a knob at the top of the rise, leaving for us that convenient pull-out.

After passing Lakes Massawippa and Te Ata, Route 6 meets Baileytown Road, which comes from Twin Lakes, on the left. There, in 1903, was the Dunderberg Lodge and a school operated by Mrs. R.H. Green. In 1851, the home of W. Van Tassel was on the north side of the road. His grandson worked for the Park in 1919, and was the last one to live in the Brooks house at Queensboro. His great-grandson Norman Van Tassel became a Park electrician and lived in the stone house at Arden Valley Road and Route 17.

A little further west, at the junction with Summit Lake Road, there is a home which is presently occupied by a Park employee. When construction of new Route 6 to the Thruway was begun on September 10, 1965, there were several houses and a service station 0.5 mile west of Summit Lake Road. All of these buildings, except one, were demolished. That one house was moved to the junction with Summit Lake Road, where it remains today. Opposite this house is a parcel of land, once owned by Elisha Stockbridge, on which a hotel was formerly located (see pp. 385-86).

Until 1967, Route 6 turned right, 0.7 mile past Summit Lake Road, and continued downhill to Central Valley (Smith's Clove). The new 1967 road goes straight ahead and, after crossing the Thruway just south of Exit 16, joins Route 17 just north of Harriman. The abandoned road now carries the Long Path down into the valley toward Schunemunk Mountain.

Route 9W

Hikers are well acquainted with the highway that passes the Bear Mountain Inn and Bridge, and crosses the Popolopen Viaduct on its way to Albany.

There was no such road in 1777, when Sir Henry Clinton's troops marched from Stony Point to Bear Mountain. Their road, then known as the King's Road, went up over the Dunderberg and down through Doodletown. The 1777 Trail now follows this route. From Doodletown, the road went down to the river level, and then continued up to Highland Lake (now known as Hessian Lake). In 1809, another road was built through Doodletown to Caldwell's Landing (Jones Point), where it met a road coming north from Tomkins Cove.

In 1907, the State built a new road around Dunderberg Mountain at Jones Point. When the new road was opened, the older 1809 road was abandoned. The *Rockland County Times* of September 23, 1909 said: "People who have never driven over the new Tomkins Cove-Highland Lake Road, and observed what a charming view of the river the new road affords, now have the opportunity." (In 1912, the road was continued down to Haverstraw.)

One man engaged in building the road around Dunderberg Mountain was John Stalter, a woodcutter who lived in Doodletown. To supply water for the construction workers, he installed a pipe from a spring (the "Stalter Spring") near the top of the mountain (see p. 221).

After twenty years, it became apparent that the 12-foot-wide river-level road was too narrow to carry the growing volume of traffic. Rather than widening that road, which would have meant closing it to traffic during construction, Major Welch in 1928 planned a southbound road higher up the slope of Dunderberg. While this new 18-foot-wide road was being built, Federal funds became available, and the "bench" was widened to 30 feet for the 2.4 miles from Iona Island to Jones Point. The southbound route to Tomkins Cove was opened in September 1931 (*N.Y. Times*, 9/27/31). Sometime later, the river-level road was closed, and the higher road was used for two-way traffic. (The river-level road is now part of the Hudson River Trail.)

When the Park was formed in 1910, the road north of Highland Lake "straggled down to a little iron bridge over Hell Hole" (*N.Y. Post*, 1/4/29). The abutments of

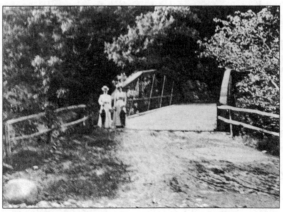

Hell Hole Bridge – 1900

that bridge are still there, on the Popolopen Gorge Trail. The Report of the Commissioners for 1914 said: "The present road (Route 3) north from Bear Mountain is one of the most dangerous in the state: coming down into the gorge of the Popolopen Creek at a steep grade, crossing the canyon in a very bad turn, and climbing up the other side of the gorge on steep grades." The report recommended that a steel bridge be built over the gorge.

One of Major Welch's first engineering projects was the construction of a new bridge across Popolopen Gorge. He started in 1915 to build the 140-foot-high steel arch, which opened to traffic on July 15, 1916 as part of State Highway Route 3 (it was renumbered 9W in 1930). In 1936, the width of the Popolopen Viaduct was doubled by building a second bridge of similar design on the west side of the 1916 bridge. In the same year, Route 9W into Fort Montgomery was straightened by the construction of still another 491-foot span over the gully just north of the Popolopen Gorge bridge.

When the Popolopen Viaduct was opened, those who strolled across the bridge could see Henry Hudson's ship, the *Half Moon*, at anchor in the mouth of the brook below.

The ship, a full-size replica of the ship that carried Henry Hudson up the river in 1609, was a gift of the government of the Netherlands. It was presented in time for the 1909 Hudson-Fulton Celebration, held in New York harbor. A replica of Robert Fulton's *Clermont* was also built, and both ships sailed up the river to Albany. On October 11, 1909, the *Half-Moon* arrived at Cohoes, just north of Albany.

After the Celebration was over, the *Half-Moon* was

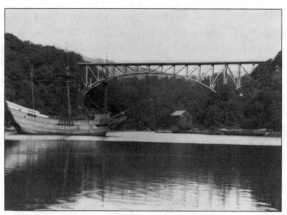

Half-Moon at mouth of Popolopen Brook

given to the Palisades Inter-state Park Commission. In July 1910, it was moored at the Englewood Boat Basin. In May 1911, it was taken to Nyack, and in 1912 it was moved to the new dock at Bear Mountain. When regular steamboat service from New York City to Bear Mountain began in 1913, the little *Half-Moon* was often found to be in the way at the dock, so it was moved to the mouth of Popolopen Brook, where Henry Hudson had anchored in 1609.

There it stayed, under the care of Park employee Captain Augustus Allen. After a few years, it began to leak, and Major Welch proposed to encase it in concrete. Then, in 1923, Daniel J. Cosgro, Mayor of Cohoes, suggested that the *Half-Moon* would be better cared for in Cohoes. He persuaded Governor Alfred E. Smith, and in April 1924 the *Half-Moon* was legally transferred to the City of Cohoes. The partly sunken ship was refloated. Its ballast was removed, and it was eased up over the West Shore Railroad tracks by two horses operating a windlass.

Before going to Cohoes, the *Half-Moon* was once again taken down the river to the Spuyten Duyvil inlet by the tugboat *Libbie Barker*. There, on September 28, 1924, a crew of ten boys from DeWitt Clinton High School, dressed as sailors, manned the ship in commemoration of the 315th anniversary of Hudson's landing at 215th Street and Inwood Hill Park.

After ten days, the *Half-Moon* was towed to Cohoes. It came to rest on Van Schaick Island, where it was surrounded by a fence. For a few years the town took pride in their historic ship. But Mayor Cosgro retired in December 1929, and he died soon afterward. The fence was broken. Teen gangs over-ran the ship. Hoboes slept below decks. Finally, on July 22, 1934, the *Half-Moon* was destroyed by fire.

An interesting epilogue to the *Half-Moon* saga occurred in March 1946. At that time, the Palisades Interstate Park Commission received a bill in the amount of $10,552.50 for duty and internal revenue on the *Half-Moon* as of July 23, 1909 (the date the ship was received in the Brooklyn Navy Yard). At that time, the ship had been accepted "on condition of bond." The bond, on file in the Custom House, apparently had been broken, so that the duty was therefore payable (Commission Minutes, 3/13/46). Exactly what happened then has not been recorded, but the minutes of the Commission meeting of October 11, 1946 state that "the Treasury Department has cancelled the bond."

In order to make the Park more accessible to the population of the surrounding region, the Commissioners also built bridges outside of the Park boundaries. In 1923, the Park built a 400-foot steel arch bridge across Tiorati Brook in Stony Point. That bridge was commemorated on May 30, 1988 by a plaque which named it the James A. Farley Memorial Bridge. Farley had been Town Supervisor of Stony Point from 1920 to

1923; National Chairman of the Democratic Party from 1922 to 1940; and Postmaster General, under President Franklin D. Roosevelt, from 1933 to 1940. In 1926, the Park built a 1,200-foot span over Sparkill Creek in Piermont, N.Y.

Another section of State Route 3 was the road around Storm King Mountain. In 1903, the State appropriated funds to build this road. But a group of financiers, disguised as a quarry company, bought the land at the river level, thus frustrating the State's plans. In 1913, under the direction of Major Welch, a new route was surveyed 400 feet above the river. Construction of the Storm King Highway began in July 1915. This highly scenic but narrow (20 feet) road was completed in September 1922. Immediately afterward, Dr. Ernest G. Stillman gave to the Park 800 acres on the south side of Storm King Mountain.

By 1937, it was realized that the Storm King Highway was inadequate, and Major Welch planned a Storm King Bypass. Construction was started in the spring of 1939, with much apprehension in the ranks of organized hikers who feared that beautiful Crow's Nest above West Point would be defaced. The present Route 9W around Storm King was opened to traffic on September 26, 1940 (*N.Y. Times*, 9/27/40).

Route 17

A road most familiar to those who hike in Harriman Park is New York State Route 17, which runs from Suffern through Arden to Harriman, N.Y.

In 1778, Robert Erskine prepared a map for General Washington which showed this road along the Ramapough River, then known as the Albany Road. A mile and a half north of Suffran's tavern, the road crossed the river (this portion of the road is now designated as Route 59), then passed Sidman's Tavern (still standing, just south of Sloatsburg — a name on the tree there is "Mapes"). It passed through Slott's (Sloatsburg), where the Eagle Valley Road went west to Ringwood. Before the Revolution, Erskine had been master of the Ringwood Iron Works.

The Albany Road crossed to the east side of the river at Greenwood (Arden). It went past June's Tavern in Smith's Clove (the site of this tavern is in the cloverleaf approach to the northbound lanes of the New York Thruway at Harriman) and Smith's Tavern in Highland Mills (on Route 32, just south of St. Patrick's Church), and continued past Schunemunk Mountain to New Windsor. Washington's troops made many trips through this valley from their headquarters at New Windsor.

Since it was the road the stagecoach took to Albany, the Albany Road was an especially significant route in the winter, when the Hudson River was closed to ships. From Suffern to Southfields, it also was the road to Goshen, the county seat of Orange County. The road to Goshen, known as the Orange Turnpike, departed from the Albany Road at Southfields, and went west, through Monroe, to Goshen.

To keep the road to Goshen in repair, the Orange Turnpike Company was chartered on April 4, 1800. Among the 67 original stockholders were Aaron Burr,

J.A. Pierson and John Suffern. In 1859, there were tollgates on the Albany Road in Sloatsburg at Eagle Valley Road, at Greenwood (Arden) and at the Houghton Farm at the foot of Schunemunk Mountain. The toll for a wagon and two horses was 6 1/4 cents.

The appearance of the valley was much changed by the building of the New York and Lake Erie Railroad. Construction began in the Ramapo Pass in 1836, and the line was opened to Goshen in September 1841.

Much of the ore used at the Greenwood Furnace (built at Arden in 1811) came from the O'Neil and Forshee Mines in the hills west of the Pass. A road from the furnace crossed to the west side of the river and turned north along the hillside. After 0.5 mile, the road went up left over the ridge to what later was named Harriman Heights Road. It reached Harriman Heights Road 0.5 mile north of its intersection with Orange Turnpike. To find the O'Neil Mine, continue north on Orange Turnpike for 0.3 mile past its intersection with Harriman Heights Road. At a turnout where the road bends, an old road goes left to the O'Neil Mine.

In 1906, when Edward Harriman began to build his new mansion, the Arden House, he wanted the Albany Road moved to the west side of the Ramapo River, so that it would be further away from his home. In August 1909, he bought from the Town of Woodbury three miles of the Albany Road, from Arden to Central Valley. In return, he gave the town part of the O'Neil Mine Road on the western hillside and two more miles of right-of-way for a new road along the west side of the river to Turner's Junction (now Harriman) (*N.Y. Times*, 8/5/09).

This newer road — which was paved in 1911 — ran parallel to and slightly above the present-day Route 17. It continued to Central Valley, where it joined the older route north. Hikers who follow it today, on the hillside west of Route 17, will note that the pavement is surprisingly good in many places. The present Route 17 was built about 1928.

When the New Jersey state roads were given numbers, sometime before 1930, our present-day Route 17 was designated as Route 2. North of Ramsey it was known as the Franklin Turnpike. It went through Mahwah and followed the Erie tracks through Suffern and Hillburn. In 1932, a new highway was built, roughly parallel to the Franklin Turnpike. This road crossed to the west side of the Ramapo River near Mahwah, and continued through Hillburn to Ramapo, where it met the old road (now known as Route 59). In the early 1990s, Route 17 was relocated to follow the New York Thruway from the state line to just north of Route 59, and the road through Hillburn now serves local traffic only.

New York State Thruway

The Thruway is the modern Albany Turnpike through the Ramapo Pass. Construction of the 14-mile section from Suffern to Harriman was begun in the spring of 1953, and it was opened to traffic on May 27, 1955. Needless to say, the Thruway brought many changes to the hikers' familiar trails.

In Sloatsburg, the northern branch of Johnsontown Road to Dater's Crossing (now known as Washington

Avenue) was cut off, and the road was relocated to pass under the Thruway. In Tuxedo, the Kakiat Trail had crossed the Ramapo River on a footbridge south of the railroad station, and had gone directly uphill, south of the Italian Village. After May 1955, the approach to the Ramapo-Dunderberg, Tuxedo-Mt. Ivy, Kakiat and Triangle Trails was through the underpass on East Village Road.

At Southfields, the old footbridge which carried the Nurian Trail over the Ramapo River had been washed away in 1946. In 1950, the Park built a steel bridge across the river, only to have the trail cut again in 1953 by the Thruway. Through the efforts of the Trail Conference, a footbridge was finally built, and it was formally opened on July 15, 1956 (see pp. 86-87).

At Arden, the new highway remedied a long-existing deficiency of Arden Valley Road, which carried the Appalachian Trail. When first built in 1930, the road followed a roundabout route which went *under* the Erie tracks and *through* the river on a concrete-paved ford (see pp. 421-22). The overpass, built in 1954, remedied that situation. Also, until 1953 the Arden-Surebridge Trail (A-SB) had come south from the Arden station, using Harriman's Arden Road. That road was cut by the new Thruway, so A-SB was rerouted along the west side of the tracks, and up the old road to the new overpass. (That route was abandoned in 1970.)

Route 106 (Old Route 210)

The road which crosses the middle of Harriman Park was formerly designated New York State Route

210. In 1982, the state turned over to the counties the responsibility for maintaining the road. The road is now known as Route 106.

Our Route 106 was chartered in 1824 as a "New Turnpike" from Monroe to Haverstraw (in those days, Southfields was called Monroe). The New Turnpike started at Roger Parmelee's slitting mill (nail factory), and it crossed the Ramapo River on a wooden bridge. (The site of this bridge is just north of the present Nurian Trail bridge over the Ramapo River — the old abutments are still visible.) The road went south about a mile, around the end of the ridge, and passed Car Pond (now Lake Stahahe). This road from Southfields is still used by hikers, who sometimes think that it was built by Edward Harriman. In fact, Harriman's Level Road (the Old Arden Road), which was built in 1894, went *north* from Southfields (see pp. 205-06).

The New Turnpike passed Little Long Pond, then went through the village of Sandyfield (Beaver Pond). Until 1870, there was a tollgate where the road started downhill (near the crossing of Minisceongo Creek) and, heading east from there, the road was known as Gate Hill Road. Downstream from the tollgate, the road divided: the right fork (now known as Old Gate Hill Road) went down to Willow Grove, where it joined the Old Turnpike to Haverstraw. The left fork, which later became Route 210, joined the road from Cedar Ponds (Lake Tiorati) and went to Stony Point (King's Ferry).

In the early part of this century, the New Turnpike was a gravel road which was known as County Highway 416. When the Park was formed in 1910, the part of the New Turnpike leading to Southfields was called

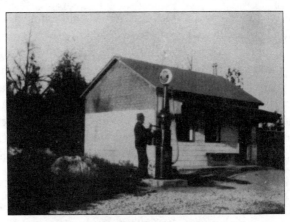

Fred Odell's gas station at Sandyfield – 1930

the Southfields Road. In 1913, it became part of the road to Bear Mountain which was later named the Seven Lakes Drive. The western section of the road was rerouted by the County in 1915 to its present end at the Wildcat Bridge. The older route, around the mountain to the railroad station at Southfields, was abandoned. The girder bridge at Southfields was disassembled and re-erected at its present location.

In 1923, a new road was built west to Greenwood Lake Village, replacing the older Warwick Turnpike. Now known as Route 17A, it was opened in May 1926.

Route 202

Route 202 is often used by hikers to reach the Kakiat and Tuxedo-Mt. Ivy Trails and the Long Path. The modern road goes northeast from Suffern to Ladentown, and then continues on a more easterly course to Mt. Ivy and Haverstraw. On old maps, it was called the Suffern-Haverstraw Highway.

General Robert Erskine's 1779 map shows a military road going northeast from "Suffran's," but after crossing the Mahwah River (near Viola) it turned east (on the present Grandview Avenue) to the hamlet of Kakiat (settlers from Long Island later changed the name of Kakiat to New Hempstead). From there the road (our Route 45/202) went north to Mt. Ivy and east to Haverstraw and King's Ferry (Stony Point).

A country road ran parallel to the Mahwah River from Viola to a crossroads where Michael Laden opened a store and tavern in 1816. That store was acquired in 1902 by Pincus Margulies of Brooklyn. In the years that followed, Margulies held various offices in the town, and bought the baskets and woodenware made by the folks who lived in the nearby hills. He died on November 15, 1952, but his daughter Hazel continued to live in the old building until she died in 1993.

In 1820, an improved road was built from "Suffran's" through Ladentown to Mt. Ivy, where it joined the older military road to Haverstraw. When roads were first given numbers, that road became N.Y. State Route 61. In 1934, it became Route 122, and in 1936 it became Route 202.

Arden Valley Road

This two-lane road runs for 4.8 miles between Tiorati Circle and Route 17 at Arden. The Ramapo-Dunderberg Trail goes up the road from the Circle for 0.35 mile to join the Appalachian Trail, which crosses the road at this point. At 0.5 mile, at a sharp left turn, the Long Path crosses. The woods road which leaves to the right was the route of Arden Valley Road until 1917. At that turn, too, an even older road once went north to Central Valley.

At 0.9 mile, a rocky path on the right leads to the large Bradley Mine. Further downhill, Upper and Lower Cohasset Lakes are passed. Then, at 1.85 miles, the road turns sharp left. Here, on the right side, a dirt road, blocked off by a gate, leads into the Harriman Estate. Until 1930, this estate road was the public road from the Erie Railroad station at Arden. After Roland Harriman gave Island Pond to the Park in 1927, a new Park road was planned. This road, opened in 1934, goes along the southern boundary of the lands retained by the Harriman family. It passes the entrance to Island Pond and further down goes by the Elk Pen hikers' parking area.

Things looked different in 1934. The road had to cross the Erie Railroad and the Ramapo River. That problem was solved by making an underpass under the Erie tracks, at the point where Arden Brook joins the Ramapo River. A ford was built there, paved with concrete. The tracks above were supported by a bridge built of steel beams which had been removed from the Tallman Mountain quarry. Stepping stones were provided for walkers.

One can still follow that 1934 road: From Route 17, go to the stone cabin near the Thruway bridge. Across from the cabin, a grassy old road goes downhill to the river level, where it turns under the culvert. The concrete pavement in the river is still visible. Now the

Thruway is on the other side of the ford, but before it was built in 1953 the road turned south for 0.5 mile, went up a bank and swung north again to the present line. The area there now used for hikers' parking was part of the old 1930 road. The wire fence of the Elk Pen can still be seen there.

Toward the end of 1919, Major Welch received from Yellowstone Park a herd of 75 elk, male and female. Actually, many had died en route, and more died soon after arrival. The surviving elk were kept in a great wire pen, between Arden and Southfields, built by Park Forester Raymond Adolph. Despite considerable efforts to care for them, the elk did not thrive. Their numbers gradually dwindled. Some could still be seen in 1935, but by 1942 they were all gone.

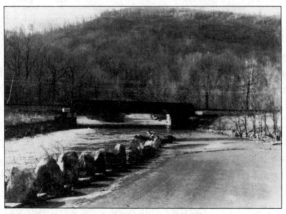

Arden Valley Road ford at Ramapo River, after storm –
March 31, 1951

Johnsontown Road

Johnsontown Road starts in Sloatsburg at the first left turn after Seven Lakes Drive passes under the New York Thruway. It goes northeast from there for 1.6 miles, parallel to the Seven Lakes Drive but on the west side of Stony Brook. The paved road presently ends at a circle (where there is ample parking), just beyond the Park boundary. The Blue Disc Trail goes up to the left just before the end of the road, following the right-of-way of the Columbia Gas Transmission Company.

Johnsontown Road once was a main Park drive which continued past the site of the present New Sebago Beach to end at old Route 210 near Little Long Pond. From the 1920s to 1962, the road was shown on Park maps as Stony Brook Drive. On November 10, 1962, after the new Seven Lakes Drive had been opened, the road was closed beyond the circle. We will describe the old road, which still is walkable.

Proceeding northeast from the circle, the road is now marked with the white blazes of the White Bar Trail. After 0.3 mile, the Kakiat Trail comes in from the left, runs along the road for 300 feet, then leaves to the right. Just beyond this point, a stone wall begins to run along the right side of the road. Here, the Matthew Waldron family once had their home and blacksmith shop. At 0.5 mile, the old road forks. The left fork, followed by the White Bar Trail, goes to the Dutch Doctor Shelter and beyond. The right fork is Johnsontown Road. It is necessary to cross the Parkway here and follow the old road on the other side. A path on the *west* side of the Parkway, carrying a buried telephone cable, once was the camp road which led to the American Canoe Association (ACA) Camp and the ADK Camp Nawakwa on Lake Sebago. A quarter mile up the camp road, on the right, was the home of the William Lewis Becraft family.

Now the old Johnsontown Road is on the east side of Seven Lakes Drive. 0.5 mile north of the Kakiat Trail crossing, the old road approaches the new Drive, but immediately swings east again. At this point, on the right, there is a wide path that leads up to the ridge above Stony Brook. In a clearing on the ridge is the cellar of a home that was built there in 1935 by Fred Koerber. In 1960, when the Park condemned his land, he had his house moved down the road and re-erected at its present location — 125 Johnsontown Road.

The old Johnsontown Road goes around a small hill and again crosses Seven Lakes Drive. 0.4 mile further

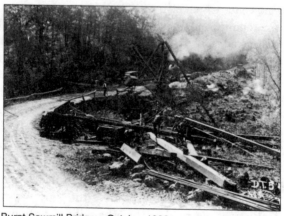

Burnt Sawmill Bridge – October 1923

on, it crosses the road to the ACA camp and follows the shoreline to the Drive, where it crosses over the dam. Before the dam was completed in 1925, the road crossed the brook on the Burnt Sawmill Bridge.

After the dam was built, the road ran along the top of the dam, then went through an area where Old Sebago Beach was built in 1932. At the same time, a car-camping area, which included a comfort station and picnic tables, was built near the brook below Sebago Dam. Today, the old road goes along the top of the hikers'/fishermen's parking area. North of the parking area, a red-blazed ski trail uses the old road. The road continues across the entrance to the Sebago Cabin Camps (formerly, the NYU camp) through a grove of young trees, and crosses the Drive 250 feet south of the gate on Pine Meadow Road. The old road crosses Pine Meadow Road, and 0.2 mile farther re-crosses the Drive and continues along the Park road leading to Baker Camp.

The old Johnsontown Road follows the Baker Camp Road for 0.3 mile, until the road makes a sharp left turn. Here, the old road continues straight ahead, past a boulder barrier. It is now a wide, grass-covered highway which ends above a cut of the modern Seven Lakes Drive. A woods road, known as the High Hill Trail, once started here. Its beginning is now marked by a cairn atop a large boulder on the east bank (see p. 296).

Scramble down now, and follow the new road around to the entrance to Sebago Beach (opened on May 24, 1952). We now are approaching old Johnsontown, where the new beach is now. But first, walk along the Drive for about 0.1 mile beyond the road leading to the beach. There, down left, in a grove of pines, is one of the Johnsontown cemeteries. There are perhaps 150 graves, many marked with plain fieldstones. Only a few have inscriptions, the most recent being the gravestone of Mary Johnson, who died on February 11, 1884, aged 75 years.

Go back and make a right turn onto the beach road, then take the first left turn. This road passes the other Johnsontown cemetery. Most of the stones here have inscriptions, the latest being Louise Johnson, 1858-1957. Now, go back to the beach road, and follow it to the parking area beyond the beach. There are several picnic tables on the hillside on the right edge of the large parking area; these tables are sitting on the old Johnsontown Road. Just north of those picnic tables, there is a short stone staircase on the right, and beyond that is a driveway that leads around to a cellar hole near a great hemlock on a knoll. This was once the home of Fred Johnson, who sold it to the Park in 1918. It was not demolished until the 1940s.

Up the road 0.25 mile from the parking area, a camp road from Lake Skenonto joins on the left. To make a circular hike of about nine miles, take this road to the Victory Trail, turn left onto the Victory Trail and follow it to its end at Black Ash Swamp, and then return to Johnsontown Circle via the Blue Disc Trail. Beyond the road to Lake Skenonto, old Johnsontown Road continues northerly for another 0.8 mile. It ends at a gate on Route 106, just west of Little Long Pond.

In 1907, the County Superintendent of Roads reported: "One new section of road was taken on during last year, that leading from Johnsontown to the Burnt Sawmill Bridge, which is known as the Diamond Valley Road. This is one of the most picturesque drives in our county, although it is little used, owing to the condition of the road. This was nothing but a poor wood road, but since it became a county road the bad places have been stoned in, and it has been widened out in many places" (Rockland County Board of Supervisors Proceedings, 4/25/07).

Johnsontown Road was described in 1923 in the first *New York Walk Book* as "a good dirt road through farming country." On the first Park trail map in 1920, the Park boundary crossed Johnsontown Road 0.3 mile south of the present Sebago Dam.

In the valley along Stony Brook close to Sloatsburg were two large farms, owned by Robert Reeves and by George Grant Mason. The Reeves' farm line started on the north side of Stony Brook, opposite the point where Reeves Brook joins Stony Brook. From there the property line went northwest to Johnsontown Road where the circle is at present. Taking in land for 0.1 mile west of the road, Reeves' line proceeded southwest for 0.55 mile, then crossed back to the brook. *All* of Reeves' land was north and west of Stony Brook.

The meadow on the southeast side of the present-day Seven Lakes Drive, where the Reeves Meadow Visitor Center is now located, was once part of a farm owned by George Grant Mason. (What is nowadays called Reeves' Meadow actually was Mason's Meadow!) Mason was a wealthy man who lived in Tuxedo Park. Born in 1868 of Scottish parents, he married Marion Peak in 1897. In 1907, Mason, who then lived in Mason City, Iowa and was superintendent of the Jim River Division of the Chicago, Milwaukee and St. Paul Railroad, learned of the death of his uncle James Henry Smith (Silent Smith). Smith had inherited $56,000,000 from *his* uncle George Smith. The fortune included a large holding in the Milwaukee Road (as the railroad was commonly known). Silent Smith who, about 1890, had built a mansion in the new (1886) Tuxedo Park, was on his wedding trip when he died in Kioto, Japan (*N.Y. Times*, 3/28/07). In his will he left $12,000,000 to his nephew George Grant Mason, and $6,000,000 to George's brother William Smith Mason. George got the Tuxedo Park home (photo in *N.Y. Times*, 9/8/07), and William got a farm in Sloatsburg which Silent Smith had bought in 1903 from a local man named Nicholas Rose. Rose had owned it since 1865. For reasons unknown, in 1908 George Mason bought his brother's farm, and used it to raise pedigreed cattle, and also fish. When his farm superintendent became ill in 1919, he decided to give his farm to the Park if they would dam the brook and create a lake for children's camps. He did give the 125-acre farm to the Park in 1921, and it was valued at $25,000 (Commission Minutes, 4/26/21).

The plan to build a lake was opposed by his neighbor Robert Reeves who, in 1915, helped form the Ramapo Mountains Water Supply and Service Co., which acquired the land north to Lake Sebago and east up to Pine Meadow. Their plan to draw water from their property collapsed when the Park began proceedings to condemn the land east of Johnsontown Road. However, because of Reeves' opposition, the Park never did build a lake on the former Mason property.

Before his death on April 30, 1955 at age 86, George Grant Mason, together with banker George Baker, endowed a new Tuxedo Park High School. Their portraits hang in the school auditorium. Mason had a daughter, Margaret Peabody, and a son, George, Jr. (1904-1970), who was a founder of Pan American Airways.

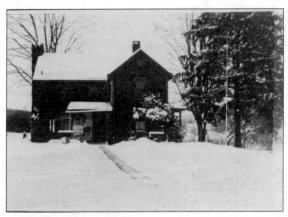
Mason farmhouse – 1925

During the years after 1922, the Mason farmhouse was occupied by Chief Park Ranger Bill Gee, who had joined the force in 1914. He continued to operate a fish hatchery there for the Park. He retired in 1941 and died in 1943, aged 74 years. After that, the farmhouse was home to John and Grace Snyder until it was demolished in 1953. The cement bridge over Stony Brook leading to the farm was demolished in 1993.

The old Reeves' farmhouse is still at 115 Johnsontown Road. It was first built about 1760 by Heinrich Bosch, a native of Leyden, Holland. Before 1917, it had belonged to Thomas Donovan. Robert Reeves bought it at auction, and eventually sold it in 1946. Since then, the 110-acre farm has passed through several owners, and is now much smaller in area.

Going north along the old road, one passes several more farm sites: the Waldron blacksmith shop (at the circle where the paved road now ends); the Becraft place (where the camp road starts); and two Waldron farms (near the entrance to Pine Meadow

Road). To the left of the ski trail as it goes through a hemlock grove is the tombstone of Abram Waldron (1819-1897). In 1917, Mary Waldron sold both family farms to the Park. Her home, which was demolished in the early 1930s, stood on the old road overlooking the present Sebago Cabin Camps. Her granddaughter Alpha and grandsons Avery and Grant are buried in the Sloatsburg Cemetery.

In 1962, the old Johnsontown Road was cut, where it turned westward, by the new Seven Lakes Drive. At the intersection where Lake Welch Drive now starts, the Johnsontown Methodist Church (built in 1872) formerly stood. The church was razed in 1950. Its last minister was Reverend Austin W. Conklin.

The village of Johnsontown was located where the beach is now, on the edge of a great swamp. In 1870, there were 30 homes, some up towards Little Long Pond, others east towards St. John's Church. (The road leading east to St. John's Church was also called Johnsontown

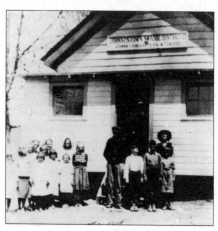

Johnsontown school – 1921

430

Road.) There were also three stores and a school. Many residents sold out to the Park in 1913; others stayed until the lake was built in 1924. Two residents who left then were Henry and Sherman Youmans. They moved to Garnerville. A story was told about Sherman, that he once agreed to "rassle" a performing bear. After a while, Sherm was heard to say, "Get this damned bear off me, or I'll kill him." The family of Muzz Jones, the last to live in Johnsontown, finally sold out in 1952.

Johnsontown was first settled about 1750 by James Johnson, of English/French descent, whose family came to New York about 1700. They made a living by cutting tall trees for ship masts. In the years that followed, the eldest son always was named James. In 1930, Jim Johnson was the construction foreman for the Park. He lived across the road from Spring Pond, just east of the Kanawauke Circle. In 1917, his daughter Mary Bessie married John Tamsen who later became Park Superintendent. They are buried in St. John's Cemetery.

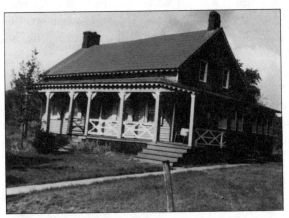

James Johnson home – 1937

Lake Welch Drive

Lake Welch Drive is a 5.6-mile road which starts from Seven Lakes Drive near the entrance to Sebago Beach, and ends at Exit 16 of the Palisades Interstate Parkway. It was opened to traffic on June 26, 1971.

At 1.0 mile from Seven Lakes Drive, a paved road on the right goes to Camp Lanowa at Breakneck Pond. That road once was part of the Old Turnpike (pre-1824) from Haverstraw to Southfields. On its way west, the Old Turnpike joined the road from St. John's Church (known as Johnsontown Road), then passed through Johnsontown (now Sebago Beach). The older road, still visible, was abandoned after Lake Welch Drive was built in 1967. At 1.45 miles, St. John's Road, which passes St. John's Church and ends at Route 106, goes off to the right. Lake Welch Drive then goes over Route 106, passes picnic areas on the right, above the lake, and, at 3.3 miles, reaches the entrances to the beach. Before the new Drive was built, the beach was reached by a road which turned off Route 106 just west of St. John's Road (that road is still open to traffic, and it provides an alternate route to the lake).

Continuing northwest from the lake, Grape Swamp is visible on the left, and the road descends a mile-long valley. The road here obliterated the Suffern-Bear Mountain Trail which once went around Grape Swamp and down this valley to Tiorati Brook. Tiorati Brook Road joins from the left, and then Lake Welch Drive ends at the Palisades Interstate Parkway.

Palisades Interstate Parkway

The Commissioners of the Palisades Interstate Park, led by George W. Perkins, were determined to make it possible for large numbers of people to reach and enjoy the Park — first in New Jersey, and later in the Hudson Highlands. In 1909, they proposed a scenic drive along the top of the Palisades. In 1914, they planned a road from Fort Lee to Storm King Mountain (*N.Y. Times*, 3/29/14). Because most of the land along the top of the Palisades was still privately owned, these plans could not immediately be implemented. In 1916, though, the Park built the eight-mile Henry Hudson Drive between the ferry landings at Edgewater, Englewood and Alpine.

In 1933, Major Welch gave the Civilian Conservation Corps the task of building a pair of roads from Queensboro south through the Beechy Bottom valley between Black Mountain and West Mountain. The north/south lanes were to join at Tiorati Brook Road and go down to Route 9W at Stony Point. Parts of those roads (which roughly parallel the present-day Parkway) were built, and are occasionally used by hikers (see pp. 217-18). Before they could be finished, however, the Corps was disbanded and the project suspended.

When John D. Rockefeller in 1935 gave the Commission 700 acres on top of the Palisades, it was possible once again to plan a highway from the George Washington Bridge to Bear Mountain (*N.Y. Times*, 6/7/42). By 1946, the surveys had been completed. Both New York and New Jersey appropriated funds, and construction began in 1947. In 1951, the first southern mile was opened, and on November 30, 1953 the section from Mount Ivy to the Bear Mountain Bridge was opened. (From the Queensboro Circle to the Bear Mountain Bridge, the new Parkway incorporated the route of the older Popolopen Drive.) On June 22, 1957, with the help of Governors W. Averell Harriman and Robert B. Meyner, the New York and New Jersey sections were joined. The final 5.2 miles, from Orangeburg to the New York Thruway, were opened on August 28, 1958. The 38-mile road had cost $47,000,000.

During those years, hikers followed the construction of the road with mixed feelings. Indeed, hikers all through the years had protested the building of roads in the Park because the construction created such scenes of destruction, and changed the familiar course of the hiking trails. For example, in 1960, as a result of the construction of the Parkway, the Timp-Torne Trail was rerouted entirely away from Bear Mountain.

As part of the Parkway project, the Anthony Wayne Recreation Area was created in 1951. The original 35 acres for bathing, picnicking and playfields were opened by Governor Harriman on Saturday, June 18, 1955. The area was expanded in 1958, but the swimming pools have been closed for the last several years.

The New York section of the Parkway is patrolled by state troopers; the New Jersey section by the Palisades Interstate Park police.

Perkins Memorial Drive

The Perkins Memorial Drive is popular with Park visitors because it enables them, with little effort, to reach the top of Bear Mountain and enjoy its views and picnic areas.

The road starts from the Seven Lakes Drive, 1.0 mile east of the Palisades Interstate Parkway. In 2.0 miles the road climbs 650 feet to the elevation 1,280 feet, where it circles the Perkins Tower (the actual summit, elevation 1,305 feet, is 600 feet north of the Tower). Just east of the Tower, a side road, now known as the Scenic Drive, descends gradually for 1.0 mile to a dead-end viewpoint. That side road once was a part of Perkins Drive, when it was a one-way loop extending from the Seven Lakes Drive to Popolopen Drive on the north side of the mountain (see below).

On the way up the road, the Appalachian Trail joins from the left at 0.35 mile. Here, on the east side, is the abandoned route of the Drive, which extends for 0.6 mile to the dead-end turnaround where the Scenic Drive presently ends. Opposite, on the same side as the Appalachian Trail, the abandoned road continued down 0.7 mile to Popolopen Drive.

At 0.85 mile, the Appalachian Trail leaves the road and goes up to the right. Here, too, the Major Welch Trail comes down from the right. At 1.4 miles, the ascending route of the Major Welch Trail crosses the road. Near the trail at this point is a stone marker which shows the 1910 boundary of the new Bear Mountain State Park. At that time, the West Point Military Academy owned a pie-shaped 50-acre piece of the north side of the mountain, across Popolopen Brook from the Torne. In 1942, the Park acquired that piece and the Torne, in exchange for land on Long Mountain and Turkey Hill which they had bought in 1928 from the Fort Montgomery Iron Corporation (see p. 79).

Perkins Drive was built as a memorial to George Walbridge Perkins, Sr., the first chairman of the Palisades Interstate Park Commission (he served in that capacity from 1900 until his death in 1920). The initial survey was made in 1923 (*N.Y. Post*, 11/5/23). The plans were drawn up by Major Welch, and the construction was directed by John J. Tamsen, Superintendent of the New York Division of the Park. The work did not actually begin until November 21, 1932, when Temporary Emergency Relief Administration workers from New York City and Orange and Rockland Counties became available. During the first year, 1,520 men worked on the project, and 764 men worked for another 18 months. The work was 95% hand labor, and the men were paid an average of $12 per week.

The 4.5-mile-long road was dedicated on October 31, 1934 by two grandsons of George W. Perkins, Sr.: George Edward Freeman and George W. Perkins 3rd (*N.Y. Times*, 11/1/34). The entrance then was on Popolopen Drive, about 0.25 mile west of the crossing of the Timp-Torne Trail (which had been blazed in 1921). The exit was on Seven Lakes Drive (as it is today).

At the same time that the road was built, a memorial Tower was constructed on the summit — a gift of George W. Perkins' widow and son. A steel fire tower which had been on that spot was removed and re-erected on Diamond Mountain in 1935. For nineteen years, until it was closed on May 23, 1953, Perkins Tower was used as a weather station and fire lookout.

In 1990, George W. Perkins' daughter-in-law and other members of the Perkins family donated $100,000 to defray the costs of producing new exhibits for installation in the Tower, and also agreed to donate $650,000 over a period of years to provide an endowment for maintaining the Tower and its exhibits (Commission Minutes, 9/24/90, pp. 16-20). The new exhibits visually relate the visitor to the surrounding topography, and also graphically recount the history of the Park and the role played by its founders. The renovated Tower was rededicated on September 18, 1992.

In 1950, Perkins Drive was closed by rock slides. In rebuilding the road, the Park engineers took into consideration the effect of the new Palisades Interstate Parkway, which was started in 1951. They rebuilt Perkins Drive as a two-way road, with a single entrance on Seven Lakes Drive. It was reopened to the public in the spring of 1952.

Popolopen Drive

Popolopen Drive is now part of the Palisades Interstate Parkway (1953) and of U.S. Route 6.

When Bear Mountain State Park was opened to the public on July 5, 1913, there was an old woods road which went around the north side of Bear Mountain, high above Popolopen Creek. The Park's first trail map in 1920 called this the Queensboro Trail. In 1923, the new Appalachian Trail went up this road for 0.5 mile from the bridge approach (the bridge was opened on November 27, 1924), then turned up the mountain on the route now called the Major Welch Trail.

Early in 1925, the Park Commission decided to build an entirely new road around the north side of Bear Mountain to meet the Seven Lakes Drive and the Long Mountain Parkway at Queensboro (*N.Y. Times*, 2/8/25). The 18-foot-wide road opened to traffic in 1927. During 1933-34, it was widened to 30 feet (3 lanes), with the help of the Works Progress Administration.

On November 30, 1953, Popolopen Drive, having been widened to four lanes, became part of the new Palisades Interstate Parkway.

Seven Lakes Drive

In 1912, after Major Welch joined the Palisades Interstate Park, he made plans to build a road west from Bear Mountain through the recently acquired Harriman lands to Southfields. Construction of the "Southfields Road" was started in September 1913, and the road was opened in August 1915. Ten and one-half miles of 10-foot-wide gravel road had been built from Bear Mountain to County Route 416 (now Route 106), where Lake Kanawauke was created in 1916. From there, the Southfields Road (which was soon renamed Seven Lakes Drive) continued west along County Route 416. The lakes it passed at that time were: Hessian, Queensboro, Nawahunta, Tiorati, Kanawauke, Little Long Pond and Stahahe. Until 1915, when the present route and the Wildcat Bridge over the Ramapo River/Erie Railroad were built, the Seven Lakes Drive turned north after Lake Stahahe, and went around the mountain to Southfields. In 1933, the Drive was widened to 30 feet.

In October 1961, bulldozers began clearing a new 75-foot-wide road north from Sloatsburg, parallel to the older Johnsontown Road (known as Stony Brook Drive from the Park boundary near Sloatsburg to the Kanawauke Circle), and crossing it in several places. When this new road was opened in September 1962, it was named Seven Lakes Drive (today, it passes nine lakes). Stony Brook Drive was closed at the Park boundary, two miles from Route 17. The remaining part of this road is now, once again, known as Johnsontown Road.

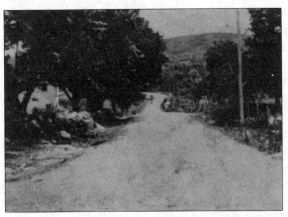

Seven Lakes Drive looking west from Kanawauke Circle – 1919

St. John's Road

Presently, St. John's Road branches from Lake Welch Drive 1.4 miles east of Seven Lakes Drive, and goes 0.75 mile to a junction with Route 106.

At the junction with Lake Welch Drive, the Long Path crosses. Further along St. John's Road, on the left, is St. John's Cemetery, and just beyond is St. John's Episcopal Church (known since the 1920s as St. John's-in-the-Wilderness). This is a mission church of the Protestant Episcopal Diocese of New York.

In 1870, an orphanage known as the House of the Good Shepherd was built in Tomkins Cove. Soon afterward, Ada Bessie Carey came to the orphanage from Guernsey, Channel Isles. She was a teacher who, in her spare time, rode a white horse into the nearby mountains to gather botany specimens. She found that there were many mountain children who could not get to a school. By 1874, Ada Carey had started a school in a log cabin for the mountain children.

This touching story was seen in a New York City newspaper by Margaret Zimmerman. She invited Ada Carey to New York City to talk about possibly building a church and school in the mountains as a memorial to her husband, who had died in Palestine in 1876. Advised by Ada Carey, Mrs. Zimmerman purchased land, and on June 23, 1880, a cornerstone was laid. Ada Carey taught in the school and was caretaker of the church until she returned to Guernsey in 1914. Mrs. Zimmerman died in 1921; Ada Carey died in Guernsey in 1925.

The first rector (who served from 1878 to 1918) was Dr. Mytton Maury, who was editor of the well-known Maury's geography textbook.

Reverend Dr. Mytton Maury was born in Wales on January 18, 1839, and was brought to New York City at the age of ten. He took his M.A. at Columbia University in 1860. Rev. Maury became a Hebrew scholar and teacher, and served as curate of St. Thomas Church in New York City for ten years. He married Virginia Draper, daughter of John Draper, the historian. They had three children: Carlotta (1878-1938), who became a paleontologist for the government of Brazil, and a geologist for oil companies; Antonia (1867-1952), who was a research astronomer at the Harvard Observatory from 1889 to 1935; and a son, Dr. John William Draper Maury.

The next rector was Reverend Burton Lee, who served from 1918 to 1928. He also served churches in other places, such as Willow Grove and Doodletown. Reverend Lee was followed by Reverend Walter Frederick Hoffman, who served from 1928 until he died at the age of 58 on February 5, 1950. In 1952, the New York-New Jersey Trail Conference solicited contributions for a Hoffman memorial window for the church. It was during Reverend Hoffman's tenure that the hikers' Palm Sunday service was started by Frank Place of the Tramp and Trail Club (*Trail Walker*, Sept./Oct. 1971). After a lapse of several years, the Palm Sunday service was started again in 1935 by Walter Shannon of the Adirondack Mountain Club.

Several rectors came after Reverend Hoffman. At present the rector is Reverend William Dearman of Peekskill.

In the nearby cemetery, some of the names on the gravestones are: Reverend Walter Hoffman (1891-1950); Ruby Jolliffe (1882-1968) (she was Park Camps Director); John Tamsen (1892-1973) (was Park Superintendent, 1915-1940); and Frank Ballard (1918-1977) (was Police Chief of Sloatsburg, 1950-1977).

Across the road from the church are a social hall and the home of the church caretaker. Fifty yards up the road, on the right, is a path which will take hikers to the Long Path.

Before Lake Kanawauke was built in 1915, St. John's Road went west from the church, past Lily Pond, where it branched. Parts of that old road can still be walked. The right branch, known as Goodspring Road, went north along Stony Brook (which later became Lake Kanawauke) and ended at the Monroe-Haverstraw Turnpike (now Route 106). In 1917, after the lake had been built, Goodspring Road was rebuilt for 1.25 miles along the shore. In 1929, when the new Stony Brook Drive was built south from the Kanawauke Circle, that lakeside piece of Goodspring Road became a camp road. The left branch of St. John's Road was known as Johnsontown Road; it went to Johnsontown (now Sebago Beach). This left branch (as well as St. John's Road itself, west of the junction with the Camp Lanowa Road) had been part of the Old Turnpike, built before 1824 from Monroe (*i.e.*, Southfields) to Haverstraw. These roads are clearly shown on R.F. O'Connor's 1854 map of Rockland County. In 1907, the County Superintendent of Roads reported that "the road heading from Beaver Pond at the Stony Point line, through to Johnsontown, by way of the St. John's Church was widened and graveled, and is now the best gravel road, excepting none, in our county" (Rockland County Board of Supervisors Proceedings, 4/25/07).

Tiorati Brook Road

Tiorati Brook Road was once called the Cedar Ponds Road, and extended from Cedar Ponds (Lake Tiorati) to Stony Point. Presently, it runs 4.0 miles from the Tiorati Circle to a junction with Lake Welch Drive, just before Exit 16 of the Palisades Interstate Parkway. Going southeast from Tiorati Circle, the Ramapo-Dunderberg Trail goes off to the left at 0.35 mile, the Lake Tiorati dam is crossed at 1.15 miles, and the Red Cross Trail crosses at 1.5 miles. After entering Rockland County at 1.8 miles, the Beech Trail comes in from the right at 2.35 miles (parking is available here), and Tiorati Brook crosses (and the Beech Trail leaves to the left) at 2.5 miles. Tiorati Brook Road ends at Lake Welch Drive, 4.0 miles from the start. The road is closed to traffic during the winter months.

Robert Erskine, Surveyor General for George Washington, did not show Cedar Ponds Road on his 1778 map, but it is shown on David Barr's 1839 map of Rockland County. The road in those days was not a good one. One correspondent remembered that in 1900, the only way to get to Cedar Ponds was on foot, or by side-bar buggy over the old road from Stony Point (*N.Y. Post*, 1/4/29). In 1907, Calvin T. Allison, Superintendent of Roads, reported to the Rockland County Board of Supervisors: "The road from Pingyp to Cedar Pond is in poor condition for a county road. This is one of the

most neglected roads in the town [of Stony Point] . . . .
It became a county road in 1899" (Rockland County
Board of Supervisors Proceedings, 4/25/07).

In May 1915, the new Interstate Park rebuilt the
Cedar Ponds dam, and in 1916 it began improving the
road along the eastern shore, widening it to 26 feet and
surfacing it with gravel. About 1931, the road was
paved from Tiorati Circle to its junction with Route
210.

In 1953, the new Palisades Interstate Parkway was
built through this area. On its way north, the Parkway
joined Tiorati Brook Road at the foot of the Pingyp.
(Coming from the southeast, Tiorati Brook Road still
joins the northbound lanes of the Parkway at this
point.) After about half a mile, the Parkway departs
north, following Stillwater Brook.

Then, in 1971, Lake Welch Drive was opened. The
Drive "borrowed" another half-mile of Tiorati Brook
Road, and the two roads now run jointly for this
distance.

THE MINES IN BEAR MOUNTAIN/ HARRIMAN PARK

There are over 20 known mines in the Park — always good places to take a group of hikers. Several of these are really only prospector holes, and more such holes without names will be seen along the trails. Much of the following information on the iron mines in the Park comes from James M. Ransom's Vanishing Ironworks of the Ramapos *(Rutgers University Press, 1966).*

For more detailed material on the various iron mines described in this chapter, see Iron Mine Trails: A History and Hiker's Guide to the Historic Mines of the New Jersey and New York Highlands, *by Edward J. Lenik, published by the New York-New Jersey Trail Conference.*

Barnes Mine

The Barnes Mine can be easily seen on the hillside north of Lake Welch Drive, 0.2 mile east of its intersection with St. John's Road. A pile of tailings shows its location. The mine can be approached by a road going uphill from the Drive, 0.1 mile further east. An old, overgrown road goes left along the hillside to the mine, which is a rather large cavity in the hillside.

The mine is on a 17-acre parcel bought in 1846 by Isaac Barnes. It probably was he who first opened a mine there, and the place was known as the "mine lot." By 1864, it belonged to John Charleston. In 1871, he leased the mine to the Rockland Nickel Company, which operated the Nickel Mine on nearby Grape Swamp Mountain. It appears that mining operations at the Barnes Mine were suspended in 1884.

The land remained with the Charleston family and was sold to the Park by Jerome Charleston in 1938. His

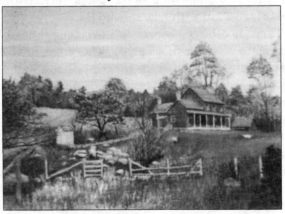

Charleston farmhouse – 1958

farm was located about where Lake Welch Drive now passes. The mine was approached through his farm yard (and that of his son Russell) from St. John's Road. That farm lane is now a private driveway just a short distance east of St. John's Church. This driveway led to a house which was owned by the Park and leased to a Park employee. Unfortunately, this house — the last remnant of the community of Sandyfield — was destroyed by fire in February 1999. Its last occupant was Dalton Stalter.

The Barnes Mine is mentioned in a book by Cornelia F. Bedell, *Now and Then and Long Ago in Rockland County* (1941).

Boston Mine

The Boston Mine is located on the Dunning Trail just east of Island Pond Road. It is 0.85 mile north of Route 106 or 0.3 mile south of the junction of the Arden-Surebridge Trail with Island Pond Road.

There is a large opening in the side of a low hill, leading to a water-filled shaft. The mine was last worked in 1880, and from the size of the dump it appears not to have been very deep. The ore was sent to the Clove (anthracite) Furnace at Greenwood (Arden) (Ransom, p. 231).

One of the "Wednesday Hikers" in 1987 told of visiting the library at Oxford University, where he asked for a book on Peter Hasenclever. There he read that ore from one mine in the Ramapo Mountains was sent to Boston, where it was made into iron products, which was then against the law.

Bradley Mine

Bradley Mine is on the north side of Arden Valley Road, about 0.9 mile west of Tiorati Circle. An eroded path goes steeply up to the mine entrance. There is no marker at the road to show the way. A vein about 10 feet wide ran for 150 feet into the hillside, then became a "pod" of rich ore about 200 feet long and 75 feet wide. The main chamber, which is at least 200 feet deep, is now filled with water.

There is a hole in the roof of the main chamber, through which light comes from above. Agile hikers can climb up there and, when they do, they discover another chamber — a limestone cave in the rock above the mine.

From 1922 to 1949, the Fingerboard-Storm King Trail went up the hillside past the mine opening and over the two summits of Bradley Mountain.

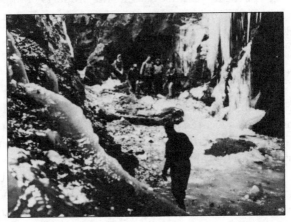

Bradley Mine – 1962

It has often been supposed that this mine and mountain were named after Richard Bradley who, in 1722, was appointed Attorney General of the Province of New York. King George II made several grants of land to Bradley and his children. These grants, however, were in the vicinity of Bear Mountain, and did not extend to Bradley Mountain.

Further study now reveals that, during the period of the American Revolution, a man named Bradley first opened iron mines on the land which in 1885 was bought by Edward Harriman (*Middletown Times Herald*, 2/24/40). Later, the land was bought at a sheriff's sale by James Cunningham of Warwick, N.Y. (Orange County Deeds, Liber N, Page 402, 9/1/1810). It was he who, in 1811, built the charcoal blast furnace which he named Greenwood Furnace.

After several further changes of ownership, the land, mines and furnace became the property of Robert P. Parrott in 1837. The Bradley Mine was worked until 1874.

Christie Mine

This mine, which is not shown on the 1995 Conference map, is located on the eastern side of Horsechock Mountain. That is the mountain to the east of Horsechock Brook, which drains the Letchworth Reservoirs.

If one follows the gas pipeline on the east side of the mountain for 0.75 mile north of File Factory Brook, another brook comes down the hill. A mine will be found in that gully, about 0.2 mile up from the gas line. A map of Haverstraw Township in the New Historical Atlas of

Rockland County (1876) shows a mine on Horse Chock Mountain, belonging to the Christie Mining Company. The mine does not appear to have been extensively worked.

In the early 1800s, the Christie family owned much land in the eastern Ramapo Mountains. They were descended from James Christie, born 1672 in Scotland, and living in Schralenburg, New Jersey about 1720.

Cornell Mine

The Cornell Mine consists of a group of mine openings at the top and on the north side of Bald Mountain. It may be reached by the Cornell Mine Trail and by the Ramapo-Dunderberg Trail (R-D). At the 980-foot level, where these two trails meet, a large depression in the earth marks the site of one of the old mine workings. Higher up, to the left of the R-D, almost at the top of the mountain, is a larger opening.

A third, much larger opening is slightly northeast of the summit of Bald Mountain, and about 80 feet down. The characteristic pile of tailings shows its location. This hole is about 15 by 20 feet in area.

The fourth opening is directly downhill from the third one, about 50 feet lower. (It is at about the same level as the junction of the Cornell Mine and R-D Trails, and may also be reached by bushwhacking a short distance west from the trail junction.) It, too, has its pile of tailings. This opening is worth a visit — it is a real tunnel, with water at least five inches deep, that goes horizontally into the hillside for about 50 feet. Bring a good flashlight!

In 1874, Minerva Herbert inherited from a previous husband a 175-acre parcel which went uphill from Pleasant Valley Road, over the top of Bald Mountain, to the cliff above the Jones Trail. This had once been a part of the 3,000-acre tract granted by King George III in 1769 to William Kempe, James Lamb and John Crum. (Minerva Herbert's grave may be found in one of the Doodletown cemeteries.)

In 1880, Minerva leased her property for twenty years to Alexander Phyfe of New York City, for the purpose of mining iron ore. In 1885, the lease was transferred to Thomas Cornell of Kingston, New York. Thomas Cornell was an affluent businessman who had been a New York State Senator in 1867-69 and 1881-83, and was president of the Ulster and Delaware Railroad. Hikers will recognize that as the railroad (now largely abandoned) that parallels Route 28 in the Catskills, from Kingston to Phoenicia, Belleayre, Arkville and beyond. In 1879, Cornell's name was given to one of the Catskill peaks by Princeton geology professor Arnold Guyot.

Cornell was also president of the Cornell Steamboat Company, which operated two dayliners and a fleet of tugboats which towed barges down the Hudson River from the Delaware and Hudson Canal (of which Cornell was a director). No doubt, Cornell wanted to carry iron ore in his barges, too.

Cornell hired a local man named Baldwin to operate the mine on Bald Mountain. Baldwin lost his eyesight in a premature explosion (this story was related by Oscar Herbert, a nephew of Minerva Herbert, who thought that the name Bald Mountain was a shortened form of Baldwin Mountain; *N.Y. Post*, 5/26/38).

Like the Doodletown Mine and the Herbert Mine, the upper two openings on Bald Mountain were probably made before 1859. The lower openings were probably made between 1885 and 1890. There is no record of how much iron ore this mine produced. It seems likely that all activity there ended in 1890, when both Minerva Herbert and Thomas Cornell died.

Cranberry Mine

On Seven Lakes Drive, 0.3 mile west of Long Mountain Circle, there is an abandoned comfort station on the north side of the road. Behind the building, a trail goes up, west, about 0.8 mile to the Cranberry Mine. To follow the trail, it is necessary to go around a gravel pit which interrupts it. The mine will be recognized by its steel door, which nowadays is open. It is a dry mine, which extends about 100 feet into the hillside.

In the early days of the Interstate Park, the mine on Cranberry Mountain was used for the storage of dynamite. Major Welch's letter to John Pratt White (then president of the New York Commission), dated April 16, 1924, described the mine: "A magazine was constructed there several years ago with a capacity of 100,000 pounds — entirely underground, dry, ventilated. The entrance is sheet iron-faced, doors of steel plate. Nearby is a corrugated steel building with a capacity of 2000 pounds." As of March 31, 1934, there were 99,500 pounds of TNT in the Cranberry Mine. In recent years, the Park's dynamite has been stored elsewhere.

Daters Mine

About 1.35 miles south of its start in Tuxedo, the Kakiat Trail turns sharply right as it goes around the southern end of Daters Mountain. A path there goes uphill from the trail, almost to Daters Mine. Climb a bit higher, and you will see a fairly large mine.

It is not known just when the mine was worked. In 1800, Abram Dater built two forges on the Ramapo River, north of Sloatsburg. The site of these forges was where the present-day Washington Avenue crosses the Ramapo River. Here, the remains of a dam, foundations and slag are visible. This bridge was once known as Dater's Crossing.

In 1812, Abram Dater was the second largest taxpayer in the Township of Ramapo (he paid $17.50 in taxes per year). He had another forge on Stony Brook, about where the Thruway now crosses the brook, and owned 2,600 acres between Stony Brook and the Ramapo River, in Rockland and Orange Counties. Abram Dater died in 1831. His grandson, George Washington Dater, operated a hardware store in 1884 across the highway from Dater's Crossing. The building is still there, occupied now by an antique shop.

Doodletown Mine

Going southeast across Doodletown Valley, the Suffern-Bear Mountain Trail leaves the Bridle Path at the foot of West Mountain. The Doodlekill is crossed 0.15 mile further southeast along the Bridle Path. About 200 feet beyond the brook, a vague old road, marked with cairns, goes uphill 0.25 mile to the

Doodletown Mine. At the end of the road, a pile of tailings may be seen on the hillside to the left. Climb this pile to reach the mine, a water-filled shaft.

Little is known about the mine. Oscar Herbert, who worked there, is mentioned in the *New York Evening Post* of May 26, 1938.

Dunn Mine

This rather small opening is located 25 yards east of the Nawahunta Fire Road, 0.3 mile from the Seven Lakes Drive. There is a hole and a short shaft in the hillside. Nothing is known about the mine except the way it got its name.

One summer day in 1973, Tom Dunn of the Westchester Trails Association was hiking in Harriman Park with his young nephew. After lunch, while Tom was trying to rest, the boy was anxious to go. Tom said: "Go find a mine or something." Not long afterward, the boy came running back, shouting: "Uncle Tom, I found one!" When that story was heard by cartographer Don Derr, the Dunn Mine appeared for the first time on the 1982 edition of the Conference map. In his *Iron Mine Trails* book, Ed Lenik calls this mine the "Lewis Mine," after the Lewis family who formerly resided on this property.

Greenwood Mine

The Greenwood Mine is located where the Appalachian Trail comes down from Fingerboard Mountain and runs along the Surebridge Mine Road. There are extensive dumps of broken stone and a large opening in the hillside. Remains of the foundation of a pumphouse can be seen near the shaft, as well as a piece of large pipe. A second pit may be seen a bit higher on the hillside.

Also called the Patterson Mine, the Greenwood Mine was worked as early as 1838, a year after Peter Parrott bought the furnace at Echo Lake (the Greenwood Furnace). The ore was used during the Civil War in both the Greenwood and Clove Furnaces. Unused from 1870 to 1879, the mine was last worked in 1880.

Harris Mine

The main complex of the Harris Mine is located on the northwest side of Arden Valley Road, 0.6 mile northeast of the gravel road that leads to Island Pond. There are two large mine openings, with piles of tailings nearby, both on private property, less than 100 feet from Arden Valley Road. This mine is not shown on the 1995 edition of the Conference map.

Older (pre-1995) editions of the Conference map showed this mine as being located southeast of Arden Valley Road, on the southern slope of Echo Mountain. Old mining roads do lead to several shallow exploratory pits in this area, but according to Ed Lenik, the main operations of the mine were north of Arden Valley Road, which was constructed long after the mine was abandoned. Lenik believes that the Harris Mine was most likely operated by the Parrott brothers to supply ore to their furnaces at present-day Arden, New York.

A column by Raymond Torrey (*N.Y. Post*, 12/29/23) was entitled, "Where Is the Harris Mine?" He confessed that he had not found it, although he did find two other mine shafts higher up on Echo Mountain.

Hasenclever Mine

The Hasenclever Mine is on the Red Cross Trail, 0.55 mile south of Tiorati Brook Road. The trail here follows the old Hasenclever Road. Peter Hasenclever traveled along that road in 1765 and discovered a deposit of iron ore. He immediately bought 1,000 acres there, including most of Cedar Ponds (Lake Tiorati). It seems likely that he had the ore transported across the Hudson to a furnace he had bought in Cortlandt, near Peekskill. In 1767, he built a dam on the brook that drained Cedar Ponds. That made one pond where there had been two, to provide power for a furnace he intended to build. Hasenclever was recalled to England before he could build the furnace.

During the Revolution and for some time afterward, the mine was operated by Samuel Brewster under lease. On June 1, 1799, Hasenclever's thousand-acre tract was bought by Jonas Brewster of Stony Point, and about 1800 he erected a furnace on Hasenclever's site. Its remains can still be seen on Tiorati Brook, above the crossing of the Red Cross Trail.

The mine changed owners many times. In 1854, it belonged to the Haverstraw Iron and Mining Company. They began to build a railroad from the mine to Stony Point. It was to run in a trench, across the road from the mine. The cars were to be loaded from the banks of the trench. The railroad was never finished, but the trench can still be seen.

The long history of the Hasenclever Mine is recited in James M. Ransom's *Vanishing Ironworks of the Ramapos* and in Edward J. Lenik's *Iron Mine Trails.* The mine, which is said to be 100 feet deep, is now filled with water.

Herbert Mine

The Herbert Mine is a sizeable pit, opened before 1859 and named for the local Herbert family. To reach it, follow Timp Pass Road up from the 1777 Trail, as shown on Trail Conference Map No. 4. About 0.2 mile from the start, a cairn will be seen on a rock to the right. From here, a road crosses Timp Brook and goes up 0.2 mile to a fork. Follow the right fork, which leads in 0.5 mile to the mine, at the 980-foot contour. Two openings can be seen above piles of tailings. The Suffern-Bear Mountain Trail is 200 feet higher on the mountain. (The left fork of the road goes through an interesting region and leads in 0.5 mile to Timp Pass.)

Hogencamp Mine

The Hogencamp Mine is on the Dunning Trail, about 0.2 mile south of its junction with the Long Path, and 0.2 mile north of a junction with the woods road coming up through the abandoned camp at Little Long

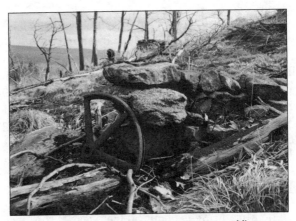

Remnants of pulley and cable above Hogencamp Mine

Pond. The largest openings are fairly narrow cuts on the mountainside. There are at least six openings, all in the line of one vein of ore. One opening is a vertical shaft about 12 feet across. Another shaft near the trail is filled with water. A six-inch pipe rises from the water. Across the trail, iron bars are fixed in a rock, and nearby is a concrete base with more bars. These were probably used to anchor machinery for pumping and hoisting.

Ore from the mine was put into buckets and hoisted over the cliff above the mine. The buckets were carried on a tramway which took them up a valley (the Long Path runs along the hill on the side of that valley) to a point on a mine road where they could be unloaded into horse-drawn carts. The stone supports of the old tramway can still be seen on the cliff above the mine, and in the valley up to the point where the Long Path joins the old mine road. Sharp-eyed hikers may also see up there pieces of the cables and pulleys that carried the buckets.

As at the Pine Swamp Mine, there was a small village near the mine. A well can be seen near the road, which was called the Pine Swamp Trail before 1943 when Joe Bartha made it part of the Dunning Trail.

The mine was worked steadily from 1865 to 1885 (Ransom, p. 237).

Mica Mine

The Mica Mine is about 50 feet west of the Beechy Bottom East Road, 0.4 mile south of the start of the Fawn Trail. It can be reached from the southernmost parking lot of the Anthony Wayne Recreation Area. From the north end of that lot, a path goes uphill toward West Mountain. Go up that path until it reaches Beechy Bottom East Road. Go south about 300 feet, then down from the trail about 50 feet. The opening is at the foot of a steep bank, just above a marshy area. Pieces of mica may be found lying about.

The mineral found around this mine is a biotite, a silicate of potassium, magnesium, iron and aluminum. It occurs in dark shining plates, often as triangular-shaped crystals.

The mine was opened in 1893. Large sheets of "isinglass" were obtained. A vein of graphite was also found there (*News of the Highlands*, 12/16/1893, 1/27/1894).

In 1920, when the Ramapo-Dunderberg Trail was being blazed, there still was a farmhouse near the

Mica Mine, the home of Park employee Paul Stout. Trail blazers E. Cecil Earle and A.B. Malcolmson boarded at the Stout farmhouse. That farmhouse had been built in 1877 by John Wesley Van Wart, who lived there until his death in 1892.

Nickel Mine

This mine is on the north side of Grape Swamp Mountain, near the crest of the ridge. It may be reached from Tiorati Brook Road by following one of the unmarked Grape Swamp Mountain Trails (see pp. 294-95). The mine is fairly large, and there are two openings, separated by about 500 feet. The east opening is larger than the west opening.

For many years, it was believed that this mine really was an iron mine owned by a man named Nichol. That was the opinion of Raymond Torrey (*N.Y. Post*, 5/26/38). The facts are different.

Before the Park was formed in 1910, Grape Swamp Mountain and Pound Swamp Mountain (where the Suffern-Bear Mountain Trail goes now) belonged to Brewster J. Allison, a resident of Stony Point. In 1871, a mine was opened on Grape Swamp Mountain on land of B.J. Allison, leased to John Sneviley of New York City. He sold his rights in 1875 to the Rockland Nickel Company. For ten years, nickel ore was taken from the mine. It was abandoned in 1884 (Cole, *History of Rockland County,* 1884, p. 330).

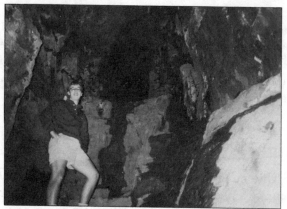
Pine Swamp Mine — passageway into hillside

Pine Swamp Mine

The Pine Swamp Mine is on the Dunning Trail, about 0.15 mile south of its junction with the Arden-Surebridge Trail, or 0.5 mile north of its junction with the Long Path. There are eight openings to the mine, the largest being the one farthest south. A dump rises about 60 feet on the hillside near the trail. By climbing over the dump, one comes to a large cut, about 25 feet wide, with high walls on each side. In the cut, there is a perpendicular shaft, now filled with water. The cut leads into a passageway tunnelled into the hillside, which runs uphill, with walls 30 feet high. An opening overhead lets some light into the passageway.

When this mine was active, there was a small village nearby, with homes, barns, stores and a saloon. The foundations of some of these can still be seen across the trail from the mine.

The mine was probably first worked in 1830 by Gouverneur Kemble, owner of the West Point Foundry at Cold Spring, New York (Ransom, pp. 141, 238).

Spanish Mine

On the summit of Black Mountain, just a bit north of the Appalachian/Ramapo-Dunderberg Trail, are two mine openings. They were first shown on the trail map issued by the Park in December 1930, and then again on the Park's 1937 map. Bill Hoeferlin named this mine the "Spanish Mine" on his June 1943 Hikers Region Map #16. (The mine is not shown on the 1995 Conference map.) Through the years it has been mistakenly called the Silver Mine, a name given in 1936 to the nearby ski hill. The legend about the Spanish seamen said that they carried out sacks of silver coins from a mine on Black Mountain (see pp. 379-80).

Surebridge Mine

The Surebridge Mine is located on Surebridge Mine Road, 0.5 mile north of "Times Square" and 0.1 mile south of the Bottle Cap Trail.

In a fairly level, tree-covered region just east of the Surebridge Mine Road there are several fairly large water-filled shafts. One is visible from the road; others are further up on the hillside. They were worked during the Civil War for the two Greenwood Furnaces. A total of 458 tons of ore was raised in 1880 (Ransom, p. 239).

THE STORY OF
BEAR MOUNTAIN

On September 15, 1609, Henry Hudson's ship, the *Half-Moon*, rode at anchor in the mouth of Popolopen Brook. His crew had to defend themselves from hostile natives — the Haverstroo Indians. After the Dutch founded New Amsterdam and Albany in 1624, Hudson's River was the route for their commerce. They named the mountains Dunderberg, Pingyp, Timp, Anthony's Nose and Bear Hill (now known as Bear Mountain).

After driving the Dutch away in 1664-67, the English began to acquire title to the lands along the Hudson. In 1683, during the reign of Charles II, Sakaghkemerk, sachem of the Haverstroos, sold for "the sum of six shillings, silver money" all of Bear Mountain, Hessian Lake and Iona Island to Stephanus van Cortlandt, the Mayor of New York City. The same Indians sold the same land in 1685 to New York Governor Dongan and his friends. It was under Governor Dongan that a representative assembly in October 1683 passed a law providing for representation and for religious liberty.

In 1743, King George II granted the 800-acre Bear Hill tract to Richard Bradley who was, at the time, Attorney General of the Colony of New York. He soon sold the tract to Theodorus Snedeker of Hempstead, Long Island. During the following years, Snedeker acquired much of the land between Haverstraw and Bear Mountain. Because he was a Tory during the Revolution, Snedeker's land was confiscated by the State of New York.

The State transferred the land on the north side of Bear Mountain to the Military Academy at West Point. The rest of the mountain was sold to Samuel Brewster on May 15, 1790. In 1849, Brewster's land at Bear Mountain became the property of the Knickerbocker Ice Company, which cut ice on Highland Lake (now Hessian Lake) and sold it in New York City. Their land passed to Alfred C. Cheny in 1874, and then to Charles E. Lambert of Perth Amboy, New Jersey.

The Formation of Palisades Interstate Park

The Hudson Highlands and the Palisades of the Hudson were a much admired feature of American landscape, popularized by the artists of the Hudson River School. They were also much admired by quarrymen who, after 1875, used Alfred Nobel's dynamite to destroy the cliffs. Between Fort Lee and the state line there were 17 quarries.

Public agitation developed in the 1890s to stop the quarrying. In 1894, New Jersey and New York passed bills which ceded 16 miles of the face and base of the Palisades to the Federal Government as a military reservation. This measure was rejected by Congress in 1895 and again in 1898. Meanwhile, the quarrymen, seeing the handwriting on the cliff, demolished more and more landmarks. In March 1898, 7,000 pounds of dynamite reduced Washington Head and Indian Head at Fort Lee to 2.5 million cubic yards of traprock.

Then in 1899 the New Jersey Federation of Women's Clubs secured passage of a bill empowering the Governor to appoint a commission which would suggest a method of preservation. A similar bill was passed in New York State with the backing of Governor Theodore Roosevelt. In March 1900, the commissioners recommended that a permanent Interstate Park Commission be given power to acquire Palisades land for recreational purposes. This proposal was voted into law by both legislatures and signed by Theodore Roosevelt for New York and by Governor Voorhees for New Jersey. The jurisdiction of the Commission extended from Fort Lee, New Jersey to Piermont, New York. In 1906, it was extended to Stony Point, including Hook Mountain.

Governor Roosevelt appointed George W. Perkins, a vice-president of New York Life Insurance Company, as President of the new Commission. When Roosevelt telephoned Perkins, the latter tried to decline, but Roosevelt said he hadn't called to *ask* Perkins, but to *tell* him the appointment had already been made.

George Walbridge Perkins, Sr., a resident of Riverdale, New York, was born in Chicago on January 31, 1862. With only a public school education, he began work as an office boy in the Chicago office of New York Life Insurance Company. After many promotions, he became a vice-president of the company in 1898. When Perkins became President of the Interstate Park Commission, the two states had provided only $10,000 to stop the quarrying. He soon learned that about $125,000 was needed. He approached J.P. Morgan, Sr. for help. Morgan replied that he would put up the whole sum, provided that Perkins would agree to become a Morgan partner. Perkins agreed, and the Carpenter Bros. quarry at Fort Lee was bought for $132,500. On Christmas Eve 1900, the blasting was stopped forever.

The Fight to Save the Highlands

In 1908, the Commission on New Prisons which had been appointed by New York Governor Higgins made known plans to build a new Sing Sing Prison at Bear Mountain. One reason for the choice of that 500-acre site was that it would yield a great deal of traprock for building new highways (*Rockland County Journal*, 2/1/08). By mid-summer, hundreds of convicts were living on the terrace above the river. On January 9, 1909, the State purchased the 740-acre Bear Mountain tract from Charles Lambert's widow.

To conservationists and lovers of the Hudson Highlands, this scheme to build a prison at Highland Lake seemed like sacrilege. They were inspired by the success of the Interstate Park in stopping the defacement of the Palisades. Foremost among those who fought for the preservation of the Hudson Highlands was Dr.

Edward Lasell Partridge, a New York City physician and medical teacher who had a summer home on Storm King Mountain.[1] In a lengthy article in *The Outlook* magazine for November 9, 1907, Dr. Partridge had advocated the formation of a national preserve, to include 65 square miles between Peekskill and Breakneck Mountain, and 57 square miles between Jones Point and Storm King.

The public interest in the upcoming Hudson-Fulton Celebration of 1909 created much opinion in favor of the Partridge proposals. A *New York Times* feature article on Sunday, September 20, 1908 urged a "Fight to Save the Hudson" and decried the State's decision to build a prison at Bear Mountain.

After long discussions, the New York State Legislature in 1909 created the "Highlands of the Hudson Forest Preserve." A state forester was appointed to oversee the preserve, and Dr. Partridge was made secretary of a commission to administer it.[2] The prison, however, was not cancelled.

---

[1] Partridge's summer "cottage," known as the Spy Rock House, was on a saddle between Storm King and Whitehorse Mountain. Hikers following the present-day Stillman Trail from the parking area on Route 9W over Storm King will encounter the ruin of that cottage on West Rocks. In 1936, the Interstate Hiking Club described that two-story house as "deserted" (*Paterson Morning Call*, 5/1/36).

[2] In 1913, Dr. Edward L. Partridge was appointed to the Palisades Interstate Park Commission. He served the Commission for many years as its treasurer and as a member of various committees until his death on May 2, 1930, at the age of 77.

Mary Averell Harriman

Fortunately for the generations to come, one of those upset by the plan to construct the prison was Mary Averell Harriman, whose husband, Edward H. Harriman, had died on September 9, 1909. The Harriman estate included over 30,000 acres in the Highlands west of the Hudson, which had been assembled over a period of twenty years. Edward and Mary Harriman had long wanted to preserve the woodlands from exploitation, and to make part of their land available to the public as a park. They were personally acquainted with like-minded persons such as James Stillman and Dr. Edward Partridge.

On December 15, 1909, Mrs. Harriman wrote to Governor Charles Evans Hughes that she would convey to New York State 10,000 acres of land in Orange and Rockland Counties for a state park, and give $1,000,000 in cash to administer the park, provided that the State of New York appropriate $2,500,000 for the Park Commission to acquire lands and build roads; that the State discontinue construction of a prison at Bear Mountain; that by January 1, 1910 a further $1,500,000 be raised by private subscription; and that the State of New Jersey appropriate such amount as the Park Commissioners deemed to be its fair share.

Before Mrs. Harriman sent her letter, George W. Perkins had begun negotiations to ensure that the desired private contributions would be forthcoming. By December 31, 1909, Mr. Perkins informed Governor Hughes that $1,625,000 had been subscribed. Among the contributors were John D. Rockefeller, Sr. and J. Pierpont Morgan, Sr., who gave $500,000 each; and Mrs. Margaret Sage, William K. Vanderbilt, George F. Baker, Sr., James Stillman, John D. Archbold, William Rockefeller, Frank A. Munsey, Henry Phipps, E.T. Stotesbury, Elbert H. Gary and George W. Perkins, Sr., who contributed $50,000 each.

In March 1910, the New York Legislature passed the necessary measures, and the New Jersey Legislature appropriated $500,000 to build the Henry Hudson Drive along the river in the New Jersey section of the Park. On October 29, 1910, on behalf of his mother, 18-year-old W. Averell Harriman presented to the Palisades Interstate Park Commission $1,000,000 and 10,000 acres of land.

The Life of Edward H. Harriman

Edward Henry Harriman, whose love of the woods and mountains made possible our great State Park, was born on February 25, 1848 in the Episcopal rectory in Hempstead, Long Island. His father was the Rev. Orlando Harriman. While a young boy, Edward spent a summer as a timekeeper at the Greenwood Furnace owned by the Parrott family. It was then that he became acquainted with the hills and lakes in the Ramapo Mountains.

At the age of 14, he left school and started as an office boy in Wall Street. When he was 22, he opened his own broker's office, and became very successful. After his marriage in 1879 to Mary Williamson Averell, Harriman became a director of his father-in-law's Ogdensburg and Lake Champlain Railroad Co. In 1883, he was made a director of the Illinois Central Railroad. He later became chairman of the executive committee of the Union Pacific Railroad (1898), and president of the Southern Pacific Railroad (1901).

Edward and Mary Harriman had three sons: Henry Neilson (1883), William Averell (1891) and Edward Roland (1895). They also had three daughters: Mary (1881), Cornelia (1884) and Carol (1889).

In 1885, Harriman learned that the Parrotts had put up their estate for sale. He learned, too, that certain land speculators intended to divide it, and to sell the lumber that still grew there. To thwart those plans, Harriman bid at the auction for the entire 7,863 acres. His bid of $52,500 was accepted, to the disappointment of the Parrotts, who believed they would have received more money if the land had been sold in pieces.

The Harrimans, who had a Manhattan home at 22 East 51st Street, took possession of the Parrott farm in the summer of 1888. They gave the estate the name Arden, which had been Mrs. Parrott's maiden name. In the next two years, Edward Harriman bought about 40 different farms and tracts — an additional 20,000 acres. To make all parts of his estate accessible, he built 40 miles of bridle paths.

Bear Mountain/Harriman Parks: 1910–1920

Although they adjoin each other and both are part of the Palisades Interstate Park system, Bear Mountain and Harriman State Parks are technically separate entities. For historical reasons, Bear Mountain State Park extends south from Brooks Lake in Fort Montgomery, and includes Popolopen Torne, Bear Mountain, West Mountain, Iona Island and Dunderberg Mountain. It contains 5,067 acres. In November 1923, the Palisades Interstate Park Commission decided that "all of the Park lying west of Bear Mountain [later, west of West Mountain] shall be designated Harriman State Park." That park now contains 46,613 acres.

In 1901, the Commission retained as consultant the eminent landscape engineer Charles W. Leavitt, Jr. (*N.Y. Times,* 10/23/01). Leavitt served as Chief Engineer from 1901 to 1912, and was responsible for the development of the park along the Palisades. In 1912, he was succeeded as Chief Engineer by Major W.A. Welch.

William Addams Welch was born in Cynthiana, Kentucky on August 20, 1868. He was educated at Colorado Springs (1882) and at the University of Virginia (1886), where he received a Master of Engineering degree. For six years, he worked for the U.S. Government in Alaska, where he assembled the first iron steamship to be built in the territory. Later he worked in the western states, in Mexico and in Bolivia

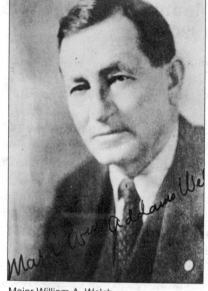

Major William A. Welch

(1906).[3] He returned to the United States in 1907, and was working for the Olmstead Brothers when he met George Perkins in 1912. Perkins persuaded him to become General Manager and Chief Engineer of the Palisades Interstate Park.

Major Welch's work for the Park won him fame as father of the state park movement. Together with Stephen Mather and Horace Albright, he was also a pioneer in the national park movement. In the years

---

[3] The legendary 228-mile Madeira-Mamoré Railway in Bolivia that Welch helped build was described in a *New York Times* feature article on November 26, 1989.

that followed, he built 23 lakes, 100 miles of roads and 103 children's camps. He helped found the Palisades Interstate Park Trail Conference, and later served as chairman of the newly organized Appalachian Trail Conference.

Work began at Bear Mountain in 1910 with the demolition of the prison and the building of a dock for steamboat excursion traffic. In 1911, the West Shore Railroad built a new station near the dock, and in 1912 a replica of Henry Hudson's *Half-Moon* was moored at the new dock. A comfort station was built at Hessian Lake, and a reservoir and water mains were constructed. Spring water was provided in ice-filled green barrels, with free cups. A park office was built from parts of the prison barracks. The Park was first opened to public use by Commissioner Perkins on July 5, 1913. Regular steamboat service from New York City was begun in the summer of 1913 by the McAllister Steamboat Company, and 22,590 passengers were carried by the boats that season. Camping was begun around Hessian Lake, and in 1913 the first Boy Scout camps were built at Car Pond (later named Lake Stahahe).

Bear Mountain Inn was completed in 1915, built of great boulders and chestnut logs. The stones for the fireplace came from old stone walls. Some hikers may remember the sections of a great 350-year-old chestnut tree which were made into chairs, a settee, a cigar case, and a cashier's cage for the upstairs dining room. The tree came from the western border of the Harriman estate, where it died about 1912 of the chestnut blight. The Inn was opened on June 27, 1915 by George W.

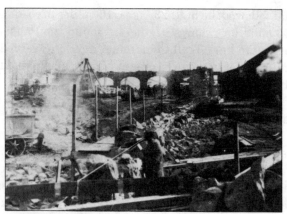
Construction of Bear Mountain Inn – 1914

Perkins, who gave a luncheon for the Governor of New York, Charles S. Whitman. Rooms at the Inn were $4.50 per day, which included lodging and three meals. In December 1927, two bronze bears were purchased to adorn the entrance to the Inn. They are still there, painted black.

In September 1913, construction was begun on a road to link Bear Mountain with the Harriman lands to the west. This road, originally called the Southfields Road and later renamed Seven Lakes Drive, was opened in August 1915. (At that time, it did not extend to Sloatsburg.) As soon as the Southfields Road was underway, Major Welch began planning a new bridge across Popolopen Gorge. In 1916, the Popolopen Viaduct to Fort Montgomery was opened. That bridge and similar ones at Stony Point (1923) and Sparkill (1926), the highway around Storm King Mountain, and the dock and railroad station at Bear Mountain, were all constructed in order to make the Park more accessible to the population of the surrounding region.

The year 1919 saw the acquisition of the steamboats *Clermont* and *Onteora*.[4] Both ships had been built in Newburgh, the *Onteora* in 1898, and the *Clermont* in 1911. The round trip from New York City on weekends was 85 cents for adults and 45 cents for children.

The Growth of the Parks: 1920–1936

On June 18, 1920, friends of the Park were saddened by the death of George W. Perkins, Sr., who had been President of the Park Commission for twenty years. In his memory, the Commission declared at its meeting of June 25, 1920:

> The Palisades Interstate Park as it now exists was the conception of Mr. Perkins, and it was he and he alone who raised the money for its acquisition and development. As the Park grew in size and usefulness, his ideas and enthusiasm grew with it, until in the latter years of his life he conceived a playground large enough and complete enough to afford rest and recreation to all the people of New York and New Jersey who lived

---

[4] Actually, these two boats were initially acquired by George Perkins in the fall of 1919, since the Commission then lacked funds to purchase them. After Perkins died in June 1920, the boats were acquired by the Commission with funds from the Laura Spelman Rockefeller Memorial Fund.

near enough to enjoy it, and where all the facilities for such enjoyment should be furnished at cost, without profit to concessionaires or others.

In 1921, the Commission decided that a proper memorial to George Perkins would be a scenic road to the top of Bear Mountain.

Winter sports began at Bear Mountain in the 1922-23 season. 1923 saw the completion of the first 16-mile section of the Appalachian Trail, from the Hudson River to Arden. The Bear Mountain Hudson River Bridge Co. was incorporated in 1922, with E. Roland Harriman as president. Opened on Thanksgiving Day 1924, the Bear Mountain Bridge was the longest span in the world at that time. The bridge became the property of the New York State Bridge Authority at midnight, September 25, 1940. The construction of Dam No. 10 for Lake Sebago was begun in 1923.

In 1925, the War Department (which owned the land) gave permission to build Hell Hole Drive around

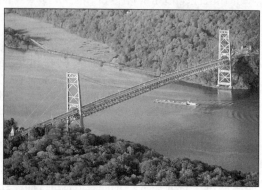

Bear Mountain Bridge

the north side of Bear Mountain. When opened in 1927, this 18-foot-wide road was christened Popolopen Drive. It was widened to three lanes in 1933-34.

In 1926, the Commission authorized Major Welch to construct three trail shelters, including the ones at Big Hill and at Tom Jones Mountain.

The Trailside Nature Museum and the Bear Mountain ski jump were opened in 1927. In 1929, a 12-inch pipe was laid along Popolopen Gorge to supply water from Queensboro Lake to Bear Mountain.

Roland Harriman gave Island Pond to the Park in 1927. In exchange, the Park built a new Arden Valley Road past the Elk Pen, so that traffic would no longer go through Harriman land, and Roland would no longer be surprised by hikers peering through his windows.

The period of the Great Depression which began in 1929 saw increased construction activity in Bear Mountain/Harriman Parks. Under Governor Franklin D. Roosevelt, New York State set up the Temporary Emergency Relief Administration (TERA), which sent unemployed workers each day to Bear Mountain on the West Shore Railroad. The TERA workers built the Perkins Memorial Drive and the Doodletown Bridle Path. When Roosevelt became President of the United States, other agencies were created to put unemployed men to work on public works projects. Men from the Works Progress Administration (WPA) built the new Administration Building (1937)[5] and a number of bridges in the Park. Between 1933 and 1942, the Civilian Conservation Corps (CCC) established nine camps in

---

[5] This building replaced an earlier one, built in 1920.

the Park (other camps were at Storm King, Blauvelt and the Palisades). Each camp employed 200 young men who stayed for 18 months. The CCC men built ten lakes: Pine Meadow, Wanoksink, Massawippa, Minsi, Owl, Welch, Silvermine, Turkey Hill, Skenonto and Skannatati. They also built many roads, such as the Beechy Bottom Road, Owl Lake Road, Summer Hill Road and Deep Hollow Road, and several ski trails.

Unfortunately, the State could not provide funds for the construction and maintenance of the children's camps which were proposed to be built on the lakes being constructed by the CCC. In a letter dated March 9, 1935 to Conrad L. Wirth, Assistant Director of the National Park Service,[6] Major Welch requested the withdrawal of the CCC workers. Despite this request, the CCC camps in the Park were not immediately disbanded. However, the workers were gradually withdrawn during the next several years, and all camps were closed in 1942.

In 1936, the first ski tow, known as the Old Silvermine Ski Tow, was built on the slopes at Lake Menomine. (In 1951, the name of the lake was changed to Silvermine Lake.)

---

[6] In 1964, Conrad Wirth became a Commissioner of the Interstate Park.

The Growth of the Parks: 1937–1999

Since its formation in 1900, the Interstate Park had been governed by ten commissioners: five appointed by the Governor of New York and five appointed by the Governor of New Jersey. Legally, there were two commissions — the New Jersey commission owned the park lands in New Jersey, and the New York commission owned the park lands in New York. Although they legally formed two separate commissions, in practice all ten commissioners functioned as one body. This arrangement continued until 1937, when a compact was entered into by both state legislatures and approved by a joint resolution of the United States Congress. It provided for *one* commission, with five members appointed by the Governor of New York and five by the Governor of New Jersey. Title to all Interstate Park property in both states now resides in the ten-member Commission. The Compact assured the permanence of the Park as an interstate undertaking.

At their meeting of August 17, 1938, the Commissioners noted that Raymond H. Torrey, for many years in charge of publicity for the Commission, had died on July 15, 1938.

In the fall of 1938, the residents of Beaver Pond (now Lake Welch) lost their last court appeal to block the Park's acquisition of their land. Their claims were finally settled, and the lake was filled with water in 1942.

In 1939, Harry Keevil of Cornwall was authorized to operate a riding academy at Bear Mountain. Riding horses were available until December 1961, when conditions in the stables were found to be unfit for the horses.

Major Welch, who had been General Manager since 1912, retired on February 1, 1940, and was followed by A. Kenneth Morgan. Morgan had worked for the Long Island State Park Commission, and most recently had been responsible for the design and operation of the 1939 New York World's Fair.

One of Morgan's first tasks was to prepare plans for a Palisades Interstate Parkway, which was to extend from the George Washington Bridge to the Bear Mountain Bridge. In February 1943, he requested $7,000,000 for the construction of the Parkway, but construction was delayed by the entry of the nation into the Second World War. During the war, the Army used the Pine Meadow and Beaver Pond areas (on weekdays only) for training personnel in ground photography. In 1945, the Navy built a water line from Doodletown Brook to Iona Island to supply the naval base there. On September 3, 1947, a contract was signed to build the first section of the Palisades Interstate Parkway, from Bear Mountain to Mt. Ivy. That section was opened to traffic on November 30, 1953. The Parkway was completed on August 28, 1958 — at a cost of $47 million. As part of the highway project, the Anthony Wayne Recreation Area was begun in 1951 and opened to the public on June 18, 1955 by Governor W. Averell Harriman.

On January 10, 1960, George W. Perkins died. He had been a commissioner since 1922 and President of the Commission since 1945, and also served as the permanent U.S. representative to NATO. Like his father, he devoted much of his life and fortune to the welfare of the Interstate Park. Perkins was succeeded on the Commission by his wife. When she resigned in 1973, Governor Rockefeller appointed her son, George W. Perkins, Jr., to the Commission. He resigned in 1988 and was succeeded in 1990 by his sister Anne Perkins Cabot.

In 1962, Lake Welch Beach was opened to 1,100 guests (it rained). In 1965, the last residents left Doodletown, and the new Long Mountain Parkway was begun. In the same year, the entire Park was declared to be a National Historic Landmark. The Navy gave up Iona Island in 1965 and transferred its title to the Park.

On August 28, 1969, after 29 years of service, A.K. Morgan retired as General Manager of the Park. He died shortly afterward. In his memory, the lodge (near the Bear Mountain Inn) that Morgan had recently built was designated by the Commission as the A.K. Morgan Overlook Lodge.

Taking Morgan's place on September 1, 1969 was Nash Castro. Born on January 14, 1920, he was educated at St. Thomas Aquinas College in New York and at George Washington University. In 1939, he began a career with the National Park Service, which culminated in his service as Director of the Capital Region (Washington, D.C.) from 1961 to 1969. Castro's service with the Commission marked a period of important growth, including the acquisition by the Commission of Minnewaska State Park.

In February 1974, construction was begun on the Doodletown Reservoir, which was designed to supply drinking water to Iona Island and to serve as a backup to the Bear Mountain supply.

On October 7, 1978, "Sammy" the bald eagle, a resident of the Bear Mountain Zoo since 1954, succumbed in an encounter with a raccoon.

In 1979, an anonymous donor gave $200,000 to pay for a youth corps for trail improvements. It was later learned that the donor was DeWitt Wallace, the founder of *Reader's Digest*. In the years that followed, the DeWitt Wallace Fund gave the Park over $1.5 million for summer youth work programs. Other donors, including the commissioners themselves, have also given gifts to the Park over the years. The Mary W. Harriman Fund makes an annual gift to bring inner-city children to the Tiorati Workshop for Environmental Learning.

The 60th anniversary of the Appalachian Trail was celebrated in June 1983 at the Bear Mountain Inn. Three hundred people heard Commissioner Mary Fisk speak about the many years of cooperation between the Commission and the Trail Conference. She then cut a six-foot-long birthday cake, with the help of her grandson.

Hikers and all friends of the Park were saddened to learn of the death of W. Averell Harriman on July 26, 1986. Born on November 15, 1891, he was an 18-year-old Yale student in 1910 when he presented to Governor Charles Evans Hughes, on behalf of his mother, a deed for 10,000 acres and a gift of $1,000,000, which led to the formation of Bear Mountain State Park. He was appointed a commissioner of the Park in 1915, when he was 24 years old (he was already a vice president of the Union Pacific Railroad). He remained a commissioner for the next 59 years (except for the period from 1955 to 1959, when he was Governor of the state). When he resigned in 1974, his daughter Mary Fisk took his place (she served as a commissioner until her death in January 1996). Averell Harriman's concern for the welfare of the Park was never failing; he often made gifts of land and money to the Commission. He was survived by his wife, two daughters, six grandchildren and six great-grandchildren.

The year 1990 brought the retirement of Executive Director Nash Castro.[7] On April 15, 1990, he was succeeded by Robert O. Binnewies, who came to the Park from the New York State Department of Environmental Conservation, where he served as Deputy Commissioner for Natural Resources. Binnewies began his career in 1960 as a ranger in Yellowstone National Park.

During Bob Binnewies' tenure as Executive Director, in February 1998, the Commission acquired nearly 14,000 acres of Sterling Forest — the culmination of many years of efforts to protect this land by a consortium of public and private organizations. Although this land is entirely in the State of New York, the State of

---

[7] During Castro's tenure, the position of General Manager was renamed Executive Director.

New Jersey contributed $10 million towards the purchase of this property, much of which serves as a watershed for the State of New Jersey. (Interestingly, in 1900, when the Commission was first created, the State of New York contributed $400,000 towards the purchase of the Palisades along the Hudson River in New Jersey, which was part of the viewshed of New York City residents across the river.)

In 1995, the jurisdiction of the PIPC in New Jersey was expanded to include Passaic, Morris, Warren, Hunterdon and Somerset Counties, in addition to Bergen County. This broadening of the PIPC's jurisdiction makes it possible for the Commission to expand its efforts in preserving environmentally sensitive lands in the New Jersey Highlands.

Bob Binnewies retired as PIPC Executive Director in February 1999, and was succeeded by Carol Ash, who previously served as the director of The Nature Conservancy of New York State.

In 1999, the Park is looking forward to its second century of service to the people of New York and New Jersey. In facing the challenging times ahead, the Commission can count on the hearty cooperation of the organized hikers of the metropolitan area, represented by the New York-New Jersey Trail Conference.

The Trailside Museum

In 1920, a new scoutmaster, Benjamin Talbot Babbitt Hyde, came to the Boy Scout camps on Lake Kanawauke. Fondly known as "Uncle Benny," he was a Patron of the Museum of Natural History. In the huge Scout headquarters building, he established the first museum in the Park, and filled it with snakes, flowers, rocks and tree specimens. By 1925, three more such museums had been created in the camps at Twin Lakes, Cohasset and Tiorati. Uncle Benny's work ended when the Scout camps left the Park in 1929.

In 1925, Dr. Frank E. Lutz, Curator of Entomology at the American Museum of Natural History, established a Station for the Study of Insects. The Park allotted him 40 acres on Wildcat Brook, on the west side of Route 17. His nature trail, which included informative signs, was soon imitated in twenty camps around the Park.

In 1926, with the assistance of a $7,500 grant from the Laura Spelman Rockefeller Foundation, plans were made for a museum and zoo at Bear Mountain, on the site of old Fort Clinton. William H. Carr, who had been Uncle Benny's assistant in 1922, was appointed the Museum's first director. Construction of the first building was completed in September 1927, and by 1934, three more buildings had been added. The museum thrived through the following years. In 1942, Daniel Carter Beard, a founder of the Boy Scouts of America, gave much of his personal memorabilia for an exhibit at the Trailside Museum.

The Trailside Museum has had six directors:

William H. Carr	1927-1944
John C. Orth	1946-1955
John J. Kenney	1955-1970
John H. Mead	1972-1987
John Yurus	1987-1988
John Focht	1988-

The New York– New Jersey Trail Conference

During the early years of the twentieth century, a number of organized groups actively promoted hiking. These groups (and the dates they were founded) were:

Torrey Botanical Club - 1868

Fresh Air Club (New York Athletic Club) - 1877

Paterson Rambling Club - September 15, 1904

Appalachian Mountain Club (N.Y. Chapter) - 1911

Tramp and Trail Club - September 11, 1914

Green Mountain Club (N.Y. Section) - 1915

Inkowa Club for Women - 1915

Nature Friends

Boy Scouts and Girl Scouts

Newspapers, such as the *New York Evening Post* and the *New York Times*, devoted much space to walking and hiking, especially after the formation in 1910 of the Bear Mountain-Harriman State Parks. Already by 1913 the Boy Scouts were camping at Car Pond (Lake Stahahe), and in 1917 they made their headquarters at Lake Kanawauke. By the time Major Welch published his first trail map in 1920, all those clubs had developed leaders who were quite familiar with hiking routes in the Highlands and Ramapos.

In the *New York Evening Post* for Friday, August 27, 1920, Meade C. Dobson of the Fresh Air Club described the new Park map and proposed to the walking clubs that they cooperate with the Park Commission to develop new hiking trails. Dobson was an engineer and Boy Scout executive who later chaired the New York Chapter of the Adirondack Mountain Club.

With the cooperation of Major William A. Welch, General Manager of the Park, a meeting was held at 8:15 p.m. on October 5, 1920, in the log cabin atop the Abercrombie and Fitch building in Manhattan. The object of the meeting was to organize a Palisades Interstate Park Trail Conference. Those present included: Major W.A. Welch; Edward F. Brown, Superintendent of Camps; Albert Britt of Outdoor Publishing Co.; Meade C. Dobson of the Boy Scouts; and Raymond H. Torrey, Editor of the *New York Evening Post* Outings Page.

Also present were representatives of the various hiking clubs and other interested parties: Appalachian Mountain Club (William W. Bell, James D. Merriman, Sidney E. Morse and Dr. Mary Goddard Potter); Fresh Air Club (Mortimer Bishop, James T. Horn, Frederick D. Ilgen and Benjamin F. Seaver); Green Mountain Club (J. Ashton Allis, Major William D. Ennis, Prof. Will S. Monroe and George F. Parmelee); Tramp and Trail Club (Elizabeth G. Baldwin, E. Cecil Earle, Frank Place, Jr. and A.B. Malcolmson); Associated Mountain Clubs (LeRoy Jeffers); League of Walkers (Dr. George

J. Fisher) and New York State College of Forestry (Dean F.F. Moon).

Albert Britt was asked to act as chairman of the meeting. He spoke briefly on the need for new trails, and then appointed Meade C. Dobson as secretary. After much discussion of the need for trails, and suggestions for trail requirements, Dr. George Fisher moved that the chairman appoint a committee to study the problems and report back with definite proposals. The committee later appointed by Mr. Britt included J. Ashton Allis, William W. Bell, Albert Britt, Meade C. Dobson, Dr. George J. Fisher, Frederick Ilgen, LeRoy Jeffers, Dean F.F. Moon and Edgar D. Stone.

The chairman was empowered to appoint a chairman of a Committee on Camps and Shelters. Dr. Monroe was later appointed to this post. It also was decided to have a Committee on Ways and Means.

Because the fall was the best time for scouting and blazing trails, the new Conference got busy immediately. They elected Major Welch as their permanent chairman and Raymond H. Torrey as secretary. The first trail to be tackled, proposed by Major Welch, was the one from Tuxedo to Jones Point, later called the Ramapo-Dunderberg Trail (R-D). On May 6, 1921, Torrey reported that the trail was practically complete. A second trail, from Mt. Ivy to Tuxedo, was proposed for the summer of 1921 (it was started in 1923). Actually, the next Conference trail was the Timp-Torne Trail (built in the fall/winter of 1921-22), which was regarded as a branch of the R-D. Another branch, started in the summer of 1922, was the Fingerboard-Storm King Trail.

During the years 1920-23, the Boy Scouts, under Chief H.A. Gordon, and led by Archibald T. Shorey of Brooklyn, were building their 35-mile White Bar trail system.

The next big event in Trail Conference history was the proposal by Benton MacKaye to build a trail from Maine to Georgia along the Appalachian ridges. His plan was described by Torrey in the *New York Evening Post* of April 7, 1922. It was quickly adopted by the Palisades Interstate Park Trail Conference as their main project.

Because the new trail would go through two states from the Connecticut line to the Delaware River, the Conference was reorganized on April 25, 1922 as the New York-New Jersey Trail Conference (*N.Y. Post*, 4/28/22). Twenty organizations became members. The officers of the new Conference were: W.A. Welch, Chairman; W.W. Bell (AMC), Vice-Chairman for New York; C.P. Wilbur (State Fire Warden), Vice-Chairman for New Jersey; J. Ashton Allis (ADK), Trails Committee; Frank Place (Tramp and Trail Club), Publicity; and Raymond H. Torrey (GMC), Secretary.

There was great enthusiasm for the new task. J.A. Allis and his Trail Committee immediately started scouting a route for the Appalachian Trail (AT). By October 7, 1923, the AT had been completed through Bear Mountain-Harriman Park (the Bear Mountain Bridge was opened on November 27, 1924), and the trail makers concentrated on extending the route north and south. During this period, the Tuxedo-Mt. Ivy Trail was marked (1923) and the Suffern-Bear Mountain Trail (1924-27) was begun.

On March 2-3, 1925, the Appalachian Trail Conference (ATC) was formed in Washington, D.C. Major W.A. Welch was elected Chairman; Raymond Torrey became Treasurer. During this period, Welch and Torrey became active in the national park movement as members of a commission to study extensions of the national parks. Because of his increasing commitments, Welch relinquished his active ATC role in 1927 to Judge Arthur Perkins. In 1928, Welch became Honorary Chairman and J.A. Allis became Treasurer of ATC.

Back in Harriman Park, hikers were becoming concerned over the lack of maintenance on the trails they had made. In 1928, Jack Spivack of the New York Ramblers (organized on October 25, 1923) suggested

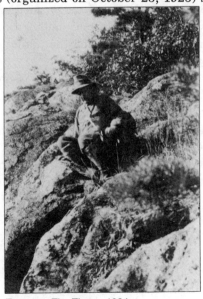

Torrey on The Timp – 1934

that trails should be assigned to hiking clubs for maintenance. Some clubs began to volunteer: the Green Mountain Club asked for the Arden-Surebridge Trail; the New York Ramblers took the Seven Hills Trail; and the Catskill Mountain Club took the Fingerboard-Storm King Trail.

On April 21, 1931, Bill Burton of the Green Mountain Club called a meeting of metropolitan hiking clubs to discuss uniform standards of trail marking. This meeting turned out to be a reorganization of the New York-New Jersey Trail Conference, which since 1925 had in effect been a branch of the Appalachian Trail Conference. Raymond Torrey was chosen as Chairman; Angelique Rivolier of the Inkowa Outdoor Club became Secretary. A committee on methods of trail marking was led by Bill Burton; another committee on allocation of trail work among the hiking clubs was chaired by Frank Place.

In June 1931, the new Conference issued its first handbook on trail building and maintenance. The color system in use by the New York State Conservation Department was adopted: red for east-west trails, blue for north-south trails, and yellow for diagonal trails.

In 1938, the Trail Conference was stunned by the death of their leader, Raymond Torrey. In that year, Frank Place became Chairman; J. Ashton Allis, Treasurer; and Richmond Barton, Secretary. Bill Hoeferlin, who became Conference Secretary in 1939, began publishing a monthly subscription newsletter, "Walking News," to replace Torrey's *New York Evening Post* column, "The Long Brown Path."

A new constitution for the Conference was adopted on February 4, 1942. On December 6, 1944, Joseph Bartha was named head of the Trail Patrol (which had been formed under J.A. Allis in 1940). He continued that activity until December 5, 1951, when he became 80 years old. He was replaced by Bill Burton, who was then 70.

In April 1958, the Conference became incorporated in New York State. In November 1963, it began publishing a newsletter for its members, which in 1965 was named the *Trail Walker*. Rosa Gottfried, who proposed this newsletter, was its first editor. Harry Nees was then the President of the Conference. The lead article in 1965 blasted Consolidated Edison's plan to build a pumped storage power plant at Storm King Mountain. That issue also announced the first Litter Day, organized by Elizabeth Levers. In 1976, the *Trail Walker* adopted the present newspaper format.

The Conference had 35 member clubs in 1969, maintaining 600 miles of trails. In that year, new by-laws provided for individual memberships (Class C members). In January 1973, the Conference took an office at 15 East 40th Street, New York City, and the following year hired Bob Parnes as part-time Executive Director. In November 1975, Jim Robinson became the first full-time Executive Director.

An early contribution to the hiking community was the *New York Walk Book* by Torrey, Place and Dickinson, first published in 1923. Revised editions appeared in 1934, 1936, 1951, 1971, 1984 and 1998.

Presidents of New York–New Jersey Trail Conference

1.	1920-1931	Major William A. Welch (1868-1941)
2.	1931-1938	Raymond Torrey (1880-1938)
3.	1938-1941	Frank Place (1881-1959)
4.	1941-1945	William Burton (1881-1966)
5.	1945-1947	Murray H. Stevens
6.	1947-1950	Ridsdale Ellis (1887-1955)
7.	1950-1951	Mortimer Bloom
8.	1951-1953	Ridsdale Ellis (1887-1955)
9.	1953-1955	John Coggeshall (d. 1960)
10.	1955-1956	Carl Geiser
11.	1956-1961	Samuel Wilkinson (d. 1973)
12.	1961-1964	Harry Nees (d. 1989)
13.	1964-1970	George Zoebelein
14.	1970-1972	Elizabeth Levers (d. 1998)
15.	1972-1974	John Danielsen (d. 1998)
16.	1974-1975	George Zoebelein
17.	1975-1976	Arthur J. Paul (d. 1988)
18.	1976-1978	Walter D. Houck
19.	1978-1984	Donald B. Derr
20.	1984-1987	Richard J. Kavalek
21.	1987-1999	H. Neil Zimmerman

At present, the office of the Trail Conference is at 232 Madison Avenue, Room 802, New York, New York 10016. The Conference, which now includes over 85 outdoors and hiking clubs and over 10,000 individual members, maintains over 1,300 miles of marked trails extending from the Connecticut border to the Delaware

Water Gap. Conference activities are carried out almost entirely by volunteers who work together

–to build and maintain trails and trail shelters in New York and New Jersey
–to promote the public interest in hiking and conservation
–to protect wild lands, wildlife and places of natural beauty.

Current projects of the Conference include extending and relocating the Long Path in New York, and local management planning for the Appalachian Trail in New York and New Jersey. The Conference has also been active in the relocation of portions of the Appalachian Trail off roads and onto a protected trail corridor, and in the preservation of Sterling Forest.

Conference publications include the *New York Walk Book*, the *New Jersey Walk Book,* the *Appalachian Trail Guide for New York-New Jersey*, *Guide to the Long Path*, *Hiking Guide to Delaware Water Gap National Recreation Area*, *Scenes and Walks in the Northern Shawangunks*, *Iron Mine Trails*, *Health Hints for Hikers*, and maps for Harriman/Bear Mountain Trails, North Jersey Trails, East Hudson Trails, West Hudson Trails, Kittatinny Trails, South Taconic Trails, the Shawangunks, the Catskills and the Hudson Palisades. It also publishes the *Trail Walker*, a bi-monthly newspaper for members.

ABOUT MEASURING TRAILS

Back in 1943, the Trail Conference made plans to measure by surveyor's wheel all the unmeasured marked trails in Bear Mountain/Harriman Park (*Walking News*, Nov. 1943). The measurements were made on 25 day trips between March and June 1944 by Bill Hoeferlin, Joseph Bartha, Paul Schubert and others. The result of their efforts was Bill Hoeferlin's *Harriman Park Trail Guide*, published in October 1944. Seven editions of Bill's guide were issued through 1976. It served Harriman hikers well.

When the present author first planned a book on Harriman trails, it was clear that many changes had taken place in the trails, and that the measurements in Bill Hoeferlin's guide could no longer be relied upon. To avoid all the work of remeasuring the trails, the author simply measured the trails on Conference maps #3 and #4.

When Dan Chazin, the editor, received the text of the book, the trail lengths set forth in the manuscript had been computed by map measurements. Now the editor (bless him!) is a man who places great importance on precision. He himself had previously measured the Appalachian Trail with a wheel, and my map-measure was over 2.5 miles less than his wheel figure. So, as part of the editorial process, Dan Chazin, together with other volunteers he recruited, have measured many of the trails, using surveying measuring wheels. For this edition, all of the marked trails have been measured, as have many of the unmarked trails. The following table sets forth the names of those who measured each trail:

Anthony Wayne Trail – Bill and Mary Ann Pruehsner; Robert and Lois Pruehsner

Appalachian Trail – Daniel Chazin

Arden-Surebridge Trail – Daniel Chazin

Beech Trail – Bill and Mary Ann Pruehsner

Blue Disc Trail – Dianne Philipps and Duane Nealon

Bottle Cap Trail – Daniel Chazin; Bill and Mary Ann Pruehsner

Breakneck Mountain Trail – Daniel Chazin

Conklins Crossing Trail – Bill and Mary Ann Pruehsner

Cornell Mine Trail – Bill and Mary Ann Pruehsner

Diamond Mountain-Tower Trail – Daniel Chazin; Bill and Mary Ann Pruehsner

Dunning Trail – Daniel Chazin

Fawn Trail – Bill and Robert Pruehsner

Hillburn-Torne-Sebago Trail – Daniel Chazin

Hurst Trail – Daniel Chazin

Kakiat Trail – Dianne Philipps and Duane Nealon

Lichen Trail – Bill and Mary Ann Pruehsner

Long Path – Wayne Richter, Daniel Chazin and Doug Broadbent

Major Welch Trail – Bill Pruehsner

Menomine Trail – Daniel Chazin

Nurian Trail – Daniel Chazin and Torey Adler

Pine Meadow Trail – Torey Adler

Popolopen Gorge Trail – Bill and Mary Ann Pruehsner

Raccoon Brook Hills Trail – Daniel Chazin

Ramapo-Dunderberg Trail – Bill and Mary Ann Pruehsner

Red Arrow Trail – Daniel Chazin

Red Cross Trail – Daniel Chazin

Red Timp Trail – Daniel Chazin

Reeves Brook Trail – Daniel Chazin

Seven Hills Trail – Dianne Philipps and Duane Nealon

Suffern-Bear Mountain Trail – Daniel Chazin; Bill and
  Mary Ann Pruehsner

Timp-Torne Trail – Daniel Chazin; Bill and Mary Ann
  Pruehsner

Triangle Trail – Daniel Chazin; Dianne Philipps
  and Duane Nealon

Tuxedo-Mt. Ivy Trail – Daniel Chazin and Torey Adler

Victory Trail – Torey Adler; Bill and Mary Ann Pruehsner

White Bar Trail – Daniel Chazin; Bill and Mary Ann
  Pruehsner

White Cross Trail – Torey Adler

1777 Trail – Bill and Mary Ann Pruehsner

1777E Trail – Bill and Mary Ann Pruehsner

1777W Trail – Bill and Mary Ann Pruehsner

1779 Trail – Bill and Mary Ann Pruehsner

Arden Road – Bill Pruehsner

Beechy Bottom East Road – Bill and Mary Ann Pruehsner

Bockberg Trail (part) – Daniel Chazin

Bockey Swamp Trail – Daniel Chazin and
  Jonathan Goldstein

Buck Trail (part) – Daniel Chazin

Crooked Road – Daniel Chazin; Bill and Mary Ann
  Pruehsner

Dean Trail – Daniel Chazin

Hasenclever Road – Torey Adler

Iron Mountain Trail (part) – Torey Adler

Island Pond Road – Daniel Chazin

Jones Trail – Daniel Chazin

Pine Meadow Road (part) – Daniel Chazin

Sherwood Path – Daniel Chazin

Sloatsburg Trail – Dianne Philipps and Duane Nealon

Stony Brook Trail – Torey Adler
Surebridge Mine Road – Daniel Chazin
Woodtown Road – Daniel Chazin
Cranberry Mountain Trail –Daniel Chazin
Hasenclever Mountain Trail – Daniel Chazin
Rockhouse Mountain Trail – Daniel Chazin
North "Ski" Trail – Daniel Chazin
North-South Connector – Daniel Chazin
South "Ski" Trail – Daniel Chazin
Timp Pass Road – Daniel Chazin
Doodletown Bridle Path – Bill and Mary Ann Pruehsner

Photo Credits

Doug Broadbent – page 459

Doris Collver – page 354

Clarence Conklin – pages 16, 359, 429

Larry Davies – page 157

Ralph Ginzburg – page 75

Bob Goetschius – pages 259, 260

Al Mastrodonato – pages 97, 399

Tom Melaccio – page 379

Bill Myles – pages 30, 94

Lou Odell – pages 229, 383, 419, 430, 431, 439, 447

Frank Oliver – pages 89, 141, 449, 493

Palisades Interstate Park Commission – pages 147, 155, 317, 328, 330, 331, 335, 362, 372, 375, 403, 409, 411, 422, 424, 474, 476

Ken Richardson – pages 43, 462

Rockland County Historical Society – page 258

Lou Tenace – pages 369, 396

Michael Warren – pages 4, 12, 14, 25, 26, 74, 76, 80, 100, 113, 134, 150, 174, 182, 224, 322, 327, 356, 392, 478

INDEX

A

Abbott, William P. 352

Addisone Boyce Camp
122-23, 125-26, 158-59,
187, 213, 312

Addisone Boyce (A-B) Trail
122, 213, 312

Adirondack Mountain Club
109, 162, 167, 180, 373,
375-76, 394, 441

Adolph, Raymond 17, 143,
328

Agony Grind 15

Air sampling stations 221

Albany Road 414-15

Allen's Pond 92

Algonquin gas pipeline 138,
264

Allis, J. Ashton 21, 73, 108

    Allis Trail 73

    Allis Short Trail 21

    Appalachian Trail 492

    Arden-Surebridge Trail
    20-21

    Fingerboard-Storm King
    Trail 73-74

    HTS Trail 50

    Ramapo-Dunderberg
    Trail 108, 111, 115

    Red Cross Trail 122

    Seven Hills Trail 132

    Victory Trail 174

Allison, Brewster J. 461

Almost Perpendicular 28-30,
178

American Canoe Associa-
tion camp 167, 375, 424

Anderson's file factory 244,
293

Anthony Wayne Recreation
Area 5, 216, 434, 482

Anthony Wayne South Ski
Trail 203-04

Anthony Wayne Trail 3-5

Appalachian Mountain Club
111, 115, 154

Appalachian Trail 6-17

    early years 9-10, 12-13,
    15, 492-93

    on Bear Mountain 78

Appalachian Trail Confer-
ence 493

Archbold, John D. 471

Arden 472

Arden House 72, 415

Arden Road 205-06, 417-18

Arden-Surebridge Trail
18-22

Arden Valley Road 15, 111,
417, 420-22, 479

Arthur's Falls 24-25

Askoti, Lake 70, 350

B

Bailey family 207-09, 248, 387, 393-94

Bailey, Jeremiah 336

Baileytown Road 205, 207-09, 393

Baker, George F., Sr. 376, 428, 471

Baker Camp 376, 425

Bald Mountain 115, 187, 219-20, 451-53

Bald Rocks Shelter 43, 109

Ballard, Frank 442

Bambino, Roland 332

Barnes Lake 350-51

Barnes Mine 447-48

Barrie, Gertrude 332

Bartha, Joseph 8, 45, 79, 109, 118, 147, 163, 495

Beach, Art 25, 169

Beard, Daniel Carter, 192, 487

Bear Mountain 8, 77-80, 435-38, 465-66, 475-77

Bear Mountain Aqueduct 100, 153, 196, 479

Bear Mountain Bridge 7, 9, 478

Bear Mountain Bypass 8

Bear Mountain Inn 475-76

Bear Mountain State Park 473-75

Beaver Pond 396-97

Beaver Pond Brook 69, 352

Becraft family 57, 178, 424, 429

Bedford, Isaac and Mary 282

Beech Trail 23-26

Beechy Bottom Brook 10, 114, 203-04, 210-11, 317

Beechy Bottom East Road 210-13, 215-18

Beechy Bottom Shelter 114

Beechy Bottom West Road 122, 214-18

Bell, William W. 111, 154

Bentley Place 57

Beveridge, John 321

Big Green Swamp 168, 243

Big Hill Shelter 68, 141, 479

Big Swamp 173, 381

Binnewies, Robert O. 485-86

Black Ash Brook 107-09, 172-73

Black Ash Mountain 108

Black Ash Swamp Road 107-09, 172-74

Blackcap Mountain 76

Black Mountain 11, 113-14, 378-80

Black Mountain Trail 113, 122, 198, 309-10

Black Mountain II (Trail) 310

Black Rock Mountain 88

Blanchard, George 375

Blauvelt Mountain 177

Your Invitation to Join the
NY-NJ TRAIL CONFERENCE
GPO Box 2250 • NY, NY 10116

Hikers and friends who wish to support the efforts of the Conference to maintain and protect 1,300 miles of marked foot trails in the NY/NJ area are invited to join as members. Dues include a subscription to our bi-monthly *Trail Walker,* 20-25% discounts on our publications (and 10% discounts at dozens of local outdoor stores and trail area lodges), and use of our extensive library...*and, above all, the opportunity to protect the hiking trails and to get involved!*

Name (s) _____

Address _____

City _____ State _____ ZIP _____

Phone (s) Day _____ Evening _____

Email _____ (Please PRINT clearly)

Check ✔	Individual	Joint/Family
Regular	❏ $21	❏ $26
Sponsor	❏ $45	❏ $50
Benefactor	❏ $95	❏ $100
Student	❏ $15	❏ $20
Senior	❏ $15	❏ $20
Limited Income	❏ $15	❏ $20
Life	❏ $400	❏ $600 (2 adults)

Do you belong to a hiking or outdoor club(s)? If yes, please list:

_____

❏ Mailing: Check box to left if you do ***not*** want your name exchanged with others (hiking clubs, etc.)
Membership rates as of 1999.